WAR SURGERY 1914–18

Edited by
Thomas Scotland and Steven Heys

Helion & Company Ltd

Helion & Company Limited
26 Willow Road
Solihull
West Midlands
B91 1UE
England
Tel. 0121 705 3393
Fax 0121 711 4075
Email: info@helion.co.uk
Website: www.helion.co.uk
Twitter: @helionbooks
Visit our blog http://blog.helion.co.uk

Published by Helion & Company 2012
This paperback reprint 2013

Designed and typeset by Farr out Publications, Wokingham, Berkshire
Cover designed by Farr out Publications, Wokingham, Berkshire
Printed by Lightning Source Ltd, Milton Keynes, Buckinghamshire

Text © Thomas Scotland and Steven Heys
Images © as shown
Front cover: 'The Operating Theatre, 41st Casualty Clearing Station, 1918',
painting by Lobley J. Hodgson dated 1918. (Imperial War Museum ART 3750).
Rear cover: A sketch by Henry Tonks of Harold Delph Gillies operating. (The Hunterian
Museum at the Royal College of Surgeons).

ISBN 978-1-909384-40-8

British Library Cataloguing-in-Publication Data.
A catalogue record for this book is available from the British Library.

For details of other military history titles published by Helion & Company Limited
contact the above address, or visit our website: http://www.helion.co.uk.

We always welcome receiving book proposals from prospective authors.

Dedicated to

Corporal C. Reilly 9498 1st Battalion, Royal Scots Fusiliers
Killed in Action near Ypres 1st March 1915 Age 23

Private George McNamee, 277574, 2nd Manchester Regiment,
who survived the Western Front.

Contents

List of Figures

List of Tables

List of Contributors

Contributors are listed in the order in which their work appears within this book.

Thomas R Scotland

Born in St. Andrews and brought up in the East Neuk of Fife, Tom was educated at Waid Academy in Anstruther. He graduated in Medicine from the University of Edinburgh in 1971, becoming a Fellow of the Royal College of Surgeons of Edinburgh in 1975. He developed his interest in the Great War whilst a student, when there were still many veterans alive. He trained in orthopaedic surgery in Aberdeen, and after spending a year as a Fellow in the University of Toronto, returned to take up the position of Consultant Orthopaedic Surgeon with Grampian Health Board and Honorary Senior Lecturer at the University of Aberdeen. His particular interests were knee surgery, paediatric orthopaedics and tumour surgery, and for three years he was lead clinician for the Scottish Sarcoma Managed Clinical Network. Over the years he has been a frequent visitor to the Western Front, and has found cycling the best way to visit different places. He has explored many areas of the Western Front with family and friends, and since retiring from the National Health Service in 2007 has kept in touch with former colleagues by leading cycling expeditions to the Western Front. He has pursued his interest in the Great War by making a particular study of Aberdeen surgeon, Sir Henry Gray, who played a pivotal role in the development of surgery on the Western Front, and has given various lectures on the development of surgical services during the Great War. In retirement he has completely re-invented himself as a cycling orthopaedic historian.

Steven D Heys

Born in Accrington in Lancashire and educated in England, Australia and Scotland, Steve graduated in Medicine from the University of Aberdeen in 1981 and undertook surgical training in the North-East of Scotland. He is a Fellow of the Royal Colleges of Surgeons in England, Edinburgh and Glasgow and underwent research training at the Rowett Research Institute in Aberdeen, obtaining a PhD in 1992. He specialised in general and breast cancer surgery for many years before latterly concentrating on breast cancer surgery together with his research interests in the role of nutrition in the causation of cancer, and has responsibilities for medical education both locally and nationally. He has published more than 200 scientific papers and written many book chapters on different aspects of surgery and played many national and international roles in surgery and the provision of surgical services. His interest in the Great War was sparked by the stories of the Accrington pals and the Lancashire Fusiliers, by his time as a member of the RAMC(V), serving for six years in the 51st Highland Brigade, and by Tom's famous cycling tours around the Western Front where he has the dual role of bicycle mechanic and, because he is a keen bagpipe player, has been appointed as Piper to the tours!

E Ann Robertson

Ann Robertson graduated MBChB from the University of Birmingham in 1975. After registration she specialized in anaesthetics and became a registrar at King's College Hospital in London after returning from a year in Nepal. She became a Fellow of the Royal College of Anaesthetists in 1979 and progressed to senior registrar jobs at King's, rotating to Brighton.

After marrying Graeme, whom she met whilst doing some enforced research at King's, she eventually moved to Scotland where she held consultant jobs first at Hairmyres Hospital and then at Aberdeen Royal Infirmary. An interest in Tropical Medicine led her to take the Diploma in Tropical Medicine of the Royal College of Physicians in 2010.

She worked for many years with Tom Scotland, one of this book's editors, and was persuaded to cycle the Western Front on the first trip to include women. This led to an interest in anaesthetic developments during the Great War, and the writing of Chapter 3. She has a particular interest in the developments taking place in the understanding of physiology at the time and the characters that played a part in the "Shock Committee" convened in 1917. She is married with two grown-up sons.

Robin Reid

Robin Reid was born in Consett, County Durham. He graduated BSc in Molecular Biology and MBChB, both at the University of Glasgow. He trained in pathology at the Western Infirmary, Glasgow, becoming MRCPath in 1984, and gained further experience at the Nuffield Orthopaedic Centre, Oxford. He spent the rest of his career in the Western Infirmary as Senior Lecturer in Pathology then Consultant Pathologist with particular interests in the diagnosis of tumours of bone and soft tissue; he chaired the Scottish Bone Tumour Registry for over 20 years.

He has published over 70 papers, mainly on orthopaedic pathology, and four textbooks. He was President of the Association of Clinical Pathologists from 2010-2011. Retired from clinical practice, he is a member of NHS Greater Glasgow and Clyde Health Board. His historical interests range from ancient, through mediaeval to World War I.

Alexander MacDonald

Sandy MacDonald was born in 1929, and went to school at Perth Academy (1941-1947). He went to Edinburgh University, graduating MBChB. He pursued a career in radiology, and says he is old enough to remember some of the early pioneers in the specialty. He took the DMRD in 1959, and MRCPE in 1961. He became a Fellow of the Faculty of Radiologists in 1962, and became FRCR in 1970 (ish) and FRCP.

After graduating, he did his early jobs in London and Edinburgh, and was appointed Consultant Radiologist in Aberdeen in 1964, where he pioneered neuro-radiology in Aberdeen. Sandy retired in 1992, and re-invented himself, gaining a Scot Vec award in 1995, in Musical Instrument Technology. During this time, he buried himself in the part by growing a ponytail.

His wife Joan was a radiographer, who wisely decided she could not work with her husband, so changed career and became a music teacher instead. They have a grown up family. Sandy was a very keen "amateur footballer" in his day, which meant he was never to be messed with.

David Currie

David Currie graduated in Medicine at the University of Edinburgh in 1974. After posts in Orthopaedic Surgery, Gynaecology and General Surgery he trained in Neurosurgery. He was appointed to the post of Consultant Neurosurgeon at Aberdeen Royal Infirmary in 1986, providing services to the North-East of Scotland, the Highlands and the Northern and Western Isles. He is the author of *The Management of Head Injuries*, part of the Oxford University Press Emergency Medicine series.

His grandfather interrupted medical studies in Edinburgh to enlist in the Royal Flying Corps in 1914. He was shot down twice in France but survived until the armistice and was awarded the DFC. His grandmother trained as a nurse and cared for the wounded during the Great War in East Africa. His other grandfather was quartermaster to the Royal Nyasaland Volunteer Reserve during the Great War.

John David Holmes

Born in 1949 in Cheltenham, Gloucestershire, John Holmes trained at Queens' College, Cambridge and St. Bartholomew's Hospital in London, qualifying in 1974. Junior surgical jobs were undertaken all over the UK and he became a Consultant Plastic Surgeon in Aberdeen in 1993, having met his future wife while working there in the early 1980s.

Professional interests included hand surgery, especially the management of congenital hand deformity. Regular collaboration with his orthopaedic colleagues in Aberdeen in the reconstruction of defects caused by trauma and large tumour excision was a highlight of his career. Serving on the Editorial committee of the *British Journal of Plastic Surgery* for six years, he was a member of various other professional bodies and also an ATLS Instructor. He retired from his NHS post in 2010 and continues his interest in trauma education by teaching First Aid for the British Association of Ski Patrollers to outdoor groups. He is also able to indulge his passion for skiing by working as a part-time ski-patroller in Scotland.

Foreword

*How wide and varied is the experience of the battlefield and how
fertile the blood of warriors in raising good surgeons.*

Sir Clifford Allbutt, 1898

It is a privilege which I greatly prize to contribute a foreword to this volume, which should be in the hands of all whose concern is with injuries of war and conflict. The importance of the First World War to the development of surgery should not be underestimated nor should the relevance of the pioneering work of surgeons of that epoch be forgotten.

The Great War marked a watershed in the history of civil and war surgery. In a conflict of unparalleled ferocity, 19th Century surgical principles were exposed to the devastating effect of 20th Century weaponry. There were enormous numbers of casualties. The majority suffered fragment wounds from high explosive shell, bomb and mortar blast. These wounds were unfamiliar; invariably large, multiple, severe, and infected. Within a few months of the beginning of the war, it was plain that the surgical experience of previous wars was useless and the existing standards of surgical care were woefully inadequate. A complete revision of the surgical thinking and approach to the management of war wounds was required. *War Surgery 1914–1918* tells the story of the development of the surgery of warfare on the Western Front in the Great War, and of the many advances in the medical sciences consequent to the War.

The book is multi-authored, and co-edited by Tom Scotland and Professor Steven Heys, distinguished surgeons of the Royal Infirmary of Aberdeen, a city that can claim, as its own, Sir James McGrigor, founder of the Army Medical Services and surgeon to Wellington. The text reflects on the major changes that took place in the surgical management of casualties with abdominal, thoracic, limb, and head injury during the Great War. At the start of the war, abdominal wounds were managed expectantly and the great majority died. The observations from post-mortem studies of large numbers of cases informed the technical aspects of surgery and the development of new operations. The realisation that haemorrhage killed the wounded in the early stages post-wounding meant that early operative intervention became the accepted treatment of abdominal wounds and helped to reduce their high mortality. In a similar way, the management of chest wounds became more aggressive as confidence and experience grew. Major exposures of combined wounds of the chest and abdomen through an extensive thoraco-abdominal incision were performed and became standard practice. Further chapters highlight the rapid advances made in anaesthesia, resuscitation and blood transfusion, the pathology and microbiology of wounding, diagnostic radiology, and establishing an infrastructure of evacuation pathways and medical facilities, in particular, the Casualty Clearing Station (the equivalent of our present day Role 3 Field Hospital in Afghanistan) that would help to reduce mortality from of these wounds.

The text reviews in absorbing detail the evolution under the exigencies of the War of Orthopaedic surgery, Plastic and Reconstructive surgery, and Neurosurgery as independent surgical specialties. Described by Moynihan, the most influential General Surgeon of the time, as 'a war of Orthopaedic surgery', because the majority of such casualties had limb wounds with compound fractures, in the early stages of the war the poverty and neglect of Orthopaedic training in Surgery before 1914 was all too apparent. The vision and action of Sir Robert Jones in establishing the principle of segregation, unity of control and continuity of treatment of certain categories of injured soldiers on the Western Front, and the organisation of Military Orthopaedic Centres in the United Kingdom remains one of the glorious chapters of British surgery.

Disfigurement and mutilation were ubiquitous on the battlefields of the First World War. Many soldiers sustained facial wounds because they simply had no experience of trench warfare. The American surgeon Albee wrote of how 'they seemed to think that they could pop their heads up over a trench and move quickly enough to avoid the hail of machine gun bullets'. The text describes the pioneering reconstructive surgery of Harold Gillies and his team following the Battle of the Somme in 1916, and of their attempts to restore some dignity to those terribly wounded. Similarly, we learn that wounds of skull and brain represented a significant problem. By careful individual observations and the comparison of results, principles of treatment were established that were applicable to all cranial wounds and capable of modification in individual cases.

We live, as did our predecessors, in an age of war and rumours of war. *War Surgery 1914–1918* is a timely and important contribution to war surgery's literary canon, and worthy companion to the classic British monograph on war surgery, Colonel Sir Henry Gray's *The Early Treatment of War Wounds*, published in 1919. It is fitting to recall Gray's essential work on the proper preparation and selection of cases for surgery, the urgency of proper wound excision, the need for fasciotomy, the perils of closure of infected wounds, and the need for the most experienced surgeons operating on the most severely wounded casualties. His outstanding results with the British 3rd Army in the Casualty Clearing Stations of the Western Front in the latter half of the War laid the foundations of the principles and practice of modern day war surgery.

The unity of presentation and focus on the historical and clinical aspects of war surgery makes *War Surgery 1914–1918* a unique exposition and a valuable reference to the scholar, as well as the surgeon.

The thought comes to mind of how much our knowledge of war surgery already owes to Aberdeen men like Gray, Anderson, Naughton Dunn, and Gordon-Taylor who served their country with distinction in the Great War and from whom the authors of this book have derived much of their inspiration. No reader of this book will fail to realise the impact of the lessons of surgery in the Great War on the progress and advance of the science and art of Surgery itself.

Colonel Michael P M Stewart, CBE, QHS, MBChB
(Abdn) FRCS, FRCS Tr & Orth L/RAMC
Honorary Surgeon to H.M.The Queen,
Consultant Trauma and Orthopaedic Surgeon,
Lately Defence Medical Services Consultant Advisor in
Trauma and Orthopaedics to the Surgeon General
30 June, 2011

Preface

It's a long steep climb on a bike, and quite exhausting. There is no relief from aching muscles, and our lungs are gasping for oxygen. Still, it's not too hot, as it was on the 1st July 1916, so whilst we are feeling a bit thirsty, our throats are not dry and parched with the beating sun, and we don't have to carry a rifle and heavy pack. We are not cycling into a killing zone for a machine gun and we're not being blown up by high explosive shellfire. Our hearts are beating fast, but it's not because we are scared stiff; rather it reflects our varying degrees of physical fitness. Between the roaring machinery noises of respiration as our lungs work hard for oxygen, we can hear the larks singing overhead, just as they did on that Saturday morning in July 1916.

We are cycling from the valley of the River Ancre, a tributary of the Somme, up Mill Road to the village of Thiepval, along what was No Man's Land, once upon a time. The German frontline was to the left, while the British were in the margin of Thiepval Wood to the right of us. At the top of the hill, we will visit the Memorial to the Missing of the Somme, where 72,000 soldiers who died here and who have no known grave are commemorated.

The elder statesman of the cyclists is a retired orthopaedic surgeon from Aberdeen Royal Infirmary while his younger colleague and co-editor is Professor of Cancer Surgery at the University of Aberdeen. The elder of the two has been cycling round the battlefields for many years, firstly with his wife, and then with his sons before taking many colleagues and friends all around the Western Front on various trips. His interest in the Great War goes back more than forty years, when as a medical student there were still lots of veterans around, who made a lasting impression on him. His wife's uncle, whom she never knew, was an "Old Contemptible", one of the original British Expeditionary Force. He went to Flanders in 1914, and was killed in the Ypres Salient in 1915. Since retiring from the National Health Service the orthopaedic surgeon has re-invented himself as a cycling orthopaedic historian of the Great War. He maintains that there are many proper historians who know much more about the history of the Great War; he also grudgingly admits that there are many orthopaedic surgeons who know more about orthopaedics; but put the two together and he is an expert without equal!

The younger, fitter co-editor, who in fact has raced ahead on his bike to take photographs of the other members of the team as they come on at a more leisurely pace, has just been with the group to Serre, which marked the northern limit for the British 4th Army on that first day of the Battle of the Somme. He has never been to the Western Front before, and while he has been most interested in the experience, the visit to the cemeteries at Serre where the Accrington Pals, from his hometown, are buried, and his reflections in the Sunken Lane from which men of the 1st Battalion Lancashire Fusiliers went over the top on that fateful morning, have had a profound effect on his perception of the war, and what it must have been like. He is now possessed by the same passion for the subject as the orthopaedic surgeon.

Cycling towards him are other members of the group, lost in their thoughts, because the easiest way to cycle up the hill is to think of something completely different. The orthopaedic surgeon reflects that the first British soldier of the Expeditionary Force to die in the Great War was a reconnaissance cyclist called John Parr. He was killed near Mons in Belgium on 21 August 1914. Maybe if he'd had decent gears on his bike he would have got away from the German cavalry patrol he encountered. Come to think of it, if the orthopaedic surgeon had decent gears, he might not be at the tail end of the group now. The anaesthetist on the trip comes up the hill singing *A Shropshire Lad* to take her mind off her exertions. George Butterworth was a gifted musician, who set the poems of Alfred Edward Housman to music. Butterworth was killed by a sniper's bullet on the 5 August 1916 near here. His body was never found. She is going to look for his name on the Thiepval Memorial.

Most of the medical groups who have cycled this way have been orthopaedic surgeons, but there have been the occasional general surgeon, plastic surgeon, and pathologist in the groups. They must all have wondered how the medical services coped with the huge volume of badly wounded soldiers, and indeed how they would have managed themselves, and whether they would have been able to withstand the clinical stresses and demands of war that others before them had. Certainly they would all have a great admiration for what their medical predecessors achieved.

After having time to reflect, the two co-editors decided to write this book. The orthopaedic surgeon had been thinking of writing one for years, but somehow something else always cropped up. He needed the encouragement of his academic colleague to spur him on. The two complement each other, and each has harnessed the enthusiasm of the other to fix bayonets and go over the top in this endeavour.

Together, they have combined to pay tribute to the medical services during the Great War. They have done so with the help of their friends and colleagues, many of whom have cycled up Mill Road.

Acknowledgements

The battlefields of the Western Front hold a great fascination for the co-editors, and we would like to thank all those who have made this book possible. We are very grateful to Duncan Rogers of Helion and Company, who was good enough to take on this project.

We are grateful to all our colleagues who have contributed a chapter to the work – Ann Robertson (anaesthetics), Sandy MacDonald (X-rays), Robin Reid (pathology), David Currie (neurosurgery), and John Holmes (plastic surgery). We felt it was very important to get a modern perspective on the developments which were made in the various surgical and related specialties during the Great War, and to put them into context. Such insight can only be provided by experts in those particular fields.

To make the surgical achievements of the Great War relevant to modern conflict, we recognised the need to provide a link between the surgery performed then, and the problems encountered by medical personnel in warfare in the present day. We are therefore indebted to Colonel Mike Stewart, RAMC, who agreed to write the Foreword of this book. Mike has confirmed the importance of many of the surgical developments which took place between 1914 and 1918. He has made the point that the foundations of surgery of warfare were firmly established during the Great War, and they are as relevant today as they were almost one hundred years ago.

We are grateful to Mr. Gordon Stables, of the Department of Medical Illustration, University of Aberdeen, who has been of great help in the production of many illustrations and maps. Much of the background for Chapter 5 makes use of the detailed work of the late E H Burrows and the research of Adrian M K Thomas, who also gave generous advice.

We are grateful to Diane Florence (George Florence's grand-daughter) for the story and photograph of her late grandfather in Chapter 10 and to Dr Andrew Bamji for his help and permission to use the photographs (Figures 10.5–10.20) and operation notes from the Gillies Archives. Figures 10.8, 10.10 and 10.11 were adapted from the original operation notes by Seccombe Hett. Also thanks to Carolynn Morrisey in Melbourne, Australia and the Gordon Highlanders Museum in Aberdeen for the history of the 1/5th Gordon Highlanders.

We are also very grateful to the many others who have given permission to use illustrations in this book. We have made strenuous efforts to obtain permission in every case, but in some instances so much time has passed since the publication of a photograph in a book, that it has not been possible to trace the origin of every illustration or photograph. We sincerely hope we have not offended anybody by any inadvertent act of omission.

We hope this book will be read by anyone and everyone with an interest in the history of the Great War. It has been written with a general readership in mind. It is not a textbook of medicine! We are therefore very grateful to Robert (Rab) Reid, who worked under great hardship from his "dugout" in Bearsden, and proof read the chapters to ensure that they were understandable to the lay person, and that we had not become carried away by use of medical terminology.

1

Setting the scene

Thomas R Scotland and Steven D Heys

On 29 October, 1914, tired remnants of the British Expeditionary Force (BEF) were on the Menin Road, some five miles to the south-east of the Belgian city of Ypres. They were at a little village called Gheluvelt, defending the slopes of the Gheluvelt Ridge against the might of two German armies, the 4th to the north of the road, and the 6th to the south. Reinforcing these two armies was a special force called Army Group Fabeck, created for the specific purpose of forcing a way through the British defenders to the summit of the Ridge, and the city of Ypres beyond. The British would then have to retreat to the channel ports, and be knocked out of the war. By most peoples' standards the Gheluvelt Ridge is a gentle slope, and barely worthy of comment, but in the flat countryside of Flanders it represents a significant topographical feature.

The British were exhausted. A lot had happened since the two army infantry corps and one cavalry division making up the small Expeditionary Force had embarked for France from the south of England under cover of darkness on the nights of 12 and 13 August 1914. They had been fighting and marching almost continuously since Sunday

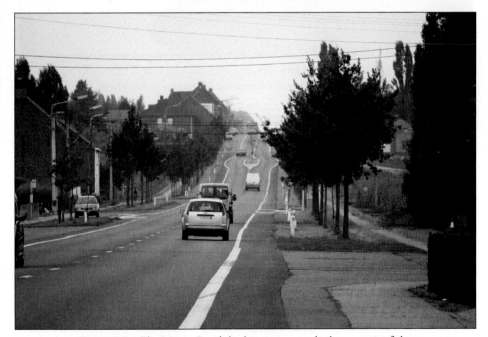

Figure 1.1   The Menin Road, looking up towards the summit of the Gheluvelt Ridge from the village of Gheluvelt. (Authors' photograph)

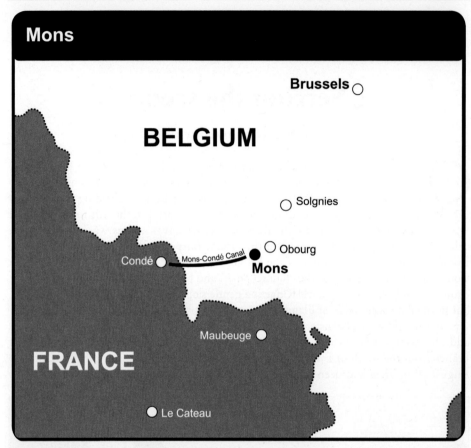

Figure 1. 2   Mons and Mons-Condé Canal, with Le Cateau to the south.
(Department of Medical Illustration, University of Aberdeen)

23 August. On that day, on the left flank of the French 5th Army, they had briefly fought the Germans at Mons and along the Mons-Condé Canal, in Belgium, before making a fighting withdrawal to the South on that Sunday evening. On 26 August at Le Cateau, General Smith-Dorrien's II Corps had turned round to deliver a stinging blow to von Kluck's German 1st Army, in a manoeuvre designed to slow down the Germans who were hard on the heels of the British forces, and not giving them a moment's respite.

The French 5th Army successfully performed a similar manoeuvre against von Bulow's German 2nd Army at Guise on 29 August, permitting the tired British to have a rest day, and tend to their blistered feet, which ached after constant marching over cobbled streets of northern France in the baking heat of late summer. Then, with their French allies on their left flank, the British pulled back to the River Marne, less than 30 miles due east of Paris. From there, General Joffre, Commander in Chief of the French forces, launched a major counter-offensive against the Germans between 6 and 9 September 1914, in what became known as the Battle of The Marne. He did so with the addition of a new French 6th Army and with the help of the British forces. It was a decisive action, and brought the German war machine to a shuddering standstill,

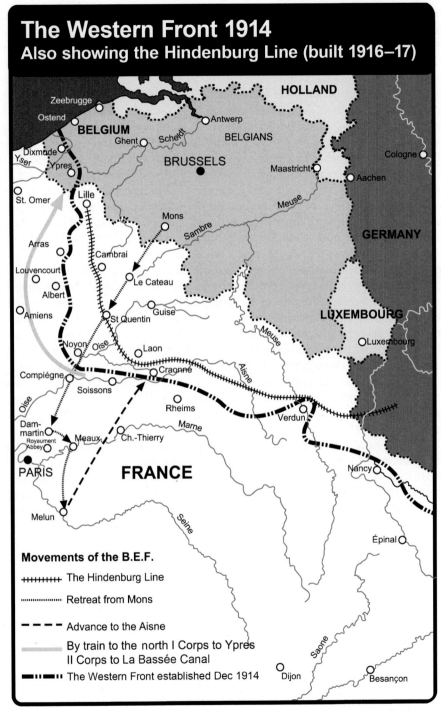

Figure 1.3   The Western Front 1914, also showing the Hindenburg Line (built 1916–17) (Department of Medical Illustration, University of Aberdeen)

pushing it into reverse. Now it was the Germans' turn to withdraw, with the French and British in pursuit.

The British had marched for more than one hundred and fifty miles since the Battle of Mons, under constant severe pressure, and now at last they had an opportunity to attack. Re-invigorated by the prospect, they and their allies pursued the enemy as they crossed the River Aisne. They had anticipated continuing the pursuit after the crossing, but instead the Germans dug in on the north bank and retreated no further. Another fierce engagement, which would become known as the Battle of the Aisne was fought between 12 and 15 September 1914 and many casualties were sustained. Each side then tried to outflank the other, in a series of moves which became known as the "race to the sea". Each tried to gain an advantage by getting in behind the enemy forces, and then "rolling up their line". These outflanking attempts were only brought to a standstill when the opposing armies reached the sandy beaches of the Belgian coast. Soon there were two lines of soldiers facing each other from the Swiss border to the Channel coast, and the Western Front came into being. A war of great movement was about to be replaced by static trench warfare, which would come to characterise the Great War. The advance to the Aisne would be the last piece of open warfare until the spring of 1918.

When troop started to move north in the "race to the sea", the BEF was transported by train in the general direction of its supply lines to play its part in the unfolding conflict. The original BEF which had fought at Mons on 23 August had two infantry corps in the field, I Corps and II Corps, each with approximately 30,000 men and a cavalry division with approximately 10,000 men. II Corps went north to fight around La Bassée, while I Corps went further north and arrived at the Belgian city of Ypres by mid-October 1914. Reinforcements to meet ever-increasing demands and growing numbers of casualties were arriving as quickly as possible. British III Corps arrived in time for the Battle of The Aisne, and IV Corps in time for the fighting around Ypres in October and November of 1914.

And so it came to be that many British troops found themselves on the Menin Road near Ypres on 29 October. Here the character of the fighting changed dramatically. The Belgian army to the north blocked access to the coastal plain in what became known as the Battle of The (River) Yser, an engagement they only won by opening the dyke sluices and flooding the flat coastal plain from the coast to Dixmuide, thus securing the northern flank of the Allied line for the duration of the war. Here, around Ypres, was the Germans' last opportunity for a breakthrough, to bring an end to fighting in the West, inflict a defeat on their hated enemy the French and knock the "contemptible" little British Army out of the war. This was to be no outflanking manoeuvre. This was to be a hammer blow of the greatest severity, to punch a hole through the heart of the British defences on the Menin Road. Only then, after first defeating the British, and then the French, would they be able to turn their full attention to deal with the Russian Armies on their Eastern Front.

It was allegedly Kaiser Wilhelm who referred to the British Expeditionary Force as a "contemptible little army". He probably had meant that it was contemptibly small, which indeed it was, rather than inferring that the soldiers themselves were contemptible. They were in fact a highly trained and hardened professional force, able to fire fifteen aimed rounds a minute using bolt-action Short Magazine Lee-Enfield Rifles. They perhaps performed best in the role of stubborn defence against overwhelming odds, as they were about to prove. There was something symbolically appropriate about the name "Old Contemptible" which the survivors of that small Professional British Army proudly called themselves as 1914 drew to a close.

The British had to call on all their experience to prevent a catastrophic breach of their lines by the Germans. By 31 October, they had been forced to withdraw to the Western, downward slope of the Gheluvelt Ridge, with the city of Ypres to their rear. There they stopped, and there they remained. The Germans never did get into Ypres just two or three miles down the road, and it would be almost four years before the British would re-occupy Gheluvelt.

As a result of this action (which became known as the Battle of Gheluvelt), and other engagements by the British, French and Belgian forces, the Allies came to hold a roughly semi-circular area of ground, bulging out against the German positions with the city of Ypres as a centre point, and with a radius of approximately 4 miles. Thus was born the infamous Ypres Salient. The Germans held the higher ground, on the ridge, and they looked down on the lower and more disadvantageous positions held by the Allies.

A salient is simply a line which protrudes outwards against the enemy position. Fighting in a salient meant that enemy artillery could be sited all round the perimeter, and defenders could be fired at from the front, from the sides, and even from the rear. There were many examples of salients throughout the length of the Western Front, but when men talked about "The Salient", they invariably referred to the killing zone around Ypres.

Opposing forces spent four years killing and maiming each other in the confined area of The Salient. There were three major engagements around Ypres, which subsequently

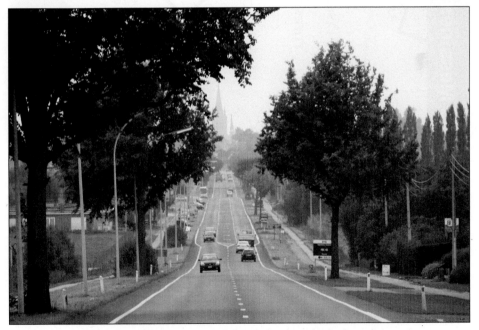

Figure 1.4   Western slope of the Gheluvelt Ridge looking down
towards the city of Ypres. (Authors' photograph)

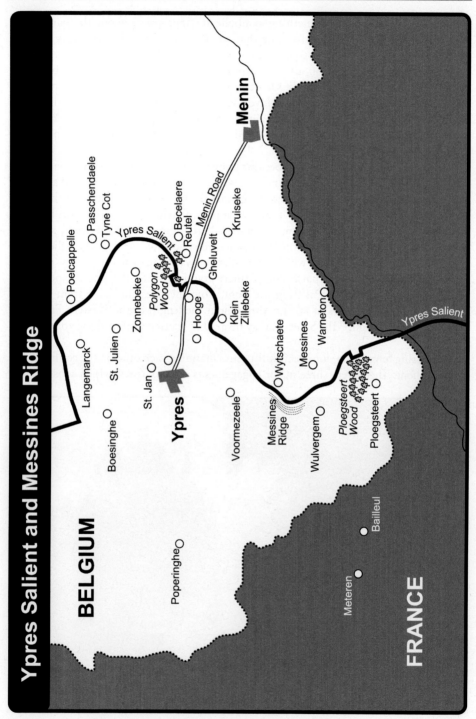

Figure 1.5   Ypres Salient and Messines Ridge (Department of Medical Illustration, University of Aberdeen)

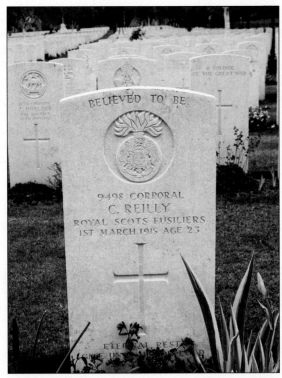

Figure 1.6   An "Old Contemptible" – he had fought at Mons, Le Cateau, the Marne and 1st Ypres. He died on a day when "nothing of importance" happened on the Western Front. (Authors' photograph)

became classified as battles, although there was fighting here every day for the duration of the war. Even when "nothing of importance" happened, men were killed or wounded in the Salient. The heavy fighting around Ypres in the closing weeks of 1914 became known as the 1st Battle of Ypres and resulted in the formation of the Ypres Salient. British casualties amounted to 58,155 killed, wounded or missing.[1] Adding casualties from prior engagements at Mons, Le Cateau, the Marne and the Aisne, it is estimated that by the end of 1914 only 1 officer and 30 other ranks remained of each battalion of 1,000 strong which had gone to France in August 1914.[2] The loss of these men was a severe blow, because they were a highly trained force of hardened professionals of great experience. In that sense they were irreplaceable, and it would be a long time before their successors acquired a matching level of ability.

There were two other major battles around Ypres. On 22 April 1915, the 2nd Battle of Ypres began when the Germans used poison gas for the first time on the Western Front. Chlorine was discharged from gas cylinders late in the afternoon of the 22nd, between the villages of Poelcapelle and Langemarck, a few miles from Ypres. This resulted in a complete collapse of the northern segment of The Salient, which became saturated by chlorine gas. French colonial troops occupying the trenches here fled, leaving a huge gap. Fortunately, the Germans had made no preparation to fully exploit the advantage gained, and so things were not as bad as they might have been, thanks to the men of the Canadian 1st Division, who had recently arrived on The Salient, and whose quick thinking and rapid deployment saved the day. While this was a crisis for the Allies, they retrieved the situation and The Salient contracted down to a tight defensive position round Ypres, making it easier to defend. The 2nd Battle of Ypres lasted approximately a month and British losses amounted to 59, 275 killed, wounded and missing. This figure includes losses sustained by the Canadian 1st Division and the Indian Corps.[3]

The 3rd Battle of Ypres began on 31st July 1917. The British strategic aim was to break out from The Salient and capture the Belgian ports of Ostend and Zeebrugge. This would deny their use to the Germans as U-boat bases. This was wishful thinking, and the offensive became completely bogged down in the mud at the village of Passchendaele in November 1917, where men fought and died in the most appalling conditions. This battle involved Australian, New Zealand and Canadian Divisions as well as British and South African troops. Total losses were 244,897 killed, wounded and missing, according to Neillands.[4] According to Prior and Wilson the losses were 275,000, with 70,000 killed.[5] The reality is that no one knows precisely how many died and sank forever into the mud.

As will be seen in Chapter 2, figures exist for numbers of casualties admitted to, and treated by, the various casualty clearing stations during the 3rd Battle of Ypres. The numbers of wounded are staggering, and one may wonder how on earth the medical services coped with so much work. If a surgical team working in a modern fully equipped hospital of today had more than twenty patients admitted during a 24 hour period, it would consider itself busy. Casualty clearing stations during 3rd Ypres were regularly dealing with 200 to 300 admissions a day, before passing the "on call" on to an adjacent clearing station while working through the caseload of admissions.

More than a quarter of a million British and Commonwealth soldiers died in the confined area of the Salient during four years of the Great War. There are approximately 150 British Military cemeteries within a five-mile radius of the city of Ypres. Some are small and secluded, with only a few dozen burials, while others are huge with several thousand graves. After the war, many tiny cemeteries and isolated graves were relocated to designated "concentration" cemeteries, to allow reclamation of the land. There were dead buried almost everywhere on The Salient, and squads of men searched the battlefield methodically, digging up the scattered dead, and taking them to be reburied in a chosen concentration cemetery. The biggest British military cemetery in the world, and an example of a concentration cemetery, is located near the village of Passchendaele at Tyne Cot, where there are 11,908 graves.

Because of the ravages of time, and the destructive nature of shellfire, 8,366, or 70% of the soldiers (or what remained of the destroyed bodies) buried in Tyne Cot are unidentified. "A Soldier of the Great War Known unto God" was the epitaph given by Imperial author, poet and Nobel Laureate, Rudyard Kipling, whose only son John had been killed at the Battle of Loos in September 1915, and his body never found. The bodies of a great many of those who died were never found, and the Menin Gate at Ypres has the names of 58,000 soldiers who have no known grave inscribed on its stone panels. There wasn't enough room for all the names here, so a further 34,000 are commemorated on a wall at the back of Tyne Cot British Military Cemetery.

To the south of Ypres, swinging away from the city and towards the nearby French border is Messines Ridge (see Figure 1.5). It was here on 31 October 1914 that the first

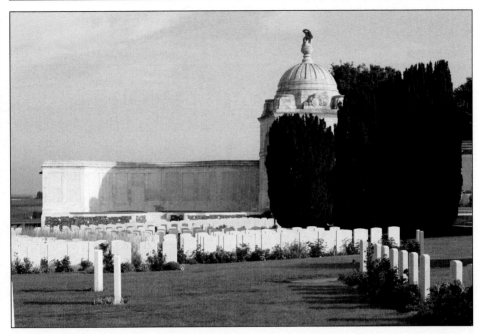

Figure 1.7   Tyne Cot British Military Cemetery, the biggest British military cemetery in the world. Part of the wall can be seen at the back of the cemetery, inscribed with the names of 34,000 soldiers who died in the "Salient" and who have no known grave. (Authors' photograph)

Territorial battalion to be involved in the Great War went into action. At the same time as the Germans were fighting the British on the Menin Road, they were also trying to get the British off the high ground to the south of Ypres at Messines Ridge. The Expeditionary Force was running severely short of men, and men of the 14th Battalion, County of London Regiment (London Scottish) were rushed into battle on 31 October, 1914 at Wytschaete, in the central part of the Messines Ridge. The London Scottish suffered heavy casualties, in no small part due to the fact that their Lee-Enfield rifles, SMLE Mk 1, were incapable of taking the new Mk VII ammunition. Their rifles jammed unless they were loaded with single rounds fed into the breach by hand, therefore seriously reducing the effectiveness of their weapons.

The destruction of the small British professional army in late 1914 resulted in Territorial divisions being sent to the Western Front in significant numbers. When the Territorial Force first came into being, the original concept was that it would guard Britain's shores in the event of the Expeditionary Force having to go overseas. Casualties in 1914 were so heavy that soldiers of the Territorial Army were invited to sign up for posting overseas and when the British took over more of the front line from their French allies in 1915, and their commitment to fighting increased, territorial troops went to France in increasing numbers, partly as battalions to reinforce depleted divisions already in France, and partly as entire divisions to take part in British offensives of 1915.

In addition to having to defend on the Ypres Salient in April and May 1915, the British conducted offensives between March and September in northern France at Neuve Chapelle, Aubers Ridge, Festubert, and Loos, all very much at the instigation

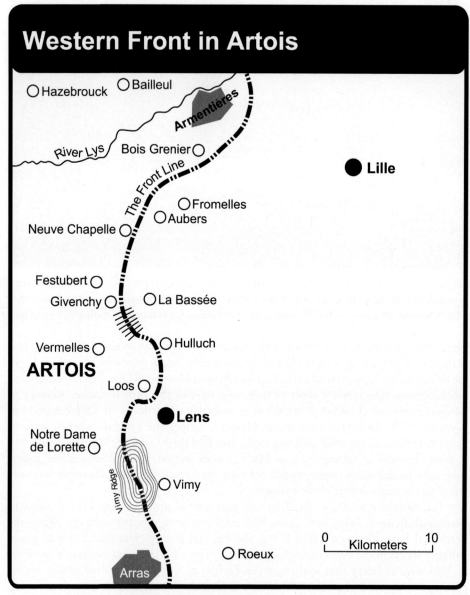

Figure 1.8   The 1915 battlefields in Northern France. (Department of Medical Illustration, University of Aberdeen)

of their French allies who wanted British support while they (the French) attacked the Germans further south.

By April 1915, there were six Territorial divisions in France, the 46th (North Midland), 47th (London), 48th (South Midland), 49th (West Riding), 50th (Northumbrian), and 51st (Highland).[6]

The first of Kitchener's Volunteer divisions had also arrived on the Western Front by 1915, and they were to play a major part in the fighting over the next two years. Lord Kitchener, Secretary of State for War, had little faith in the Territorial Army, harbouring a quite illogical prejudice against it. Kitchener was one of the few who did not believe that this war would be "over by Christmas." Realising that it would be a long and costly conflict, he instigated a recruiting campaign to persuade men to volunteer for service in the British Army. Posters appeared with Kitchener's stern face and pointing finger, challenging whoever stopped to look to join up. Men flocked in their thousands to enlist. Two of the first resulting service divisions of Kitchener's "New Army" were in the field by mid 1915, in time to take part on the first day of the Battle of Loos on the 25th September 1915. It just so happened they were both Scottish Divisions. The 9th (Scottish) and 15th (Scottish) Divisions were two of a total of six divisions which went over the top and into battle on 25 September 1915. Men forming these two divisions came from all over Scotland, as shown in Table 1.1.

Table 1.1
Scottish battalions in the 9th and 15th Scottish divisions at Loos, 25 September 1915

9th (Scottish Division)		15th (Scottish Division)	
Brigade	**Battalion**	**Brigade**	**Battalion**
26th (Highland)	8th Black Watch 7th Seaforth Highlanders 8th Gordon Highlanders 5th Cameron Highlanders	44th (Highland)	9th Black Watch 8th Seaforth Highlanders 10th Gordon Highlanders 7th Cameron Highlanders
27th (Lowland)	11th Royal Scots 12th Royal Scots 6th Royal Scots Fusiliers 10th Argyll and Sutherland Highlanders	45th	13th Royal Scots 7th Royal Scots Fusiliers 6th Cameron Highlanders 11th Argyll and Sutherland Highlanders
28th	6th King's Own Scottish Borderers 9th Scottish Rifles 10th Highland Light Infantry 11th Highland Light Infantry	46th	7th King's Own Scottish Borderers 8th King's Own Scottish Borderers 10th Scottish Rifles 12th Highland Light Infantry
Pioneers	9th Seaforth Highlanders	Pioneers	9th Gordon Highlanders

Based on Ewing, J., *The History of the 9th (Scottish) Division 1914-1919*. London: John Murray, 1921, p.398 and Stewart, J. & J. Buchan, *The 15th (Scottish) Division 1914-1919*. Edinburgh: William Blackwood and Sons, 1926, pp.286-7.

An infantry division was made up of 3 brigades, and each brigade had 4 battalions. At full strength there were nearly 1,000 men in each battalion. Thus each division had approximately 12,000 infantry, and the two Scottish divisions, in battle for the first time, sustained appalling casualties. The respective statistics for casualty figures are taken from their divisional histories[7, 8], and are summarised in Table 1.2. The figures shown refer to losses sustained over three days between 25 and 27 September, 1915.

Table 1.2
Casualty figures for the 9th and 15th (Scottish) divisions at Loos, September 1915

Division	Officers killed, wounded, missing	Other Ranks killed, wounded, missing
9th (Scottish)	190	5,867
15th (Scottish)	217	6,406

Based on Ewing, J., *The History of the 9th (Scottish) Division 1914-1919*. London: John Murray, 1921, p.398 and Stewart, J. & J. Buchan, *The 15th (Scottish) Division 1914-1919*. Edinburgh: William Blackwood and Sons, 1926, pp.286-7.

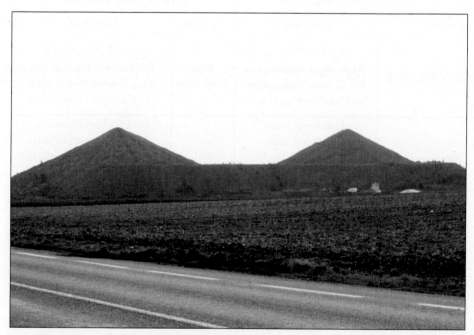

Figure 1.9   The "Double Crassier" marking the southern limit of the battlefield at Loos, so typical of this industrial region of Northern France. (Authors' photograph)

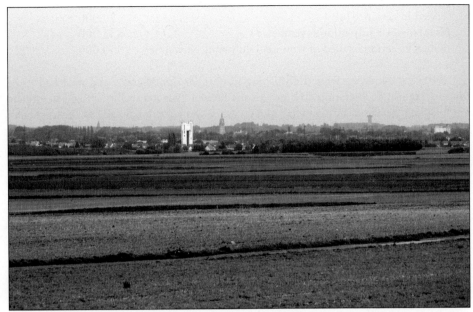

Figure 1.10   The battlefield at Loos looking north towards La Bassée. The
northern limit of the battlefield was the La Bassée canal. The town of La
Bassée was behind the German lines. (Authors' photograph)

Indeed, the Battle of Loos can justifiably be described as "a very Scottish battle", because in addition to the 9th and 15th Divisions, there were Scottish battalions in the three regular divisions that took part at Loos. The Battle of Loos was fought over ground which was partly industrialised, with slag heaps called crassiers, from coal mines, and partly over flat and featureless open country with no natural cover.

The battle was fought against the better judgement of the High Command, who were pressurised into supporting French offensives further to the south at Vimy Ridge and Champagne. Because of a severe shortage of artillery pieces and ordnance, reliance was placed on poison gas to compensate for these deficiencies. It was the only occasion during the war that a battle was fought relying strategically on gas rather than artillery to procure a successful outcome. It failed miserably. The wind such as it was, was blowing in the wrong direction over much of the battlefield, so that on the front of the 1st Division men became victims of their own gas.

It would be at the Battle of the Somme in 1916, however, when Kitchener's Volunteers would be present in a majority of participating divisions on the first day of battle.

The Somme will forever be associated with heavy and tragic loss. The 1st July 1916 was in absolute terms to be the worst ever day in British military history as Table 1.3 only too clearly illustrates.[9]

Table 1.3

Summary of losses at the Battle of the Somme, 1 July-mid-November 1916

Total casualties 1 July	60,000

Killed in action 1 July	20,000
Total losses 1 July-mid November	432,000
Killed in action or died of wounds 1 July-mid-November	150,000

By 1915, volunteers were diminishing in number significantly, and men had to be found to maintain battalion strength in the face of ever mounting casualties. By late 1915, all men between the ages of 15 and 65 years who were not already in the forces had to register to notify the authorities which trade they were in. In October 1915 Lord Derby was appointed to the position of Director of Recruiting. He then proceeded to encourage all those between the ages of 18 and 40 to either enlist or to attest with an obligation to enlist if called. The carrot to encourage enlistment, if it can be called that, was the assurance of a war pension in the event of being killed or wounded. Not surprisingly, this encouragement did not have the desired result, and consequently conscription was brought into effect in the Military Services Act in January 1916.

Many recruits from the Derby Scheme or young conscripts would first see action in 1917. The two principal battles in 1917 were the Battle of Arras, in April and May 1917, and 3rd Ypres, from the 31st July to the 10th November 1917. Losses at Arras were approximately 158,660, of whom 29,505 were killed.[10] Losses at 3rd Ypres have already been mentioned. By mid-1917 therefore, until the end of the war, the ever-expanding British Army, excluding those from the Dominions, would be a mixture of remnants of the original British Expeditionary Force, men from the Territorial Army, Kitchener's Volunteers and conscripts.

The Germans too were feeling the strain. They suffered very severe losses in 1916, both on the Somme and at Verdun, where they had fought a prolonged battle of attrition against the French from February to December 1916. As a result of losses sustained in these two battles, they withdrew to a prepared defensive line which effectively shortened the length of their front by eliminating a broad-based salient. This was called the Hindenburg Line by the British.

Beginning on 21 March 1918, the Allies had to withstand a series of five German offensives launched from the Hindenburg Line, between March and July, as they desperately tried to bring the war to a conclusion. In February 1917, the Germans had introduced unrestricted U-boat activity against neutral merchant ships supplying the allies, resulting in the sinking of American ships. This proved to be the last straw, bringing the United States of America into the war in April 1917. It would be many months before Americans would be fighting in France, but the German High Command knew that ultimately they would bring in overwhelming numbers of men with appropriate materials from their almost unlimited resources. On the 16th December 1917 the leaders of the Bolsheviks – Lenin, Trotsky, and Stalin – sued for peace with the Central Powers, and an armistice was declared. A peace treaty was signed on 29 March 1918 at Brest-Litovsk, and Russia was out of the war.

Massive numbers of German troops moved from what had been the Eastern Front across to the Western Front in preparation for major offensives in the spring of 1918. The aim was simple – to end the war before overwhelming numbers of Americans arrived and brought about the inevitable defeat of Germany. Mobile warfare was back to stay, and the British were pushed back to the very outskirts of Amiens before the first of the German offensives, codenamed "Michael", was halted. There followed a further four

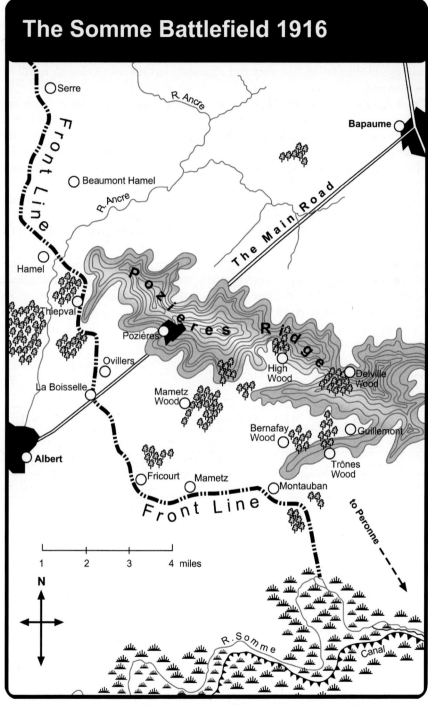

Figure 1.11   The Somme Battlefield 1916 (Department of
Medical Illustration, University of Aberdeen)

offensives, one against the British in the north, pushing up through Armentières and Messines Ridge from the south towards Ypres and the railway junction of Hazebrouck, and three against the French around Rheims. While much ground was lost to the enemy in these offensives, the Allied lines were never breached, and the attacks petered out. The German gamble had failed, and they had effectively lost the war, although it still had a long way to run.

On 8 August 1918 the British launched a major counter-offensive at the Battle of Amiens, and after 100 days of crushing victories, the war was over. Men who had gone to war in the warm summer of 1914 would not have recognised the army of 1918. It had been transformed by sophisticated artillery, able to locate German batteries accurately by sound ranging, and by new high explosive shells which were the equivalent of a modern day cruise missile by comparison with what had been available in 1914. Infantry attacks went in behind scientifically calculated creeping barrages to protect the advancing troops, and by late 1918 the British Army had become an unstoppable force.

Losses however were still very heavy. The official figures for battle losses in 1918 on the Western Front are shown in Table 1.4.[11] The very large number of prisoners of war reflects the rapid gain of ground made by the Germans during their Spring Offensives, when they made huge inroads, advancing many miles, and capturing many demoralised and confused troops. The Germans of course experienced a similar pattern of losses during the last hundred days. In 1913, before the outbreak of the war, the approximate total strength of the British Army at home and overseas was 212,355. By 1918, that number was 4,796,088.[12]

Table 1.4
Battle casualties 1918

Battle Casualties	Officers	Men	Total
Killed	5,111	75,365	80,476
Died of Wounds	3,044	43,040	40,084
Missing	1,317	62,324	63,641
Prisoners of war	3,749	103,898	107,647
Total wounded less those who died of wounds	25,733	552,669	578,402

(Modified from Mitchell, T.J. & G.M. Smith, *History of the Great War based on Official Documents. Medical Services. Casualties and Medical Statistics.* London: HMSO, 1931, p.168)

The medical response and how the medical service developed in the years leading up to the Great War

The maintenance of health, prevention of disease and the provision of medical care to wounded military personnel, from the battlefield to complex modern hospitals during times of conflict are essential in any military force. Historically, the first medical officers were appointed to the army of Charles II with the position of Regimental Surgeons. Each was provided with an assistant surgeon and a basic hospital facility. However, it was in 1812 that the first attempt was made to organise a medical service when the Duke of

Wellington and his men were fighting the armies of Napoleon in Spain and Portugal. The Chief of Medical Staff for Wellington's army was Sir James McGrigor, a graduate of the University of Aberdeen[13], who went on to become Director-General of the Army Medical Services between 1815 and 1851. He is regarded as the father of army medical services.

During the long interval of peace between the final defeat of Bonaparte in 1815 and the outbreak of the Crimean War in 1854, many of the medical lessons learned during the Napoleonic Wars were lost, which partly explains the dismal performance of the medical services during the Crimean War.

Another important factor contributing to this unsatisfactory state of affairs was the lack of authority and low status which was accorded to doctors. They were regarded as little better than camp followers. Doctors did not have a military rank. They did have some, but not all, of the privileges that would have gone with rank. Whilst provision of servants, living accommodation, financial compensation for wounds and pensions for doctors and their families were comparable to those of other officers, they usually received less pay. As a result of this inequality, there was much unrest and dissatisfaction amongst army doctors which led to considerable debate in the medical press. Some expressed the view that military rank was unnecessary and had no meaning for a doctor. His Royal Highness the Duke of Cambridge went further and argued that his "military instincts could not carry the idea of giving medical officers military titles or rank".[14] Others thought that the lack of military rank could result in doctors having disciplinary problems with soldiers in hospitals.

Each regiment had a surgeon and assistant. Whilst there was an overarching Army Medical Department, there was a lack of coordination and cohesion in the provision of services. Their low status and lack of authority within the overall army structure meant that doctors could not play any part in driving the medical agenda for the benefit and well being of soldiers. His low status meant that a medical officer was not even permitted to dine with other officers. All these factors combined to foster feelings of great resentment and discontent.

The Crimean War was a major disaster in terms of medical care of the wounded and the sick. The provision of drinking water and the disposal of sewage were inadequate. Drinking water was contaminated by harmful bacteria, and communicable disease was rife amongst the soldiers who lived in cramped and unhygienic conditions. Many more soldiers died from disease than succumbed from wounds. The figures for the Crimean War are shown in Table 1.5 where five times as many men died from disease (predominantly cholera and typhus in British, French and Russian troops with French troops also dying from scurvy). In subsequent wars, this ratio decreased, although even by the Boer War (1899-1902), typhoid fever killed many more British troops than enemy action (see Chapter 2). It would not be until 1914-1918 that deaths from wounds would greatly exceed deaths from disease, and that state of affairs would only come about after a major shift in policy regarding the role of doctors in the planning and provision of health care amongst soldiers.

Florence Nightingale worked in a military hospital at Scutari, near Istanbul, arriving there in November 1854. She found wounded soldiers being badly cared for by overworked medical staff in appalling conditions and in the face of official indifference. She quickly and inevitably came into conflict with Sir John Hall, the head of army medical services in the Crimea, who described her as a "petticoat *imperieuse*" since she was fiercely critical of him and of the hospital facilities.

Table 1.5
Deaths from those with wounds and from those with disease in different wars

War	Years	Ratio of deaths due to disease compared with that due to wounds
Peninsular War	1808-1814	7.5:1
Crimean War	1854-1856	5:1
Second Boer War	1899-1902	2:1
Russo-Japanese War	1904-1905	1.6:1

Florence Nightingale believed that the high death rates were due to poor nutrition and exhaustion of the soldiers, and this point of view brought her into conflict with another strong-willed and uncompromising figure, Dr. James Barry.

Barry was a graduate from the University of Edinburgh, who had a great interest in the role that nutrition, exercise, hygiene and sanitation played in the maintenance of good health. He was a skilled surgeon, and is credited with performing one of the first caesarean sections in South Africa when both mother and child survived in around 1820. He attracted controversy, and was recognised as being opinionated and argumentative, and he displayed lack of respect for military regulations. It is said that he spoke with a high-pitched voice and was "effeminate". He was inclined to seek confrontation with his military superiors and although frequently reprimanded he continued with his work regardless.

At the outbreak of the Crimean War, Barry had been posted to nearby Corfu, where many of the wounded were treated. Indeed, Barry's method of nursing sick and wounded soldiers evacuated from the Crimea was so successful that the recovery rate was the highest for the whole Crimea campaign. Hearing of events in Scutari, Barry applied to go there. His application was ignored, but Barry decided he was going anyway, and this brought him into conflict with Florence Nightingale. These two strong-minded individuals did not get on well together. There was a public confrontation. Barry believed that disease was caused by poor hospital sanitation and bad ventilation. He left Florence Nightingale in no doubt that poor hygiene was the cause of disease and that she had not addressed the problem. Barry scolded Nightingale for her unclean practices. She responded strongly, and in her words, Barry was "a brute" and "the most hardened creature I ever met throughout the army". Many years later after Barry's death in 1865, she said:

> As Mr. Whitehead once remarked, I will mention that I never had such a blackguard rating in all my life – I who have had more than any woman – than from this Barrie sitting on (her) horse, while I was crossing the Hospital Square, with only my cap on, in the sun. (He) kept me standing in the midst of quite a crowd of soldiers, commissariat servants, camp followers, etc., etc., everyone of whom behaved like

a gentleman during the scolding I received, while (she) behaved like a brute. After (she) was dead, I was told (he) was a woman.[15]

A Sanitary Commission was sent out to inspect the hospital facilities in Scutari, flushed out the sewers in the hospital, and improved ventilation, as a result of which death rates from infectious diseases fell dramatically with Nightingale's help.[16]

It seems unfortunate that two such single-minded individuals as James Barry and Florence Nightingale did not see "eye to eye". They were both determined to improve matters, and although they held different views as to the cause of the high mortality amongst troops they were both on the right lines for tackling the same problem from their respective approaches. Had they combined their skills, instead of being at loggerheads, the outcome for many soldiers might have been more favourable.

After the Crimean War they both returned to England, but there was a twist in the tale. Nightingale received praise and was recognised for the remarkable reduction in deaths due to infectious disease, and she continued to work tirelessly for health reforms.[17] Such praise and fame probably had an element of "Victorian spin," focusing public attention on the "lady with the lamp," while at the same time diverting the nation's focus away from the awful and embarrassing reality of the Crimean War. By way of contrast Barry was forced to retire from the army against his will in 1859. He died six years later from influenza, with very little money and in relative obscurity. After his death in 1885, despite having left strict instructions to be buried in the clothes in which he died and for there to be no post-mortem, it was revealed that he was a woman, and may even have had a child as evidence by striae gravidarum (stretch marks) on his abdomen. However, this can happen in males also if they have certain types of hormonal disturbance, e.g. Cushing's disease.

Barry's life is still the subject of mystery, and rumours of affairs with nobility persist – there are more questions than answers concerning this doctor.[18] However, Barry had lived life as a male to be able to pursue an ambition to enter medical school, had studied surgery and had made a major contribution to health in general and military surgery in

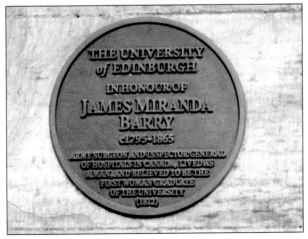

Figure 1.12   Plaque commemorating James Barry, Old College,
University of Edinburgh. (Authors' photograph)

particular. Perhaps James Barry could lay claim to being the University of Edinburgh's first female graduate and the first female from Britain to become a doctor.

Following the medical disaster of the Crimean War, a Royal Commission was set up in 1857 to look at the various problems, very much at the instigation of the British Medical Association and Florence Nightingale. It highlighted problems associated with poor sanitation, and ways of dealing with the sick and the wounded. It addressed the problems of poor medical training, and inadequate surgical experience displayed by doctors in the Crimea. It made a number of suggestions, such as the formation of an army medical school, and that medical officers should be given authority to give advice to commanding officers on matters relating to the health and well-being of the troops.

The Army Medical School was opened at Fort Pitt in 1860, moving to Netley, near Southampton, in 1863. Netley was close to, and within easy access of the port of Southampton, where hospital ships arrived, and was specifically intended for the reception and treatment of returning wounded soldiers. The site had been bought for the sum of £15,000 and Queen Victoria laid the foundation stone in 1856, beneath which were laid the plans of the hospital, the first Victoria Cross to be made and a silver Crimea Medal. When the hospital was demolished in 1966 the Victoria Cross was retrieved from beneath the foundation stone. It may now be found in the Army Medical Services Museum and is called "The Netley VC".

There were many faults with the hospital at Netley, such as lack of ventilation, and the Army medical school was subsequently moved to Millbank in London in 1907 (via temporary accommodation in London in 1902). Netley continued to function as a hospital for many years, being used by the USA in the Second World War as such. Millbank was not only a place for doctors to be trained but it also functioned as a research centre, pushing forward the frontiers of military medicine and surgery.

For a doctor to join the army in addition to being qualified in medicine, he had to be unmarried, have dissected a whole body, and observed 12 midwifery cases. Then he had to be successful in a further series of examinations including meteorology, geography, zoology, botany and not forgetting of course, medicine and surgery!

The report of the 1857 Royal Commission led to the Warrant of 1858, which introduced the first elaborate code for the medical services, but still left it weak. While it ensured that doctors now had a rank, albeit a combined medical/military one, and pay and conditions became equivalent to non-medical officers, the new combination rank (e.g. " surgeon captain") was not generally accepted by non-medical officers. The medical department was rarely consulted on matters relating to health. Medical officers spent all their time with their regiments, and had little opportunity to improve their knowledge. They were regarded exclusively as "treaters of disease." There were even separate regimental hospitals, and however many regiments were in a garrison, each had its own facilities, which was hopelessly inefficient.

In 1873, the regimental hospital system was abolished, and replaced by garrison establishments complete with laboratories, libraries, and expert instruction, which was at least a step in the right direction. This change was opposed by many senior officers, who were then granted the concession of retaining the services of a particular medical officer for ten years. Thus different battalions were cared for in different wards but all under the same roof. At least this "centralisation of services" created the potential for a coordinated medical plan for the first time in the event of a war.

Heavy casualties in the Franco-Prussian War of 1870-71 led to the establishment of a system with a regimental medical officer and a team of sixteen stretcher-bearers, based on the Prussian model, for early treatment of the wounded.

Nevertheless, while all this was happening, a life in the army was not an attractive proposition, with little perceived benefit compared with civilian practice. Recruitment continued to be difficult. Whilst conditions for medical officers may have appeared to have changed for the better, in practice nothing had altered. Army doctors were still held in low esteem, and were regarded in the same way as before. The opportunities and benefits of working in a civilian practice far outweighed those of being in the army, both in terms of status and financial remuneration.

In 1884, the medical military ranks, such as they were, e.g. "surgeon major", were abolished, and there was much bad feeling between the medical profession and the War Office. Most medical schools refused to supply candidates for the Army, and there was a great deal of lobbying by the British Medical Association (BMA) to bring about change. The medical Royal Colleges, whilst not supportive of army careers for doctors, did emphasise that army doctors should have equivalent military rank to non-medical officers, to enable them to carry out their duties with appropriate authority. However, resistance to doctors having equivalent military rank persisted, both from the War Office and other military personnel. In spite of this, there was growing awareness within the army of the difficulties faced by doctors and an appreciation of the issues which had to be addressed to allow provision of better medical care.

Even so, things did not improve. There were no new doctors taken into the army in the two years after 1887. A parliamentary committee reported on doctors' injustices in 1890, while the campaign for equality for medical officers continued, with lobbying by the BMA and Royal College of Physicians.

By now even peace time requirements for army medical personnel were not met. Only after a long and bitter struggle did commonsense prevail, and in 1898, out of struggle and strife, the Royal Army Medical Corps was born. "In Arduis Fidelis" (Steadfast in Adversity) is their motto, and how appropriate!

Officers and other ranks providing medical care became the Royal Army Medical Corps (RAMC). The first Colonel–in-Chief was HRH the Duke of Connaught, who would later become Governor General of Canada, and whose daughter, the Princess Patricia, would become Colonel-in-Chief of The Princess Patricia's Canadian Light Infantry, the first Canadian troops to set foot in France during the Great War.

In spite of the creation of the RAMC, inequality persisted, and doctors did not see joining the army as an attractive career option. Not only were there no new doctors joining but there continued to be a boycott by many medical schools for a variety of reasons, including the uncertainty about careers within the army. Army doctors had to retire after 10 years service, and they did not have the same conditions governing leave as other officers.[19]

During the Boer War, mortality from infectious disease, especially typhoid fever, significantly exceeded deaths sustained during fighting. Medical officers still had little "clout" in managing health issues, while the higher command regarded such matters as beneath their dignity.

A key figure in the development of the RAMC, and in bringing about a change in the medical officer's standing, was Sir Alfred Keogh, who had joined the Army medical services in 1880. Keogh was a doctor of exceptional ability, gaining the highest marks during his time at the Army Medical College. As his career developed, he distinguished himself in the Boer War and rose rapidly through the ranks, becoming Director-General Army Medical Services in 1904. Medical officers had experienced difficulties with other officers during the Boer War, who showed lack of respect for their commitment and professional skills. There was a suggestion that the Victoria Cross should not be awarded to doctors (no matter what their acts of bravery) and their terms and conditions were still not equivalent and appropriate. This situation could not be allowed to continue and another Royal Commission was set up to make recommendations to bring about the necessary changes to put an end to this long-standing inequality.

Alfred Keogh made important contributions in the RAMC to improvements in hygiene and to the reorganisation of the service during his tenure of this post until his initial retirement from the army in 1910.[19, 20] Poor hygiene and communicable diseases had been a cause of substantial morbidity and mortality during the Boer War. The Army School of Hygiene was established by Lt-Col Richard Firth. As Professor of Hygiene, he particularly addressed such issues as good sanitation, clean water supplies (chlorination), effective typhoid vaccine, and the education of soldiers in matters pertaining to their health and well-being. These measures were vital to ensure that the problems resulting from poor hygiene in the Boer War were not repeated in the Great War. Keogh ensured that different hospitals in existence were reorganised to create larger, fit for purpose military hospitals where appropriate expertise and facilities for treating the wounded was to be found.[21, 22]

In 1906, Richard Haldane was appointed Secretary of State for War, with a remit to modernise the British Army in preparation for a European war. He was arguably the most capable Secretary of State for War that Great Britain has known, and his achievements are discussed in detail in Chapter 2. Like any politician, Haldane was very aware of financial restraints. He knew that the army had lost too many men to various preventable diseases in previous campaigns. It was very much in his interest to ensure that the soldiers received the best possible medical care, minimising losses from disease, and maximising the fighting capability of the troops. In Alfred Keogh, he found a very supportive ally, and at long last, medical officers were to play a significant role in the health and well-being of their charges, with due attention being given to proper sanitation and appropriate education of medical personnel.

While Haldane was creating the Territorial Force, Keogh was instrumental in the development of sanitary companies in that Force, and he keenly supported the Territorial hospitals, which he saw as a key component of the provision of medical care in time of war or disaster. Needless to say, he was given every support necessary by his political ally to make all this happen.

However, there was still a problem with the number of medical officers. It was recognised that in the event of war there was an insufficient number to service an expeditionary force. To deal with this, an additional 179 medical officer posts were created.[23] The work of Haldane in planning the reorganisation of the non-regular army into Special Reserve and the Territorial Force and the Officer Training Corps provided a framework upon which Keogh could develop the medical systems. Keogh used his initiative in recruiting medical officers, going around the country to meet and consult with civilian doctors who were interested in, and understood the requirements for medicine as practiced in the army. He listened to their advice and acted upon it. His endeavours were successful, because Territorial medical units rapidly became established and by 1910 had full or near-full complements of doctors. During his tenure he actively worked with medical schools to provide a reserve of doctors who would be called upon in time of war. The Officer Training Corps (another of Haldane's reforms) was established in the Universities with the intention of encouraging an army career. This was very successful because almost 2,000 medical students gained military experience through the Officer Training Corps before the start of the Great War.

Although Keogh had retired from the army in 1910 he was recalled in October 1914 and played an important role in the Great War, taking up the post of Director-General Army Medical Services in the War Office. His work and planning formed the basis of the rapid mobilisation of Territorial hospitals at the start of the Great War and they worked with the regular hospitals very effectively. On the Western front, Sir Arthur Sloggett became Director General Medical Services (DGMS), which split responsibilities to make a manageable workload for both of these men. Interestingly, Sloggett had been at the Battle of Omdurman in 1898, had been shot through the chest, and was thought to have been killed. A closer inspection revealed that he was still alive. He was "revived", by whatever means, and survived the experience, going on to achieve great things!

At the outbreak of the Great War there was an estimated need for 800 medical officers to be attached to the British Expeditionary Force. The available doctors to the entire British Army at that time were as follows:[24]

- 406 regular army medical officers
- 119 reserve list medical officers
- 248 special reserve medical officers

In order to increase the number to the desired level, and acknowledging the need to increase numbers over and above the immediate requirements, the Central Medical War Committee in England and Wales conducted a recruiting campaign for civilian doctors. In Scotland, a Scottish Medical Service Committee had already been set up and was responding well to the needs of the military, while ensuring that the medical requirements of the civilian population were being met. Both these committees were successful and initially more than 5,000 civilian doctors were enrolled. It was planned that medical officers would stay with the army for either 12 months or until the end of the war.

Perhaps of some concern was the fact that more than 2,000 doctors had been in the Territorial and reserve units and were not available for practices in the UK. Various measures were employed to reduce the impact on the civilian population, these being of some assistance. Territorial medical officers would be kept close to their practices, exchange with other doctors or stay in a home-based unit if the unit they had been with was sent overseas. However, in many situations doctors were removed from their practices to serve and with a lack of time to sort out their civilian practices before leaving.

By the beginning of the war the required number of doctors for posting overseas had been reached and there seemed few concerns about having sufficient numbers for the war effort. That said, the medical profession itself questioned the need for so many. There were financial implications associated with joining up, with loss of income from leaving lucrative civilian practices. Furthermore, the costs of getting a locum to look after practices could be high and act as a disincentive. Attempts were made at a national level to prevent doctors who stayed at home from benefiting financially. Not only were army doctors required for overseas but fighting units still at home in the UK required an adequate number of doctors who had many tasks to ensure the maintenance of optimal health amongst their men.

A medical officer had two responsibilities. One was to the individual soldier, and the other was to the army and nation. His responsibility to the soldier was to ensure that he provided the best possible treatment in the event of that soldier being wounded, and do his utmost to save his life and mitigate his suffering. His responsibility to the army was to ensure minimum wastage of manpower. He had a duty to make a soldier fit again as quickly as possible after being wounded, and to prevent the spread of disease in a force, thereby minimising losses through disease and illness. One of the principal duties of medical officers in the forward areas was to retain soldiers with minor wounds in the forward area, preventing their loss to base hospitals and delaying their return to the front line.

The war situation was changing all the time. Large numbers of wounded on the Western Front, conflicts in other theatres of war, and the deaths of many doctors, led to a re-evaluation of the situation. It was realised by the end of 1915 that although about 25% of all doctors in the UK had already joined the army, there was going to be a shortfall. Another 100 doctors would be needed by the start of 1916. A variety of measures were adopted to allow doctors to leave their practices without disadvantaging themselves or their civilian patients. In spite of this, and in spite of increasing numbers of medical personnel from other combatant nations, there were still not enough doctors.

Lord Derby's scheme (the 17th Earl, Edward Stanley), which was started in 1915 to provide manpower for the war effort was also applied to doctors. Those doctors who volunteered for service would only be called when necessary, and those who were married would only be asked to serve in the absence of available single men. The Derby scheme was not a successful exercise, and led to the Military Service Act, 1916, which meant that doctors also were liable for conscription. There was still the problem to ensure that whilst there were adequate numbers for the ever-increasing demand of the military, there were sufficient doctors for the civilian population. To achieve this balance, and to decide where doctors would be of most use, the Central Medical War Committee, the Scottish Medical Service Committee and a Committee of Reference composed by the Medical Royal Colleges would make the necessary decision.[25]

By the later stages of the war, in the regular and Territorial Forces there were more than 12,000 medical officers and the age at which they could be called up had increased to 55 years. The official figures for the number of medical officers in 1914 and for 1918 are shown below, and reflect a striking increase in numbers to meet military demands:[26]

- Strength of RAMC in August 1914 – 1,279 officers and 3,811 other ranks
- Strength of Territorial Force in August 1914 – 1,889 officers and 12,520 other ranks
- Strength of RAMC in August 1918 – 10,178 officers and 100,176 other ranks
- Strength of Territorial Force in August 1918 – 2,885 officers and 30,923 other ranks

The scale of the problem facing the medical services

In September 1914, the Director-General of Army Medical Services, Sir Alfred Keogh, adopted the idea of gathering medical statistics which would document the scale of the problem and provide information from which appropriate plans could be made and might also allow development of better medical care. The Medical Research Committee (now the Medical Research Council) offered the services of their statistical staff to collect data (really for planning for future conflicts), and this offer was accepted by the Army Council on 17 November 1914.[27] The original undertaking was based on the assumption that the war would be short. The sheer magnitude of the Great War meant that all existing methods of record keeping fell short of what was required for complete success, and so consequently data collection was not always accurate. With huge numbers of troops in different parts of the world, and with forces in many theatres of war constantly moving, it proved very difficult to keep track of things. An index card system was employed as a record keeping mechanism.

These index cards were kept officially by stationary and general hospitals. After every six months, the cards were sent to the statistical department of the Medical Research Committee, to be used at the end of the war as data for statistics relating to medical aspects of the conflict. Mistakes were very common, however, because fighting units were very often scattered over a wide and constantly moving area in distant theatres of war. Frequently the wrong cards got sent to the wrong units, and by the time it all got sorted out, the units had often moved on. The result was that only the British Expeditionary Force in France kept records of any value. In other forces, the cards were either not used, or, if used, were of little value. The shortcoming of the medical statistics will be illustrated in the course of subsequent chapters.[27]

Casualties were either battle casualties when caused by enemy action, or non-battle casualties when caused by injury or disease. This book is about the surgery of warfare, so it will deal almost exclusively with battle casualties, although a brief mention of non-battle casualties, particularly from the important perspective of preventative medicine, will be made in Chapter 2.

Battle casualties were sub-divided into temporary and permanent "losses". Reference to Table 1.4 will demonstrate this point. Death is an extreme example of permanent loss. Other examples of permanent loss, as far as the army was concerned, were those who were missing, and those who were prisoners of war. From a military standpoint, it did not matter whether soldiers had been killed, were missing, or had been taken prisoner. If they were not able to stand in a trench with a rifle at the ready, then they were of no use to the army. Obviously, these three categories of permanent losses did not come under medical care. They constitute 26.19% of all battle casualties.[28]

It was how the medical services dealt with non-permanent losses that would determine how they were judged. Between 1914 and 1918, the medical services in France and Flanders dealt with 1,989,969 battle casualties.[29] Of the 1,989,969 battle casualties who reached the medical services, 151,356 or 7.6% died.[29] Most of the discussion in the following chapters will relate to developments in surgery in France and Flanders. Contemporary medical literature deals predominantly with wounds sustained on the Western Front.

In absolute terms, the number of troops engaged, and consequently volume of work and surgical experience gained by those medical personnel working on the Western

Front, was greater than in other theatres of war. The close geographical proximity of the Western Front to the United Kingdom meant the easy transfer of medical personnel and medical correspondence backwards and forwards between hospitals in the United Kingdom and the base hospitals and casualty clearing stations in France and Flanders. Consequently, it was in the casualty clearing stations in France and Flanders where most surgical progress was made. Only data from France and Flanders was of a reasonably reliable quality, while communications with personnel working in distant theatres was more difficult and data collection much less reliable. The percentage deaths of wounded and of those dying of disease in various theatres of war are illustrated in Table 1.6.[30]

Table 1.6
Deaths from those with wounds and from those with injury or disease

Theatre of War	Year	Army	% deaths of wounded	% deaths sick or injured
France & Flanders	1914-1918	All troops	7.61	0.91
Italy	1915-18	British	1.22	1.48
Macedonia	1915-18	British & Dominion	7.14	0.78
Dardanelles	1915-16	British & Dominion	6.45	2.84
Egypt & Palestine	1915-18	British & Dominion	7.45	1.19
Mesopotamia	1914-18	All troops	8.95	2.04
North Russia	1918-19	British & Dominion	4.54	1.26
East Africa	1917-18	All troops	9.07	2.55
South-West Africa	1914-15	Dominion	9.82	0.73

Modified from Mitchell, T.J. & G.M. Smith, *History of the Great War based on Official Documents. Medical Services. Casualties and Medical Statistics.* London: HMSO, 1931, p.16.

The percentage of soldiers who died after being admitted suffering from disease on the Western Front was low at 0.91% of admissions. As might be expected the percentages of soldiers dying from disease was higher in Mesopotamia, the Dardanelles and East Africa where they were exposed to tropical diseases and dysentery. Nevertheless, when one compares this with the percentage mortality of 3.39% of the sick admitted during the Boer War, the percentage figures for the Great War, even in "unhealthy" locations, compare favourably

One figure which really stands apart and is difficult to explain is the very low percentage of deaths from wounds in the Italian campaign at 1.22%, compared with 7.61% on the Western front. The total percentage of battle casualties killed in action was 14.7%[31] on the Western Front, while in Italy that figure was 19.46%[32], suggesting that perhaps the pattern of wounding was different, more being killed outright, and those surviving perhaps not having such serious life-threatening wounds. On the other hand, one must return to the question of reliability of data, and it may simply be that data collection was poor, and the figure may be misleading. "There are lies, damned lies and statistics!"

There is no doubt, as will become clear in the following chapters, that the medical services were caught off balance at the start of the war. The Boer War, fought out in the dry grasslands of South Africa, was the conflict on which they based past experience. Wounds sustained in the rich agricultural and heavily fertilised soil of France and Flanders behaved in a very different way. Overwhelming infection of rapid onset was to become characteristic of a conflict where wound contamination by soil rich in manure was the norm. As will be seen, the medical services had to make quick adjustments in their management of many conditions. They acquired experience in treating large numbers of casualties with many different types of wound. They were confronted by clinical situations they had not previously encountered, and they had to learn quickly from their experiences and particularly from their mistakes. They had to develop new techniques, because necessity is the mother of invention. Surgical specialties developed to keep pace with the problems surgeons encountered. Orthopaedic surgery had to resolve many acute problems on the Western Front, as well as having to deal with late problems back in the United Kingdom. The Great War led to a major expansion of orthopaedic centres in the United Kingdom. Significant numbers of facial wounds at the Battle of the Somme resulted in pioneering plastic and reconstructive surgical work on a massive scale to deal with the very difficult problems associated with these wounds.

Abdominal wounds were mostly treated by supervised neglect, or "expectant treatment", i.e. no operations were undertaken at the start of the war. It would take the observations of astute clinicians, working in a logical and methodical way, and using scientific evidence from post-mortem studies of large numbers of cases, to bring about a change in management of abdominal wounds. Thanks to this pioneering work, early operative intervention became the accepted treatment for abdominal wounds, and survival figures improved. In a similar way, the management of chest wounds became more aggressive as confidence and experience grew. Major exposures of combined wounds of the chest and abdomen through an extensive thoraco-abdominal incision were performed and became standard practice. This approach will be explained in Chapter 8. Penetrating wounds of the skull and brain had been previously regarded as not worth operating on. Application of basic surgical principles to vast numbers of head-injured soldiers saw an active policy develop, with a concomitant improvement in survival. Fighting in trenches resulted in large numbers of facial wounds, and as will be seen in Chapter 10, this brought about major developments in treating these wounds, and the birth of modern plastic surgery.

Developments in microbiology led to improvements in the understanding of infections, and a study of pathological findings at post-mortems led directly to better ways of treating many wounds, thus keeping the patients alive! Blood transfusion with stored blood helped some of the wounded to survive. A better understanding of shock resulted in improved resuscitation of the wounded prior to surgery and developments in anaesthesia led to a better chance of surviving a surgical procedure. Diagnostic use of X-rays became established in base hospitals and casualty clearing stations, helping in the planning of procedures and removal of foreign bodies, such as bullets or fragments of shrapnel. All these aspects of medical and surgical developments will be dealt with in the following chapters of this book.

References

1. Neillands, R., *The Great War Generals on the Western Front*. London: Robinson Publishing Ltd, 1999, p.136.
2. *Ibid.*, p.140.
3. *Ibid.*, p.163.
4. *Ibid.*, p.405.
5. Prior, R. & T. Wilson, *Passchendaele: The Untold Story*. New Haven: Yale University Press, 2002, p.195.
6. Neillands, R., *The Death of Glory: The Western Front 1915*. London: John Murray Publishers, 2006, p.190.
7. Ewing, J., *The History of the 9th (Scottish) Division 1914-1919*. London: John Murray, 1921, p.398.
8. Stewart, J. & J. Buchan, *The 15th (Scottish) Division 1914-1919*. Edinburgh: William Blackwood and Sons, 1926, pp.286-7.
9. Prior & Wilson, *op.cit.*, p.300.
10. Neillands, *The Great War Generals on the Western Front*, p.362.
11. Mitchell, T.J. & G.M. Smith, *History of the Great War based on Official Documents. Medical Services. Casualties and Medical Statistics*. London: HMSO, 1931, p.168.
12. *Ibid.*, p.7.
13. "Some figures in medical history: James McGrigor", *British Medical Journal* 1914, 2: pp.185-188.
14. "Naval and Military Medical Services", *British Medical Journal* 1890; 1: p.1044.
15. Scarlett, E.P., "Officer and gentleman", *Canadian Medical Association Journal* 1967: p.1415.
16. Boyd, J., "Florence Nightingale's remarkable life and work". *Lancet* 2008; 372: pp.1375-1376.
17. Gordon, S., *The Book of Hoaxes – An A-Z of Famous Fakes, Frauds and Cons*. London: Headline, 1995, pp.35-36.
18. Smith, K.M., "Dr. James Barry: military man – or woman?" *Canadian Medical Association Journal* 1982; 126: pp.854-857.
19. Blair, J.G.S., "Sir Alfred Keogh – the early years". *Journal of the Royal Army Medical Corps* 2008; 154: pp.268-269.
20. Murray, J., "Sir Alfred Keogh: Doctor and General." *Irish Medical Journal* 1987; 80: pp.427-432.
21. Blair, *op.cit.*, pp.273-74.
22. Obituary: Sir Alfred Keogh. *British Medical Journal* 1936: 2: pp.317-318.
23. MacPherson, W.G. (ed.), *History of the Great War based on Official Documents. Medical Services. General History*. London: HMSO, 1921-24, Volume 1, p.22.
24. Atenstaedt, R.L., "The organisation of the RAMC during the Great War", *Journal of the Royal Army Medical Corps*, 2006; 152: pp.81-85.
25. "Memorandum – the National Organisation of the Medical Profession in Relation to the Needs of HM Forces and of the Civil Population and to the Military Service Acts." *British Medical Journal* 1916; 1; p.142.
26. Mitchell & Smith, *op.cit.*, p.8.
27. *Ibid,* pp.ix-xii.
28. *Ibid.*, p.13.
29. *Ibid.*, p.108.
30. *Ibid.*, p.16.
31. *Ibid.*, p.108.
32. *Ibid.*, p.178.

2

Evacuation pathway for the wounded

Thomas R Scotland

Introduction

On Friday 21 August 1914, Private John Parr of the 4th Middlesex Regiment was despatched with a colleague to find the German Army, which was known to be moving in force from Brussels in a southerly direction towards the British Expeditionary Force. Parr was a reconnaissance cyclist, and as he set off towards the village of Obourg, a few miles to the north-east of Mons in Belgium, little did he know he was about to make history. Parr and his colleague duly encountered a cavalry patrol from von Kluck's German First Army, and while Parr held off the Germans, his companion set off on his bicycle as fast as he could to notify his superiors of the imminent arrival of the enemy. Parr was killed in the exchange of fire which ensued, and he became the first British soldier to die on European soil in a conflict that would last for four years.

In one of the final ironies of what became known as "The Great War" Private George Ellison of the 5th (Royal Irish) Lancers was killed at Mons on the morning of 11 November 1918, where it had all begun for the British Expeditionary Force in August 1914. Ellison was an "Old Contemptible", (which was the name that survivors of the original Expeditionary Force gave themselves by the end of 1914), a member of that original small force comprising four infantry divisions and a cavalry division which sailed for France on the nights of 12 and 13 August 1914. With artillery, and troops on lines of communication, the total number of men who sailed to France was approximately 90,000 men. They also had 15,000 horses, and 400 guns. Ellison had been at the Battle of Mons on 23 August 1914, and had survived the whole war only to die on that very last morning. He became the last British soldier to die in the conflict. Ellison was not, however, the last soldier in the Dominion forces to die. That dubious distinction belongs to Private George Price of the Saskatchewan Regiment, fighting with the Canadian Corps. Price was shot through the heart by a sniper at 10.58 am on 11 November 1918, two minutes before the armistice came into effect. The first and the last British soldiers to be killed lie buried close to one another in St Symphorian Military Cemetery at Mons.

At the outbreak of the Great War in August 1914, there was a popular and completely erroneous belief by all belligerent nations that it would "all be over by Christmas". A few soldiers would die heroes' deaths, and be buried "in some corner of a foreign field that is forever England". No one anticipated the slaughter, on an industrial scale, that was about to take place, although the Russo-Japanese War in 1904-1905 should have provided some warning of the likely casualties. Nor did anyone anticipate the appalling severity and contamination of wounds caused by bullet and particularly by high explosive shells that would result from the more advanced weaponry that would be used in this conflict.

As the Great War unfolded, it became all too clear that this was to be first and foremost an artillery war, with high explosive and shrapnel being responsible for the majority of wounds. It might be argued, indeed, that the main role of the infantryman in the Great War was an entirely passive one – to stand in a trench and defend it, and in so doing to endure being shelled, mostly by the enemy.

During the 3rd Battle of Ypres, which began on 31 July 1917 and ended on 10 November 1917, when the Canadian Corps finally grasped the muddy wasteland of the Passchendaele Ridge, an attempt was made to analyse the various causes of wounds sustained by soldiers admitted during a twenty four hour period. On 21 September 1917 a snapshot of admissions to casualty clearing stations near Ypres was documented for the causes of all wounds that had occurred.[1] The findings are illustrated in Table 2.1.

Table 2.1

Causes of wounds sustained in the Great War – a twenty-four hour 'snapshot' during the 3rd Battle of Ypres

Wounding Agent	Number of wounds	Percentage
High Explosive	3,867	35.8%
Shrapnel	2,142	19.9%
Bullet	2,933	27.2%
Hand Grenade	77	0.70%
Bayonet	17	0.16%
Gas	209	1.94%
Uncertain	1,544	14.3%
Total	10,789	100%

Data taken from Macpherson, W.G. (ed.), *History of the Great War based on Official Documents. Medical Services. General History.* London: HMSO, 1924, Volume 3, pp.170-171.

The majority of wounds were caused by high explosive or shrapnel (55.7%). Developments in artillery technology would exert a decisive influence on the outcome of the war by 1918. When soldiers went "over the top", they exposed themselves to rifle bullets, and particularly to machine gun fire. Two well placed machine guns, with interlocking fields of fire, each firing 500 rounds a minute, could wipe out an entire battalion of just under 1000 men in a matter of seconds. Bullets were thus an important cause of wounds during an offensive, accounting for 27.2% of all wounds. When men occupied enemy trenches, one of the most effective ways of gaining adjacent segments of trench was by the use of bombs and grenades, moving from one segment of a trench to the next. Such close quarter fighting resulted in wounds caused by these devices (0.70%). Bayonet wounds were conspicuous by their absence (0.16%), either because bayonets were not particularly useful in the confined space of a trench, or perhaps because such wounds were lethal, and consequently soldiers with bayonet wounds never reached the medical services.

This "snap-shot" finding is backed up by a larger series of 212,659 cases admitted to casualty clearing stations and recorded in *History of the Great War Medical Services: Casualties and Medical Statistics* by Mitchell and Smith, published in 1924. High explosive and shrapnel shells were responsible for 58.51% of wounds, bullets for 38.98%, bombs and grenades for 2.19% and bayonet for 0.32%.[2]

War wounds were very contaminated, particularly when caused by pieces of shrapnel from a high explosive shell. Frequently, fragments of clothing and other foreign material were forced into the depths of a wound, and heavy bacterial contamination of soil by the organisms responsible for tetanus and gas gangrene ensured an ideal environment for overwhelming infection, with attendant serious risk to limb and life. The magnitude of the problem facing medical services on the Western Front was great, and is illustrated by the following official figures in Table 2.2 for the British Expeditionary Force in France and Flanders 1914-1918. These figures are for British soldiers, and do not include men from Dominion forces.[3]

Table 2.2

Breakdown of battle and non-battle casualties on the Western Front 1914-18

	Officers	Other Ranks	Total	% Officers	% Other ranks	% Total
Battle Casualties						
Killed	22,346	357,915	381,261	9.48	5.99	6.13
Died of Wounds	8,458	142,898	151,356	3.43	2.39	2.43
Missing	4,265	140,633	144,898	1.73	2.35	2.33
Prisoners of war	6,648	168,278	174,926	2.70	2.82	2.81
Wounded (not including those who died)	76,224	1,761,389	1,837,613	30.95	29.49	29.55
Non-Battle Casualties						
Died of disease or injury	1,257	30,841	32,098	0.51	0.52	0.52
Sick or injured not including those who died of disease or injury	126,046	3,370,342	3,496,388	51.19	56.43	56.23
Total overall numbers	246,244	5,972,296	6,218,540			

Based on data from Mitchell, T.J. & G.M. Smith, *History of the Great War based on Official Documents. Medical Services. Casualties and Medical Statistics.* London: HMSO, 1931.

From the figures in the table, it can be seen that personnel of the Royal Army Medical Corps had to fulfil two important roles. They had to deal with the wounded, and they had to treat disease. The subject of this book is the development of surgery of warfare, but it would be an omission if the important role of preventive medicine is not mentioned, albeit briefly. During the Boer War, which took place only fifteen

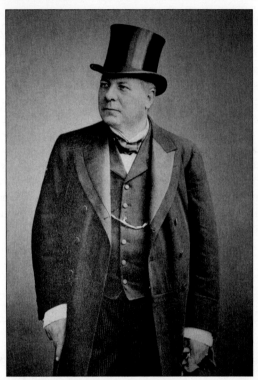

Figure 2. 1   Richard Haldane (1856-1928), Secretary of State for War 1905-
1912, Minister responsible for army reforms. (Private collection)

years before the First World War, 7,994 British soldiers were killed in action or died
of wounds. 14,048 died of disease, mostly typhoid fever, brought about by insanitary
conditions.[4] In other words, of all the deaths sustained by British troops in the Boer War,
64% were the result of disease, and 36% were the result of enemy action.

As Minister of War in 1906, Richard Haldane brought about major reforms in the
British Army. He prepared it for a European War by creating the British Expeditionary
Force. He established the Imperial General Staff, the Territorial Army, and the Special
Reserve. He was also responsible for starting the Officer Training Corps, thereby ensuring
a plentiful supply of young officers, including medical officers, to fill the vacancies in the
expanding army to meet the demands of the Great War. Haldane realised that effective
sanitation was a very important way of improving the health of army personnel, leading
to greater efficiency by reducing troop losses from the effects of preventable disease.[5]
Illness as well as wounds could prevent men from taking up arms. Officers were educated
in health matters, something beneath their dignity during the war in South Africa, and
a manual of army sanitation was produced (discussed in Chapter 1).[6]

Haldane was determined that the organisation of the Territorial Army should be as
complete as possible. He encouraged his very capable Director of Army Medical Services,
Surgeon-General Sir Alfred Keogh, to arrange for the mobilisation of the medical
resources of the country in the event of war. Sir Alfred not only greatly improved the
regular medical services of the Army, but he persuaded large numbers of doctors and

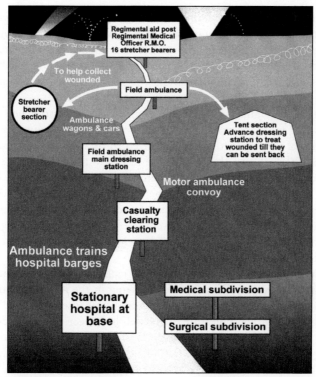

Figure 2.2   Schematic representation of the evacuation pathway that a casualty would
follow from the point of wounding to the base hospital. (Author's collection)

surgeons to join the Territorial Army. He organised a whole network of hospitals covering
the whole country, ready to deal with the casualties of war, established a Territorial Force
Nursing Service, and created the Voluntary Aid Detachments.[7]

One of the most significant steps in combating disease was the development of a
vaccine effective against typhoid fever by Sir Almroth Wright. At the outbreak of the
Great War, Kitchener encouraged men to be inoculated before being despatched to the
front. As a result of this specific measure, and others aimed generally at improvement in
hygiene and troop welfare, 96.4% of the deaths on the Western Front were attributable
to enemy action, and 4.5% due to disease, a marked contrast to the figures from the war
in South Africa.

The Regimental Aid Post

The first treatment available to a wounded soldier at the front was at the hands of the
regimental medical officer. Each battalion had a regimental medical officer. It was his
duty to treat the wounded in his regimental aid post, close to the front line, during an
offensive, and to be responsible for the general health and well being of the battalion at
other times. He had sixteen stretcher-bearers, increased to thirty-two during an offensive,
whose job it was to go out into No Man's Land and retrieve the wounded, and bring
them back to the regimental aid post.

The best time to do this was found to be the time between the battalion reaching its objective and the enemy's almost inevitable counter-attack to regain lost ground. Capture and retention of strategically unimportant trenches by one side, and their immediate recapture by the other, was one of the illogical activities of the Great War. These activities resulted in many casualties. The regimental aid post was the furthest point to which regimental stretcher-bearers carried the wounded.

Equipment in the regimental aid post included a supply of stretchers and blankets, a means of heating food and water, and a number of Thomas Splints, usually ten, for treating fractures of the femur (thigh bone). Invented by a Welsh surgeon, Hugh Owen Thomas, in the 19th Century, the Thomas Splint was to revolutionise the management of the fractured femur in the Great War. There were also shell dressings, in addition to the regulation medical and surgical equipment of a battalion.[8] A shell dressing was a medicated dressing having a cotton-wool pad 6 inches by 8 inches, wrapped in gauze, and stitched to a bandage 4 inches by several feet. It was compressed and packed in butter paper, ready to be burst open by soldiers in action and used in cases of major wounds and bleeding as an emergency dressing.

One of the major problems confronting the regimental medical officer was shock due to blood loss. In this condition, soldiers arriving in the regimental aid post would be cold and clammy and often in a state of circulatory collapse. The pulse would be very rapid, although initially blood pressure might well have been normal because fit young men are able to compensate for blood loss by constricting their peripheral blood vessels and increasing their heart rate to maintain blood flow to vital organs. Eventually, this compensatory mechanism would fail, and the blood pressure would crash, with a rapid and often imperceptible pulse. Today this is known as hypovolaemic shock and is discussed in more detail in Chapter 3 but some key features are shown in Table 2.3. In the early

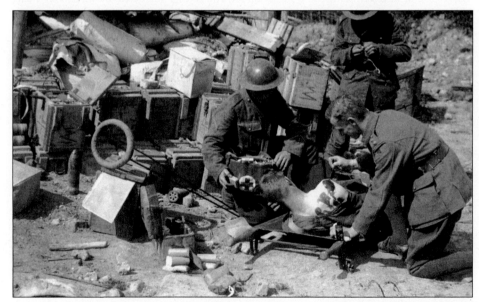

Figure 2.3   Photograph of a regimental medical officer treating a wounded man at a makeshift regimental aid post. A Thomas Splint lies nearby. (Imperial War Museum Q5916)

years of the war, blood transfusion to replace lost blood was not readily available. While direct transfusion between one individual and another had been practiced since before the war, it was quite impractical on the Western Front with overwhelming numbers of casualties being treated in makeshift conditions in a forward position. Stored blood was not available till the Battle of Cambrai in late November, 1917, but again it was not a practical proposition to administer it in such a forward position.

Warmth was very important to maintain the core body temperature, thus helping to combat shock. Keeping a supply of warm, dry blankets was a simple, yet effective measure which was employed by the regimental medical officer. When possible hot water bottles were also supplied and were of value.[9] Another cause of circulatory collapse was due to overwhelming infection, known today as septic shock and was all too common in horribly infected wounds so common in the Great War. Table 2.3 illustrates the clinical features of shock caused by blood loss, and shock secondary to overwhelming infection.

Table 2.3
The two different types of "shock" which would be encountered in casualties

Type of shock	Features	Treatment
Hypovolaemic shock	Due to lack of an adequate volume of circulating blood in the blood vessels. The casualty would be cold and clammy, sweating with a rapid pulse and a low blood pressure.	Stop the bleeding, increase the circulating blood volume with more fluid which would be either intravenous saline or fluids given into the rectum where they are rapidly absorbed, and then later blood transfusion.
Septic shock	Due to a severe infection in the body where toxins produced by bacteria cause damage and the blood pressure is very low. The toxins may be absorbed into the body and cause damage to the vital organs, e.g. heart, lungs and kidney which then may all fail.	Requires treatment of the underlying cause of infection, antibiotics and needs an intensive care unit to support functions of the heart, kidneys and lungs whilst recovery may occur. This was not possible during the Great War and so these patients invariably died.

When the British army went to war in 1914, it did so with a variety of inadequate splints for the treatment of compound gunshot fractures of the femur, a wound which was associated with a very high mortality of around 80% in 1914 and 1915.[10] The use of the Thomas Splint overcame many of the problems of this particular wound, and during the Battle of Arras in 1917, the Thomas Splint was used exclusively by the British 3rd Army. All regimental medical officers were taught how to apply the splint after first applying a field dressing to the wound. The Thomas Splint was subsequently used widely by all British armies. The correct application of the splint by regimental medical officers greatly improved the outcome of this wound.[11] Much more will be said about the compound fracture of the femur in Chapter 6, dealing with developments in orthopaedic surgery.

Partly because of close proximity to the front line, and partly because of a tendency to go out with their stretcher-bearers, regimental medical officers suffered a high mortality. The death rate amongst regimental medical officers and regimental orderlies was 40 per 1,000 per month in 1917.[12] During the Battle of The Somme, the mortality amongst medical officers in various stages of the evacuation chain between 25 June and 14 November 1916 is shown in Table 2.4.[13]

Table 2.4
Losses in medical personnel during the Battle of the Somme, 1 July-mid-November 1916

	Killed or died of Wounds	Wounded	Missing	Total
Regimental Medical Officers	43	149	4	196
Field Ambulance Medical Officers	20	65	0	85
Artillery Medical Officers	9	18	0	27
Administrative Staff	1	2	0	3
Casualty Clearing Station Medical Officers	0	6	0	6
Sanitary Officers	1	1	0	2
Totals	74	241	4	319

Data taken from Macpherson, W.G. (ed.), *History of the Great War based on Official Documents. Medical Services. General History.* London: HMSO, 1924, Volume 3, p.53.

Undoubtedly the most famous regimental medical officer of the Great War and most probably of all time was Captain Noel Chavasse, attached to the 10th King's (Liverpool) Regiment, a territorial battalion otherwise known as The Liverpool Scots. He won a Victoria Cross on The Somme in 1916, when the battalion was attacking the village of Guillemont in early August. He won a second Victoria Cross on the Ypres Salient in 1917 during the 3rd Battle of Ypres, which began on 31 July. Alas, he was mortally wounded, sustaining a penetrating abdominal wound from an exploding shell. Such wounds were associated with a high mortality rate, as will be seen in Chapter 7, dealing with abdominal wounds. Chavasse was taken to Casualty Clearing Station Number 32 at Brandhoek, which specialised in abdominal surgery. He underwent an emergency laparotomy (exploratory abdominal operation), but he died of complications on 4 August 1917 and was buried in Brandhoek New Military Cemetery. His second VC, therefore, was awarded posthumously.

Because of losses due to enemy action, there was a shortage of qualified doctors as the war went on.[14] This was particularly true for the younger medical officers who served with regimental and field units and who were well within shelling range from enemy batteries. By 1 January 1918 it was estimated that there were only 11,482 doctors left in civil practice in the United Kingdom, in contrast with 12,720 in military service.[15]

When the United States of America declared war against Germany, the situation was made easier. Six base hospitals complete with medical and nursing personnel, and an additional 112 medical officers, were despatched by the United States to the Western Front, and put at the disposal of British medical services, thus freeing up British personnel for other duties.[16] As well as general medical personnel, a group of twenty orthopaedic surgeons was sent.[17] The American contribution to orthopaedic surgery will be discussed in detail in Chapter 6.

The Field Ambulance

The common perception of an ambulance is a vehicle moving at speed, siren blaring, and dodging the traffic in its haste to pick up the victim of some accident. This is the description of an "ambulance wagon" in Great War terminology. A field ambulance was an independent mobile medical unit, of which there were three to a division, one for each brigade.

A brigade had four battalions of infantry, and three brigades made up what was termed a division. If the full strength of a battalion is taken as just under 1,000 men, there were roughly 4,000 men to a brigade, and 12,000 men to a division. Thus a brigade of 4,000 men was allocated one field ambulance. Each field ambulance had 241 men, comprising medical officers, stretcher-bearers, nursing orderlies, clerks and cooks. Each field ambulance had separate equipment, including tents, surgical instruments, drugs, appliances and dressings.

The whole ambulance had a "stretcher-bearer division" whose job it was to transport the wounded from the regimental aid posts to the medical facilities of advanced dressing station and main dressing station provided by the "tent division". Each field ambulance was made up of three sections, lettered A, B, and C, each section being capable of independent action when required, and could be detached with small bodies of troops if they happened to be engaged in an action at some distance from the main body.[18]

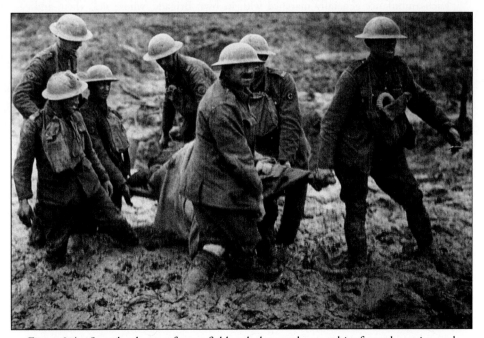

Figure 2.4   Stretcher-bearers from a field ambulance take casualties from the regimental aid post to the advanced dressing station. (Imperial War Museum Q5935)

The stretcher-bearer division and tent division were divided in equal sub-divisions between the three sections, so each section had an equal share of stretcher-bearer and tent personnel.

While the section idea was designed for mobile warfare, with small groups of troops heading off on a particular exploit, the war in France and Flanders was static for the most part, and so the sections worked together. Occasionally, when a field ambulance had to reinforce a casualty clearing station during a battle, it would despatch a section to assist the clearing station.[19] During an offensive, field ambulances were required to form a chain of medical posts between the regimental aid post and casualty clearing stations. The stretcher-bearer divisions were responsible for establishing bearer relay posts, divisional collecting posts, advanced reserve bearer posts and rear reserve bearer posts. In other words their duty predominantly involved transportation of the wounded.

One or more of the tent sub-divisions contributed to the establishment of the advanced dressing station. The tent divisions also set up the main dressing station, and were responsible for walking wounded collecting stations, sick collecting posts, and rest stations for officers and men. A rest station acted as a convalescent hospital for patients who did not need to be sent further back down the line, and who could be kept for up to a fortnight before returning to the front line.[20]

In his book *A Medico's Luck in the War*, Colonel David Rorie of the 51st (Highland) Division, and a general practitioner who practiced in the suburb of Cults on the outskirts of the City of Aberdeen, described the following arrangements used by the 51st for providing the necessary medical arrangements:

> Each ambulance generally marched with its own Brigade, whose sick, then, and in rest periods of the Division, it was responsible for collecting and treating. In a push, one of the three units, plus the bearers (nominally 100 each), ambulance cars and horse wagons of the other two, dealt with the evacuation of the wounded from the regimental aid post via the advanced dressing station back to the main dressing station run by another of the ambulances. Here divisional treatment ended and the wounded were transferred to the motor ambulance convoy administered by the Corps, and carried back to the casualty clearing station; whence by ambulance train they went to the base hospital and thereafter by hospital ship to the UK. The third of the divisional field ambulances usually ran a walking wounded collecting station in the neighbourhood of the advanced or main dressing station.[21]

The function of the advanced dressing station was to process and clear the wounded back as quickly as possible. Experienced medical personnel would triage the wounded into three broad categories of casualty. First, "lightly wounded", whose problem was not life or limb threatening, and who could be kept in the forward area before returning to the front line to fight, might well be managed by transferring them to the main dressing station. Main dressing stations helped to minimise the loss of men from divisional units. This must not be interpreted as an inference that the wounds of these men were trivial. All wounds had to be dealt with adequately, and with due care and attention to avoid serious complications, mostly relating to infection. Secondly "severe but survivable" wounds would be sent back to the appropriate casualty clearing station. Thirdly, soldiers with "non-survivable" wounds would be given pain relief, and put aside to die. They considered that there was no point wasting time on those who could not be helped, and perhaps depriving someone with survivable wounds of vital life-saving treatment. It required skill and experience when dealing with large numbers of casualties to make the right decision! An error of judgement might well have fatal consequences for the casualty concerned!

On 20 July 1916, Robert Graves, who was subsequently to become a well known author and poet, was on his way up to High Wood on The Somme, when he sustained a penetrating chest wound from a piece of shrapnel from a high explosive shell, which went in through one side of his chest and came out the other. He was taken to an advanced dressing station at the north end of Mametz Wood, where he was put aside to die. Assured that he would perish, his commanding officer wrote to Graves' mother in the usual formal letter of condolence, informing her that her son had died. Arriving back in London, Graves heard of his supposed death for the first time, and was one of the few men able to read his own obituary in *The Times*. Writing in his irreverent autobiography *Goodbye To All That*, published by Jonathan Cape in 1929, he records inserting the following notice in *The Times*:

> Captain Robert Graves, Royal Welch Fusiliers officially reported died of wounds, wishes to inform his friends that he is recovering from his wounds at Queen Alexandra's Hospital in Highgate.

They didn't always get it right!

Efficient early treatment was vital. Infection was the overriding major problem encountered by surgeons on the Western Front, and contaminated wounds with much tissue destruction provided an ideal culture medium for the bacterium responsible for

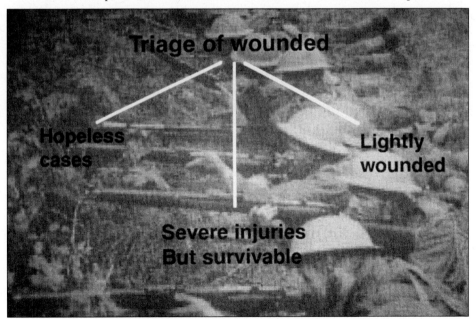

Figure 2.5   Triage of the wounded. (Author)

gas gangrene. More will be said about this in a subsequent chapter. Gangrene developed rapidly in tissue deprived of its blood supply, and wounds of the thigh, buttock and lower extremity generally were particularly susceptible.[22] Clinical shock, a condition with poorly perfused and oxygenated tissues, predisposed the wounded soldier to gas gangrene. Any unexplained, rapidly worsening pain, accompanied by a sweet offensive odour, were early clinical features of gangrene. Immediate recognition and rapid evacuation of the casualty to the appropriate casualty clearing station for early treatment might save life.[23] By the time gas was clinically obvious in the body's tissues with crepitus (a crackling sensation felt when the limb is examined and is due to the presence of gas in the tissues), it was often too late!

Reference has already been made to the warming of the wounded using dry blankets at the regimental aid post, to help maintain the core temperature and combat shock. Whenever possible, ongoing steps were taken at the advanced dressing station to maintain the patient's temperature by avoidance of exposure. A strategically placed stove could be employed with benefit. Hot air baths were also used when possible.[24] A hot air bath was made by conducting heat from a primus stove through a tin pipe into a special folding of blankets on the casualty's stretcher.[25]

Morphine was given early for pain relief. Wet clothing was removed, and hot water bottles were employed to warm the wounded soldier, who may well have been hypothermic, having lain helpless in a muddy, cold and wet shell hole for a considerable period of time before being rescued. Fluid replacement with hot drinks helped to maintain the core temperature of the body, as did fluids which were often given rectally (into the back passage) where they were absorbed into the body. Skill was employed to dress awkwardly placed wounds, and to splint fractures. The less the wounded soldier was disturbed the fewer were adverse effects on the patient's general condition induced by any painful manoeuvre and the probability of further excessive blood loss reduced.

All the above measures would help to ensure that the wounded soldier would reach the appropriate casualty clearing station in as good a clinical condition as possible. Patients too shocked to be transferred, and at risk of dying in transit, were better kept for an hour or two in the advanced dressing station, employing the various measures referred to above in an attempt to improve their general clinical condition, before sending them on the journey to the casualty clearing station.[26]

In the early years of the war, patients were given rectal or subcutaneous infusions of different things including saline, to try to restore body fluids in an attempt to combat shock, but these measures were relatively ineffective.[27] Fluids administered subcutaneously were not well absorbed, and while fluids given rectally were absorbed into the circulation, they were quickly lost again as they leaked out of the bloodstream into the tissue spaces. Intravenous infusion of gum solution was given and thought to be more effective because it increased the circulating blood volume and unlike saline did not leak out into the body's tissues, and so helped to better maintain the circulating blood volume. By late 1917, stored, citrated blood was available for transfusion at the Battle of Cambrai. It was used mostly at casualty clearing stations and fluid replacement therapy will be discussed in detail in Chapter 3.

In his book, *The Early Treatment of War Wounds*, Sir Henry Gray, Consulting Surgeon to the British 3rd Army, stressed that:

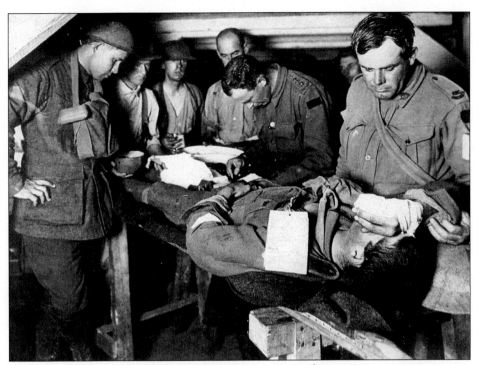

Figure 2.6   Medical officers at work in an advanced dressing station of a field ambulance. Triage of the wounded was an important role. Only in exceptional cases was surgery undertaken. (Imperial War Museum E(AUS)714).

While blood transfusion had successfully been carried out in field ambulances, it should only be undertaken by those familiar with the necessary technique.

There was little point in carrying out a blood transfusion, and causing delay in transfer, only for the patient to arrive back in the casualty clearing station with perhaps an inadequately splinted fracture causing further blood loss and with established sepsis, when earlier transfer would have been more beneficial to the patient's well being. Gray was rightly regarded as a leading authority in front line military surgery, and many of the developments in military surgery were attributable to him; his work will be referred to frequently in this, and in subsequent chapters of this book.

Surgical procedures at advanced dressing stations were performed only rarely. The forward position of an advanced dressing station meant it was well within shelling distance by the enemy, and therefore an unsuitable environment for surgery, unless intervention was required immediately to save life. Operations for life-threatening bleeding (haemorrhage), and removal of completely shattered limbs, often hanging by a thread and beyond any possibility of repair, were the only ones which were really appropriate to be carried out in advanced units.[21] The procedure of amputation could be performed using local anaesthetic infiltration. General anaesthesia in advanced areas was regarded as inadvisable. Often a profound drop in blood pressure associated with a general anaesthetic jeopardised the patient's fitness to travel down the line for life-saving surgery. Early amputation of a completely shattered limb under local anaesthetic was noted to dramatically improve the patient's general condition. This type of procedure was therefore encouraged at the advanced dressing station.[28]

Arrest of life-threatening haemorrhage was an altogether more difficult proposition, and necessitated opening the wound as much as possible to directly visualise the bleeding vessel before tying it off or applying artery forceps if suturing the vessel proved too difficult under the prevailing conditions. Arresting haemorrhage from a deeply placed vessel can prove to be a very difficult task in a modern operating theatre, with good anaesthesia, good lighting, and no shell fire! The alternative was to apply a tourniquet, if appropriate for the site of the wound, but since the casualty might not reach the operating theatre in the casualty clearing station for a few hours, a tourniquet carried the risk of further damage to already traumatised tissues and significantly increased the risk of developing gangrene. 80% of wounded soldiers whose limb blood supply had been cut off for more than three hours by use of a tourniquet required an amputation.[29]

While working in a field ambulance was not as dangerous as a regimental aid post, it nevertheless carried morbidity and mortality (Table 2.3). In 1917, during the 3rd Battle of Ypres, the 51st (Highland) Division used Essex Farm, on the west bank of the Ypres-Yser canal as their Advanced Dressing Station. Colonel David Rorie provided a vivid description of conditions at this advanced dressing station:

> Our bearers had preceded us for the A.D.S. at Essex Farm on the canal bank, a hot spot; and on the evening of our arrival four of them were killed by a shell which crashed into the shelter where they were at The Willows Collecting Post in front of this.[30]

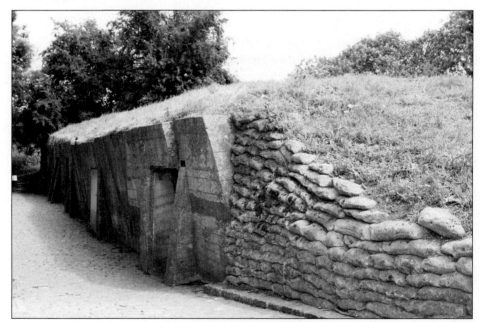

Figure 2.7   Essex Farm Advanced Dressing Station today,
much as it was in 1917. (Author's photograph)

From the advanced dressing station, wounded were transferred to the appropriate casualty clearing station by motor ambulance wagon or by light gauge railway. Motor ambulances had the advantage that they could be heated, while travelling by rail entailed an altogether colder journey. On the other hand, a light railway was smoother, while a motor ambulance lurched through potholes, potentially juddering fractures, altering the position of sharp bone ends, causing more blood loss at the fracture site and contributing to shock. For wounded soldiers with a fractured femur, suspension of a Thomas Splint from a frame minimised this disturbance ensuring that the condition of the casualties on arrival at the next medical facility was as good as it possibly could be.[31]

The wounded were usually sent to an appropriate casualty clearing station specialising in a particular wound. David Rorie, documented his experience in *A Medico's Luck in the War*:

> Here came as much work for the despatching NCOs: head cases and chest cases going to one C.C.S., fractured thighs to another, gas cases to a third, general cases to a fourth, and so on. As the nature of the casualties taken by the various C.C.S.s occasionally changed at short notice, everyone had to be alert and on the look-out to see that each class of case reached its proper destination. A large diagram of the human body was at one time hung up in the receiving room with arrows pointing from each part – head, chest, and thigh – to the name of the C.C.S. whither each special case should go. The figure being depicted as unclad bore, very properly, and after the manner of statuary, a fig leaf: and one bright morning I discovered that some brighter orderly had duly and appropriately adorned the divisions of the fig leaf with the touching legend APM.[32]

The Casualty Clearing Station

Sir Anthony Bowlby was consulting surgeon to the British Expeditionary Force. He went to France in September 1914, and realised at an early stage that many wounded soldiers were dying because it took too long to transport them back to base hospitals in France for definitive surgical intervention, as had originally been planned. Soil rich in manure often contaminated wounds, and was colonised with the bacteria responsible for tetanus and gas gangrene. Tetanus is caused by the bacterium Clostridium Tetani, which produces a potent neurotoxin (toxic to nerve tissue) resulting in the unrelenting spasm of skeletal muscle, frequently culminating in death. Gas gangrene was most commonly caused by the organism Clostridium Perfringens (formerly known as Clostridium Welchii), although infection could be caused by other related bacteria. Severe wounds with muscle destruction and tissue devitalisation provided an ideal culture medium for overwhelming infection with bacteria causing gangrene. These organisms produce a potent toxin which destroys adjacent muscle and releases gas so characteristic of this infection. Overwhelming infection led to a state of circulatory collapse which would be recognised today as septic shock, and which is associated with multiple organ failure and death.

On the evidence of the early months of the war Sir Anthony Bowlby concluded that surgery had to be performed early, and he made this clear when giving evidence to the Committee on Medical Establishments. He pointed out that wound excision should be done as soon as possible after the infliction of an extensive wound because in such

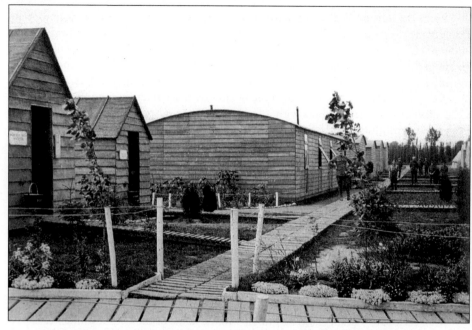

Figure 2.8   Casualty Clearing Station No 10 at Remy Siding. There
were 4 casualty clearing stations here in 1917 during 3rd Ypres – British 10
and 17 and Canadian 2 and 3. (Imperial War Museum CO 381)

cases gas gangrene may become widely spread within twenty-four hours. It was therefore
necessary to operate on such cases before the patient was sent by train to the base, as he
would seldom be surgically treated there until more than twenty four hours had elapsed
since the time he was wounded.[33]

Casualty clearing stations were for the most part situated far enough behind
the lines to be out of range and therefore relatively safe from high explosive shelling,
although some casualty clearing stations were more vulnerable than others. For example,
Casualty Clearing Stations numbers 32, 44, and 3 Australian, were responsible for
treating penetrating abdominal wounds, chest trauma, and compound fractures of the
femur, during the 3rd Battle of Ypres which began on 31 July 1917. They were located at
Brandhoek, less than 10,000 yards behind the front line – uncomfortably close![34]

They were shelled on 21 August 1917, and Staff Nurse Nellie Spindler of Queen
Alexandra's Imperial Military Nursing Service who worked in Casualty Clearing Station
44 was killed. Nellie Spindler was one of a small number of nurses who worked close to
the front in a casualty clearing station. There was a railway and munitions dump close
by, making it a likely target for enemy artillery batteries. She was struck by a piece of
shrapnel from an exploding shell, and died within minutes. Her body was taken to the
mortuary at Remy Siding Casualty Clearing Stations, and she was buried in nearby
Lijssenthoek Military Cemetery where there are 10,821 graves.

She has the dubious distinction of being the only woman buried there. Following her
death the clearing stations at Brandhoek were transferred further back to a safer position
at Nine Elms near the town of Poperinge, west of Ypres. For the most part, however,

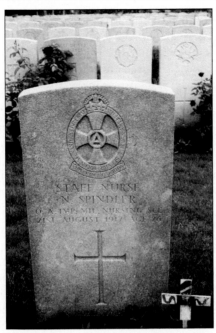

Figure 2.9   The grave of Staff Nurse Nellie Spindler at Lijssenthoek Military Cemetery
She is the only woman buried here. There are 10,821 graves. (Author's photograph)

casualty clearing stations were free from enemy fire unless deliberately targeted, and yet it was possible to transfer patients from the forward areas to a casualty clearing station fairly quickly, either by road in an ambulance convoy, or by light gauge railway. So it was at casualty clearing stations that Bowlby's directive for early wound excision was performed, and as the war progressed, an increasing percentage of casualties requiring major surgery were operated on at casualty clearing stations.

What exactly did Bowlby mean when he talked about wound excision as the single most important factor to ensure the survival of limb and life of the seriously wounded soldier? Wound excision meant radical removal, *en bloc*, of all contaminated tissue from the wound. It was a systematic procedure, excising dead skin, dead fat, dead and contused (bruised and/or crushed) underlying muscle, and, where there were fractures, removing debris and loose pieces of bone which did not have the normal soft tissue attachments, and thoroughly cleansing and irrigating the tissues. Even apparently minor looking missile wounds might be grossly contaminated on the inside of the body from the filth of the battlefield carried into the depths of the wound. Unless all dead and contaminated tissue was completely excised, and unless there was nothing left but healthy, bleeding tissue, the operation would fail, with potentially catastrophic consequences for the patient. It was also important to be able to do this in what was termed at the time the "pre-inflammatory phase", that is, before infection became established.

This surgical principle is as relevant today as it was back in 1914-18. It applies to surgery of warfare particularly, but also to high-energy civilian trauma from road traffic accidents and industrial injuries. Surgeons today ignore the lessons learned during the Great War at their peril and the foundations of today's practice were laid down by what these surgeons did. For example, orthopaedic surgeons today might see high-energy industrial or agricultural injuries, with gross contamination and destruction of muscle, often associated with an underlying fracture. This is a surgical emergency, and demands early operation by an experienced surgeon to ensure a satisfactory outcome. Inadequate treatment is potentially every bit as disastrous in the 21st Century as it was between 1914 and 1918.

This point deserves to be stressed, because it has been suggested that the introduction of an effective germicide to the recesses of an infected wound was what saved limbs and life.[35] Dakin's solution (consisting of sodium hypochlorite as its active agent) was such a germicide which cleansed by being introduced deep into the wound using the Alexis Carrel method. This delivered the solution into the recesses of the wound using a system of irrigation tubes.

Carrel was a French surgeon of great renown. Before the war he had done pioneering work on blood vessels, developing a technique to stitch severed vessels together. He was awarded the Nobel Prize for Medicine in 1912. During the war, he collaborated with English chemist Henry Dakin and used his system of irrigation tubes to deliver high concentrations of antiseptic into the deep recesses of the wound.[36] While this type of agent might well have been of help as an adjunctive measure, it was no substitute for early, radical surgical wound excision, without which, all other additional measures would fail. Furthermore, the paraphernalia of the irrigation tubes employed must have made it an unsuitable method of treatment at a busy casualty clearing station at times when pressure of work was great.

The functions and organisation of Casualty Clearing Stations

Casualty clearing stations fulfilled three roles. Firstly, and most importantly, they were the sites where major limb and life-saving surgery was carried out in the procedure of wound excision described above. Secondly, they were a site for assessment of more minor wounds, to be treated before being sent back to the front line. Thirdly, they assessed patients with wounds who were safe to be put on hospital trains, and sent back to base hospitals for definitive surgery.[37] Once those severe cases treated surgically at the casualty clearing station had recovered from their procedure, they too were sent promptly back by ambulance train to the base to create room for the next batch of casualties.

Until the onset of rapid mobile warfare, beginning with the German Spring Offensive on 21 March 1918, casualty clearing stations were almost always on a railway siding with the facility to transfer large numbers of casualties to base hospitals by hospital train making it easier to fulfil the functions referred to above. Casualty clearing stations represented the first safe haven for the wounded, and had to be kept warm in the interest of maintaining the clinical condition of the wounded. As in the regimental aid post and dressing station, attention was paid to maintaining body temperature to combat shock.

Patients were first taken to a dressing room, where thorough examinations and decisions as to further disposal were made. It goes without saying, that it required great experience and sound judgement to make the right decisions. One medical officer generally supervised eight assessment tables.[38] Those not requiring immediate surgery were re-dressed and made ready for the onward journey to base hospitals. Those requiring immediate intervention were sent to a Light Pre-Operative Ward, if their wounds were relatively minor, or a Severe Pre-Operative Ward, if their wounds were severe and potentially limb or life-threatening, before being taken to the operating theatre. Shocked wounded patients, unfit for surgery, were taken to a resuscitation ward, where they would be stabilised as much as possible. By 1918, there were "shock teams", comprising a medical officer experienced in blood transfusion, and an assistant who looked after the worst cases.[39] Warmth, absolute rest, sedatives such as omnopon, a derivative of morphine, and transfusion were the available methods for resuscitation and stabilisation of the wounded. Sisters for the resuscitation ward were specially selected for their experience.[40] Without restoration of blood pressure the probability of surviving the surgical procedure and anaesthetic would be very low.

Walking wounded soldiers at a casualty clearing station were generally dealt with by different medical officers, if these cases had not already been diverted to a special casualty clearing station dealing exclusively with walking wounded.[41]

No matter how insignificant a wound appeared, all patients were given a prophylactic dose of anti-tetanus serum (ATS). If any doubt existed in the casualty clearing station as to whether a dose had been given since infliction of the wound, then one was given. In cases where the man had been wounded for a second or third time, it was considered safer to administer in fractionated doses, since anaphylaxis, or complete allergic circulatory collapse, was a possible complication of the administration of anti-tetanus serum. Anaphylactic reactions may occur, for example after sensitised and susceptible individuals are stung by a bee.

In all serious wounds, administration of anti-tetanus serum continued for seven days or until the wound was clean and fit for closing.[42] The incubation period of tetanus varied from a few days to several weeks. This meant that sometimes the patient did not display symptoms of the disease till back in the United Kingdom. As a general rule, the shorter the incubation period, the more serious was the disease, and unfavourable the prognosis.

The routine administration of a prophylactic dose of ATS to all patients suffering from wounds, abrasions, or trench feet resulted in a significant fall in the incidence of tetanus. If the disease did develop after administration of anti-serum, it tended to run a much more benign course.[43] By the time a patient developed the full clinical picture of tetanus, the disease mortality was 70-80%. In the first series of 109 cases occurring in the British Army in 1914, the RAMC records a mortality of 73.39% falling to 26.3% by 1918.

Anti-tetanus serum could also be given therapeutically. The British Tetanus Commission, headed by Major General Sir David Bruce recommended intra-thecal (into the spinal canal directly around the spinal cord) injection of anti-tetanus serum immediately the development of the disease was suspected, supplemented by intra-muscular injections. After three days, intra-thecal injection was stopped, and either intramuscular or subcutaneous injection continued until the infection resolved.[44] How much any reduction in mortality was due to therapeutic administration of anti tetanus serum, and how much to the more benign course of the disease secondary to prior preventive administration of anti- serum is open to question.

Because of the long incubation period in some cases, again induced perhaps by administration of prophylactic ATS, there were 1,458 cases of tetanus in hospitals in the UK during the years 1914-1918. This represented an incidence of 1.2 per 1,000 of wounded treated in those same hospitals. The mortality among all cases occurring in the United Kingdom was 34.8%. The mortality of all cases occurring in France and the United Kingdom was 47%. The mortality before routine serum prophylaxis was employed was 85%.[45]

Reporting on behalf of the Tetanus Committee in the *British Medical Journal* in 1920, Sir David Bruce recorded that the mortality would have been lower if prophylactic injection in adequate dosage had always been employed. He also pointed out that many cases of trench feet succumbed from tetanus before it was realised that they should have been treated like wounded men, and been given ATS prophylaxis routinely.[46] Bruce reported the mortality from tetanus to be 55.5% in 1914, 20.5% in 1918, and 15% in 1919. Mortality was perceptibly less when there was no bony injury and it varied inversely with the duration of incubation that had been allowed before surgery was undertaken.

Each casualty clearing station had accommodation for approximately 1,000 wounded at a time. Experience of large numbers of battle casualties led to the grouping of two or three casualty clearing stations together and arranging for each to admit 150 to 200 casualties before passing the responsibility of "on call" to the adjacent station. This allowed a better way of working off the backlog without the added stress of on-going admissions streaming in.[47] The distribution of casualty clearing stations was important. Some were in a more forward position, but a distance of 12,000 to 14,000 yards was as far forward as was safe. Others were located further back, at twice the range of the forward stations. In preparation for an offensive, two stations were located in a forward position for each one positioned to the rear. The reverse positioning was applied in preparation for defence.

The personnel at a casualty clearing station comprised eight officers and seventy-seven other ranks.[48] Three chaplains were added to the establishment, and one of the

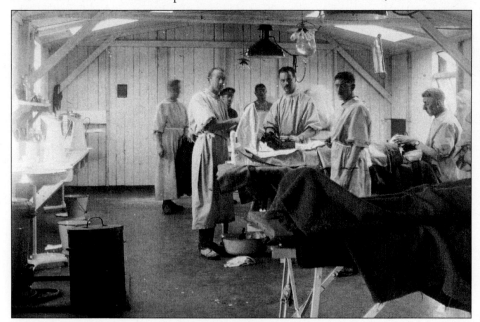

Figure 2.10 Theatre staff at work in the operating theatre of a casualty clearing station. This photograph illustrates the twin operating table system. (Imperial War Museum CO157)

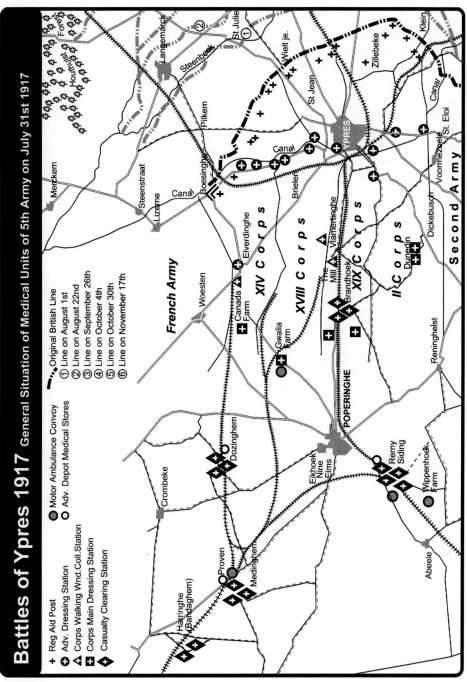

Figure 2.11   Map showing the location of casualty clearing stations for the British 5th Army, 3rd Battle of Ypres 1917. (Department of Medical Illustration, University of Aberdeen, based on material from W.G. MacPherson (ed.), *History of the Great War based on Official Documents. Medical Services. General History*. London: HMSO, 1921-24)

medical officers was appointed with dental qualifications. Nursing sisters were added in 1915, at first five, then seven. This number was satisfactory for a quiet spell, but inadequate for battle conditions. During an offensive, casualty clearing stations were reinforced by officers and men from field ambulance sections, from casualty clearing stations, from armies not involved in the offensive, and from hospitals on the lines of communication.[49]

Generally, during quiet spells, there were two surgical teams at each casualty clearing station. Each consisted of a surgeon, anaesthetist, a theatre sister, and an operating theatre orderly. When reinforcement was required, surgical teams would be sent from elsewhere. For example, by 1917, as many as six surgical teams including two formed by the casualty clearing station itself, and two tent sub-divisions of field ambulances reinforced each of the casualty clearing stations receiving the bulk of the casualties. Teams from other casualty clearing stations would bring their own operating equipment, including an operating table and surgical instruments. For the teams from base hospitals, twelve sets of equipment were kept in reserve at medical stores in Boulogne for use when required.[50]

Reinforcement of rank and file to perform the arduous tasks of unloading and loading ambulance wagons was performed by detachments of men from labour companies, unfit for front line duty. During 1917, this task was performed by fifty men convalescent from venereal disease, a small camp being pitched for them outside each casualty clearing station.[51] Operating theatres for serious cases were usually in semi-permanent wooden buildings when possible rather than tents. Using teams, it was possible for each casualty clearing station during an offensive to maintain a minimum of four and a maximum of eight operating tables in continuous use. The team system recognised the need to take full advantage of the available surgical expertise. During 1917, a twin table system was tested and proved satisfactory.[52]

The method of distributing wounded to casualty clearing stations was either geographical, according to the Corps engaged, or according to the nature of wounds. For example, during 3rd Ypres, numbers 32, 44, and 3 Australian Casualty Clearing Stations at Brandhoek took all the chest and abdominal trauma, as well as compound fractures of the femur. Remy Siding numbers 10, 17, and Canadian 2 and 3 took all other sick and wounded from the forward area. Numbers 12, 46 and 64 at Proven (Mendinghem) took all lachrymatory gas casualties, head injuries, and selected walking wounded. There was an eye centre at No 61 at Dozinghem, which also took self-inflicted wounds and those with infectious diseases.[53]

Workload of Casualty Clearing Stations

The volume of work undertaken at casualty clearing stations was staggering compared with modern day figures for accident and emergency departments. The 3rd Battle of Ypres began on 31 July 1917, employing the British 5th Army under Sir Hubert Gough. Progress was slow, and consequently the British 2nd Army under Sir Herbert Plumer was introduced into the fray on 20 September 1917, and both armies continued to fight until the capture of Passchendaele in November 1917. Casualties were heavy and conditions terrible.

Table 2.5

Summary of the personnel involved and the numbers of casualties treated at all casualty clearing stations during the 3rd Battle of Ypres, 31 July-mid-November 1917

	Data for the Second and Fifth British Armies combined (each army approximately 150,000 men)
Total Number of Casualty Clearing Stations	24
Number of Medical Officers	379
Number of Sisters	502
Number of other ranks	3570
Total number of casualties dealt with	201,864
Total Casualties Operated upon	61,423(30%)

Data taken from Macpherson, W.G. (ed.), *History of the Great War based on Official Documents. Medical Services. General History.* London: HMSO, 1924, Volume 3, pp.167-169.

During the battle, 61,423 of the wounded were operated on in casualty clearing stations. Some would be relatively lightly wounded, undergoing surgery before going back to the front line. Others would be the most seriously wounded, undergoing limb or life-saving surgery. This figure 61,423 represents 30% of the total admissions.[54]

The biggest casualty clearing stations in the Ypres area were the four at Remy Siding near Poperinge (see Figure 2.8). British Casualty Clearing Stations 10 and 17, and Canadian Casualty Clearing Stations 2 and 3 dealt with the following numbers of casualties shown in Table 2.6.[55]

Table 2.6

Summary of the numbers of casualties treated at Remy Siding Casualty Clearing Stations during the 3rd Battle of Ypres, 31st July-mid-November 1917.

Casualty Clearing Stations in Remy Siding Group	Number admitted	Number operated on	Percentage operated on
No. 2 Canadian	20,497	6,016	29.6%
No. 3 Canadian	18,721	4,673	25.0%
No 10	17,343	5,002	29.0%
No 17	17,361	5,816	30.02%

Data taken from Macpherson, W.G. (ed.), *History of the Great War based on Official Documents. Medical Services. General History.* London: HMSO, 1924, Volume 3, pp.167-169.

Smaller casualty clearing stations operated on a higher proportion of cases, because the pressure of numbers did not force them to send cases back to base that they might otherwise have operated on. For example, at the Bailleul Group, numbers 1 and 2 Australian operated on 51% and 46% of casualties respectively.[56] The documented mortality in casualty clearing stations during the 3rd Battle of Ypres was 3.7%.[57]

Cemeteries adjacent to casualty clearing stations can be readily identified by the fact that almost all those buried are named, given that the wounded survived long enough to reach the casualty clearing stations. This is in marked contrast to concentration cemeteries around the front line, where between 60% and 70% of the graves are "Soldiers of the Great War, Known unto God" and who have no name. This epitaph was the inspiration of author, poet, and Nobel Laureate Rudyard Kipling, whose only son John had been killed at the Battle of Loos on the 27th September 1915, and whose body had never been found.

Sir Henry Gray, Consulting Surgeon to the British 3rd Army was regarded as a leading authority in front line military surgery. Writing in his text, *The New Zealand Medical Services in the Great War*, Lieutenant-Colonel A. D. Carberry observed:

> The Third Army – which the New Zealanders found to be no less highly organised than our much admired Second Army – early in May re-opened its schools of instruction temporarily interrupted by the German invasion. Surgery, especially that of the front line, was a specialty of this Army whose Consulting Surgeon, Colonel H. M. W. Gray, was noted since 1916 for his work in the treatment of compound gunshot fractures. His memoranda, issued by the Third Army in 1917, formed the basis of the front line surgical practice of this and other armies, and his well-known book, *The Early Treatment of War Wounds*, published at the end of 1918, epitomised the advancing knowledge of that period. His lectures given at Louvencourt were attended by all our medical officers in turn: the problems of shock prevention at the R.A.P. and A.D.S., the best method of splinting fractures

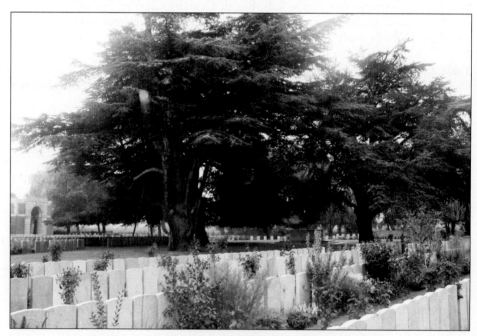

Figure 2.12   Lijssenthoek British Military Cemetery – 10,821 burials, all but 22 are named. (Author's photograph)

and the demonstration of the regulation set of splints, now carried in racks by each motor ambulance, formed the basis of these lectures which were delivered over a sufficient period to enable all our medical officers to attend in turn. This method of instruction seemed preferable to the bimonthly conferences at a C.C.S. held by the Second Army during 1917.[58]

The figures for percentage of wounds undergoing definitive surgery at casualty clearing stations reflected a growing trend that had been taking place. In 1915, casualty clearing stations only operated on 15% of cases in quiet times, and 5% when engaged in heavy fighting. In other words, at that stage in the war they were still sending the wounded back to base hospitals for definitive surgery. During the Battle of The Somme, 10% of wounded underwent surgery in a casualty clearing station.[59] By 1917 during the 3rd Battle of Ypres, 30% of the wounded were surgically treated at casualty clearing stations. Thus by 1917, the surgical role of the casualty clearing station for dealing with the most seriously wounded was well established.

More detailed examination of the surgical management of the wounded at Casualty Clearing Stations

Many with "minor wounds" were dealt with, although just because wounds were "minor" does not mean they were treated in any way other than by careful excision, conforming to the basic principle of war surgery. Minor wounds can become infected and lead to complications with relative ease! They should never be underestimated. There is a saying in operative surgery used today – "There is no such thing as a minor operation – only a minor surgeon!"

In severe wounds, the importance of early excision before infection became established has already been noted. Gray postulated excision followed by primary closure in selected wounds. After all dead and devitalised tissue had been removed and nothing but healthy bleeding tissue remained, the wound was closed by suturing.[60] Healing was then by first intention, and this greatly speeded up recovery, reducing the time necessary to spend on the patient, and avoiding the complications arising from an open infected wound.

However, this procedure required sound judgement in selection of patients, and experience in performing the procedure adequately. If the operation was incomplete, and if any dead and devitalised tissue remained, then primary closure of the wound would spell potential disaster, with pus under pressure forming in the depths of the wound, like the magma chamber of a volcano building up a dangerous pressure then suddenly exploding and spewing lava out over the mountainside. The operation would certainly fail, and the anaerobic conditions (absence of oxygen) aggravated by the build up of pressure would allow gas gangrene organisms to grow and proliferate, with potentially disastrous consequences for the patient.[61]

Nevertheless, primary suture by experienced surgeons was possible for most cases fulfilling the criteria of complete excision on early wounds. Clinical practice then and now revealed that joints always had to be closed primarily, otherwise joint destruction was the inevitable outcome. If, for example, a knee joint could not be closed, then amputation would probably be performed. Nowadays, techniques of plastic surgery can provide soft tissue cover for the exposed joint making conservative surgery the standard of care. Wounds of the brain, chest wall and abdominal wall also had to be closed primarily after wound excision. Not to close such wounds would mean the almost inevitable death of the patient.

If there was any doubt, then delayed primary suture of certain wounds could be performed after three to four days. This was a good option where the surgeon was not certain if all dead tissue had been removed. A second look after a few days would allow the surgeon to assess whether the tissues were healthy, and if so the wound safe to close.

Secondary suture was a delayed procedure, employed in soldiers with filthy infected wounds, who had perhaps lain in a shell hole for some time, and had arrived at the clearing station with established infection. It was undertaken two to three weeks after wounding when measures to clean up the wound had been successful. By this time, a velvety, bleeding tissue would have formed over living tissue. This velvety tissue is known as granulation tissue. If universally present over the wound surfaces, then the wound could be closed. If granulation had not formed, then there was still necrotic tissue in the wound and it would not be safe to close.

Sometimes, in the very worst cases, wounds had to be left open to fill up very slowly and gradually from the depths, a process known as healing by secondary intention. This process could take many months to complete.

In such instances where there was severe wound infection, antiseptic agents were used extensively during the Great War and had a place. Agents such as flavine, iodoform, boric acid, and eusol (based on calcium hypochlorite) were all employed. One method which enjoyed popularity, previously mentioned in this chapter, was Dakin's Solution.[62] The principle behind the use of antiseptics was that bacteria were killed by a chemical reaction with their proteins and other cell constituents. This reaction, however, was hindered by contamination with the proteins of blood, pus, and dead muscle, often present in large amounts in the thigh or buttock.

At the start of the war, most surgeons had anticipated that antiseptics would provide all that was necessary for the successful treatment of wounds confronting them. They had not visualised the appalling tissue destruction with sepsis they were about to encounter. The use of antiseptics alone never made up for adequate surgical treatment. They could be used as well as but not instead of, surgical excision of dead tissue.

Consider then a patient with a large soft tissue wound of the thigh without any associated underlying fracture. If that wounded soldier reached the casualty clearing station quickly, and was treated by a surgeon of experience by effective radical excision and primary closure, the wound would be healed in a couple of weeks, and the soldier ready to go back to the trenches in less than six weeks. This was the best possible outcome. If that same patient suffered severe complications resulting in his wound having to be left to heal by secondary intention, then it might take six months to a year before the soldier could resume his duties. By that time, his knee joint might have stiffened up through lack of use, and he might never have been fit for active service again.

The point of this example is to demonstrate that casualty clearing stations required the best and most experienced surgeons, who were able to make the correct decision for surgical management of every patient, depending on the clinical condition of the patient and his wound. Experienced surgeons saved limbs and lives, and could ensure the best possible outcome for the patient if the initial severity of wounding made a survivable outcome possible.

Another useful method for treating wounds with established infection at casualty clearing stations without resorting to antiseptics was hypertonic saline, using salt tablets inserted into the wound, again in conjunction with a preliminary free excision of the wound. This produced encouraging results.[63] Contaminated wounds treated in this way became clean as quickly as with any other method of treatment. Infected wounds of the buttock were invariably laid open completely, foreign bodies removed, and missile tracks excised. Such wounds were particularly predisposed to gas gangrene, and had to be treated with the greatest attention to full excision of devitalised tissue. Wounds of limbs likewise were laid completely open, and dead tissue excised till healthy bleeding tissue was universally present. Wounds were then partly closed over hypertonic saline packs. After ten days to three weeks, it was usually safe to close the wound. By this time, granulation tissue was present on all wound surfaces, and secondary closure was performed.

According to Roberts and Statham, the salt pack gave very good results, and when used in casualty clearing stations during periods of stress during an offensive, patients arrived back at base hospitals in clinically excellent condition, comparing favourably with wounded treated by other methods.[64] One of its significant advantages was that hypertonic saline dressings did not require frequent changing. With hundreds of casualties passing through a clearing station on a daily basis it was advantageous to use a dressing requiring the minimum of attention.

The worst case scenario for the casualty and the surgeon was infection and the development of gas gangrene. Prevention was obviously better than cure. Gray observed that the causative bacilli did not develop in tissues provided with a vigorous circulation of healthy blood. They thrived when the circulation had entirely stopped. The limb of a wounded soldier where the main artery had been severed provided such an environment. Long application of a tourniquet created another ideal environment for gangrene. Devitalised muscle was the key factor. Whether surgery was undertaken early, as a preventative measure or curatively, once gangrene was established, success and safety were only assured when the wounded parts were excised until definite bleeding of the cut surfaces was observed.[65]

From what has been said so far, the greatest obstacle to successful treatment of wounds in France was the virulent infection which so frequently occurred. It was also quite clear that early opening up and mechanical cleansing of severe wounds were necessary preliminaries to any other form of treatment.[66] The earlier the treatment was carried out, specifically in the pre-inflammatory phase, the better the results were likely to be.

It is interesting to look at management of sepsis today in civilian practice. Once again, this dressing, or that dressing, is used to treat infection, and instead of relying on disinfectants instilled into the wound, it is expected that antibiotics given systemically will do the same job. If civilian surgeons today were to suddenly find themselves in a war setting, they would probably have to quickly learn the same fundamental lesson that surgeons did back in the Great War, that radical wound excision was the single most important thing to do if the casualty was to survive.

Having thus dealt surgically with the most serious wounds, those cases, along with others who had been assessed and whose wounds were of a nature where surgery could be delayed until they arrived at base hospitals, were despatched. Mostly they went by

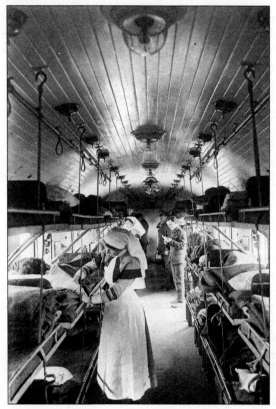

Figure 2.13   Hospital train taking wounded to base hospital. (Imperial War Museum Q8749)

hospital train, with accommodation for a combination of 400 stretcher and sitting cases. Ambulance barges provided an alternative method of transport, and were used wherever possible, although the numbers carried on a train were much greater. Barges were intended where possible for patients with wounds of the head and chest, and gunshot fractures of the femur where as little jolting as possible was desirable.

Hospitals on lines of communication and Base Hospitals

Medical establishments falling into this category were stationary hospitals and general hospitals. While initially the stationary hospitals were designed to be located somewhere between the casualty clearing stations and the general hospitals at base, in practice, there was no difference between the two other than size, and both may be regarded as base hospitals. This was due to the ever-increasing role of the casualty clearing station in the treatment of the most seriously wounded. Stationary hospitals and general hospitals may therefore be considered together.

General hospitals had a bed capacity of 520 at the beginning of the war, and stationary a capacity of 200. Both types of hospital were expanded from time to time. By 1915, general hospitals had a capacity for 1,040, and stationary for 400 patients. The Somme saw a further increase, and expansion in capacity was often in response to the crisis of a major offensive. By the end of 1917, for example, three new general hospitals were built, each with a capacity for 2,500.[67] From what has been said in the preceding sections, the role of stationary and general hospitals changed as the war progressed. Early in the war, treatment of severely wounded was progressively transferred to the casualty clearing stations. Surgeons had simply not appreciated the gross contamination of war wounds, and a major re-think in policy led to the increasingly important role of casualty clearing stations in the early radical wound excision required in these cases to avoid the development of gangrene.

The ability to use casualty clearing stations as major surgical centres in turn depended on their stable position – close enough to the front line to allow rapid evacuation of casualties from the advanced dressing station, and yet far enough away from the front line to be generally safe from enemy action. This stability was in turn of course dependent on the static warfare which characterised the Great War from November 1914 right through to 21 March 1918.

The German Spring Offensive on 21 March 1918 was a desperate throw of the dice to end the war before the United States of America had sufficient men in the field to make an impact. It resulted in British forces being pushed back from the Hindenburg Line to within a dozen miles of the city of Amiens, where the German offensive was finally halted. Soon after, on 9 April, a similar offensive south of Armentières known as the Battle of the Lys, pushed the British off Messines Ridge, and back towards the railway junction of Hazebrouck, before once again, the German offensive was brought to a standstill. Three similar attacks were launched against the French in May, June and July of that year.

As a result of this rapid movement on the front, casualty clearing stations lost their stability. They had to move back rapidly. They came under enemy attack, and consequently the important role they had fulfilled for so much of the war was suddenly curtailed. Much of the surgery undertaken had once again to be done in the base hospitals. Between 25 March and 29 March 1918, thirteen base hospitals at Étaples admitted 19,292 wounded and performed 3,698 operations, representing an operation rate of 19%.[68]

Gray's use of hypertonic saline dressings after radical wound excision in the forward areas was useful in this setting, allowed rapid evacuation of patients back from casualty clearing stations to the base hospitals for further treatment and closure of wounds by delayed primary closure. Dakin's solution was used more extensively in the base hospitals, because its administration required tubes and an irrigation system of sodium hypochlorite, which was not really possible under stressful conditions in the more advanced areas, particularly under the duress of the German Spring Offensive.

During the war, it was not practicable, with two notable exceptions, to designate base hospitals for special classes of wounds and diseases. Ambulance trains arriving from casualty clearing stations had patients with a variety of wounds requiring ongoing management. If special treatment was required then it would usually mean an onward additional journey. Firstly, casualties with compound fractures of the femur were treated in specially designated units. By the end of 1915, a memorandum had been issued that these cases should be kept in France for four to six weeks.[69] The reasons for this will be discussed in the chapter dealing with developments in orthopaedic surgery.

During the Battle of The Somme, 3,173 cases of compound fracture of the femur were admitted to base hospitals in France. Special personnel experienced in the treatment of

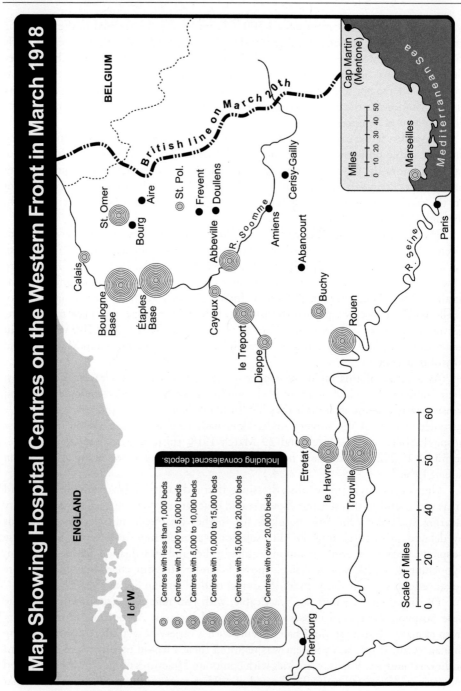

Figure 2.14   Map showing location of base hospitals in France. (Department
of Medical Illustration, University of Aberdeen, based on material from
W.G. MacPherson (ed.), *History of the Great War based on Official Documents.
Medical Services. General History.* London: HMSO, 1921-24)

this wound were employed. This allowed the application of a more uniform management policy in accordance with the best treatment available. At the beginning of 1918, beds with special fracture apparatus were set aside at selected hospitals at each centre, as listed below:[70]

- No 7 General Hospital at St Omer
- No 8 Stationary Hospital at Wimereux
- No 4 General Hospital at Étaples
- No 1 Canadian General Hospital at Étaples
- No 1 South African General Hospital at Abbeville
- No 47 General Hospital at Le Treport
- No 8 General Hospital at Rouen
- No 2 General Hospital at le Havre
- Number 9, British Red Cross Hospital at Calais was also fitted out for fractured femur cases.

Secondly, there were specialised units were for treatment of patients with venereal disease. There were no antibiotics, and treatment was prolonged, using agents with potentially serious side effects. Syphilis was usually treated by an intensive course, using a combination of arsenical and mercurial compounds given by injection. Gonorrhoea was treated by mechanical irrigation and injections of colloidal silver. Such cases remained in designated base hospitals in France until they were no longer considered infective. They did not return to the United Kingdom. Once clear of infection, they were returned to the front line. The time scale for cure or freedom from infectivity ranged from several weeks to several months, so extensive facilities had to be provided. At first, these men were sent to a stationary hospital at Le Havre, which had to be enlarged to 2,000 beds and converted to a general hospital. Soon there were other hospitals at Étaples, Rouen, Calais and St Omer for cases of venereal disease. During their convalescence, groups of these convalescent men helped with the loading and unloading of patients at casualty clearing stations.

Eye wounds were generally treated at 83 General Hospital at Boulogne, and wounds of the face and jaw were treated there as well. However, all these types of case were sent back to the UK as soon as possible. Only those patients with fractures of the femur requiring longer-term treatment in France, and patients with venereal disease who remained until they were no longer considered infective required specially designated hospital accommodation.[71]

American hospitals

In April 1917, the United States of America Secretary for War sanctioned the despatch of the personnel for six general hospitals to work as complete USA units on British lines of communication.[72] Each had 23 medical officers, 50 nursing sisters, and a complete establishment of non-commissioned officers and men. In this way, British medical personnel were released for other duties. By this stage in the war, the Royal Army Medical Corps was under significant pressure as a result of losses, and help from the United States was very welcome. By January 1918, there were 649 American medical officers working with the British forces, and were distributed as follows:[73]

Table 2.7

Distribution of American medical officers working with British forces during American involvement in the war

Location	Number
Regimental Medical Unit	122
Field Ambulances	257
Casualty Clearing Stations	5
General and Stationary Hospitals	31
USA Base Hospitals under British	211
Sick List	23

From base hospitals, casualties were sent by hospital ship back to the United Kingdom. The overall percentage figures for outcomes of the wounded soldiers after treatment are summarised as follows. 7% returned to front line duty from a front line medical unit, a dressing station or casualty clearing station. 57% returned to front line duty from a hospital or convalescent depot. 18% were fit only for administrative duties, or some form of work on lines of communication. 8% were discharged as invalids, 3% were discharged, destination unknown, and 7% of the wounded died.[74]

Notes

1   MacPherson, W.G. (ed.), *History of the Great War based on Official Documents. Medical Services. General History.* London: HMSO, 1924, Volume 3, pp.170-171.

2   Mitchell, T.J. & G.M. Smith, *History of the Great War based on Official Documents. Medical Services. Casualties and Medical Statistics.* London: HMSO, 1931, p.40.

3   Mitchell & Smith, *op.cit,* p.108.

4   Mitchell & Smith, *op.cit.,* pp.269-270.

5   "Correspondence of the War Minister on Army Sanitation", *British Medical Journal* 1906; 2: pp.157-158.

6   Whitehead, I.R., *Doctors in the Great War.* Barnsley: Leo Cooper, 1999, p.21.

7   Haldane, Maurice F., *The Life of Viscount Haldane of Clone.* London: Faber & Faber, 1937, p.231.

8   MacPherson, *op.cit.,* Volume 2, pp.16-17.

9   Wallace, C. & J. Fraser, *Surgery at a Casualty Clearing Station.* London: A & C Black, 1918, pp.16-17.

10 Gray, H.M.W., *The Early Treatment of War Wounds.* London: Henry Frowde, 1919, pp.57-64.

11 Whitehead, *op.cit.,* p.184.

12 Whitehead, *op.cit.,* p.184.

13 MacPherson, *op.cit.,* Volume 3, p.53.

14 MacPherson, *op.cit.,* Volume 1, pp.147-148.

15 *Ibid.*

16 MacPherson, *op.cit.,* Volume 3, p.53.

17 MacPherson, *op.cit.,* Volume 1, p.149.

18 MacPherson, *op.cit.,* Volume 2, pp.22-25.

19 *Ibid..*

20 MacPherson, *op.cit.,* Volume 2, pp.22-25.

21 Rorie, D.A., *A Medico's Luck in the War.* Aberdeen: Milne & Hutchison, 1929, p.5.

22 Gray, *op.cit.*, pp.8-9.

23 *Ibid.*

24 Gray, *op.cit.*, pp.18-23.

25 *Ibid.*

26 *Ibid.*

27 Marshall, G., "The Administration of Anaesthetics at the Front", *British Medical Journal* 1917; 1: pp.722-725.

28 Gray, *op.cit.*, p.42.

29 Gray, *op.cit.*, pp.43-49.

30 Rorie, *op.cit.*, pp.141-142.

31 Gray, *op.cit.*, pp.33-34.

32 Rorie, *op.cit.*, pp.143-144.

33 Whitehead, *op.cit.*, pp.206-207.

34 MacPherson, *op.cit.*, Volume 3, p.143.

35 Cooter, R., *Surgery and Society in Peace and War. Orthopaedics and the Organisation of Modern Medicine 1880-1948.* Basingstoke: Macmillan, 1993, p.111.

36 Wallace & Fraser, *op.cit.*, pp.49-57.

37 MacPherson, *op.cit.*, Volume 2, pp.42-50.

38 Gray, *op.cit.*, pp.73-79.

39 *Ibid.*

40 *Ibid.*

41 *Ibid.*

42 *Ibid.*, pp.138-139.

43 Hepburn, H.H., "Notes on Tetanus", *Canadian Medical Association Journal* 1922 May; 12(5): pp.312-315.

44 *Ibid.*

45 Bruce, D., "Tetanus in Home Hospitals", *British Medical Journal* 1920; 2: p.486.

46 *Ibid.*

47 MacPherson, *op.cit.*, Volume 2, pp.42-50.

48 *Ibid.*

49 *Ibid.*

50 *Ibid.*

51 *Ibid.*

52 Whitehead, *op.cit.*, p.200.

53 MacPherson, *op.cit.*, Volume 3, p.143.

54 *Ibid*, pp.167-169.

55 *Ibid.*

56 *Ibid*, p.170.

57 *Ibid*, pp.167-169.

58 Carberry, A.D., *The New Zealand Medical Services in the Great War 1914-1918.* Auckland: Whitcomb & Tombs, 1924, p.399.

59 Whitehead, *op.cit.*, p.201.

60 Gray, H.M.W., "Treatment of gunshot wounds by excision and primary closure", *British Medical Journal* 1915; 2: p.317.

61 Gray, Col. H.M.W., *The Early Treatment of War Wounds.* London: Henry Frowde, 1919, pp.159-165.

62 Dakin, H.D., "On the use of certain antiseptic substances in the treatment of infected wounds", *British Medical Journal* 1915; 2: pp.318-320.

63 Roberts, E.H. & R. Statham, "On the salt pack treatment of infected gunshot wounds", *British Medical Journal* 1916; 2: pp.282-286.

64 Roberts & Statham, *op.cit.*, pp.282-286.

65 Gray, H.M.W., "An essential principle in the treatment of gas gangrene", *British Medical Journal* 1918; 1: p.369.

66 Gray, Col. H.M.W., *The Early Treatment of War Wounds.* London: Henry Frowde, 1919, p.124.

67 MacPherson, *op.cit.*, Volume 2, pp.66-70.

68 Whitehead, *op.cit.*, p.211.

69 MacPherson, *op.cit.*, Volume 2, pp.74-76.

70 *Ibid.*

71 *Ibid.*

72 *Ibid*, pp.98-101.

73 *Ibid.*

74 Mitchell & Smith, *op.cit.*, p.20.

3

Anaesthesia, Shock and Resuscitation

E Ann Robertson

Historical perspective

In the year 2011 a modern anaesthetist would arrive at the equivalent of a casualty clearing station in a war zone armed with a medical degree, several years of clinical experience and probably a Fellowship in Anaesthesia (a postgraduate medical qualification) from the Royal College of Anaesthetists. He or she would have colleagues of similar status and the assistance of specially qualified technicians and nurses. The equipment would be up to date and include not only devices to measure blood pressure and monitor heart beat but also "invasive monitoring" that is plastic tubes inserted into arteries and veins that give a precise and instantaneous indication of the condition of the patient. There would be an array of anaesthetic agents including vapours that are inhaled as well as drugs that are injected along with a pharmacy containing drugs to manipulate and maintain the blood pressure. Vast quantities of fluids would be available to be given intravenously and there would be access to blood transfusion facilities.

There would be support teams that travel into the battle zone by helicopter to initiate resuscitation of the wounded, returning them speedily in good condition to the operating theatre for definitive surgery. Ventilators (machines that breathe for the patient) would be available both in the operating theatre and in the intensive care unit where the most seriously wounded patients would be looked after.

When Major Charles Corfield arrived at a casualty clearing station on the Somme in 1916 as a specially designated anaesthetist, the equipment and agents he found would have been recognizable to a doctor in the mid-19th Century.[1] He had at his disposal what he called the usual anaesthetic equipment – chloroform, ether, ethyl chloride and Schimmelbusch masks, which were simple devices made of wire that could hold gauze or lint onto which the anaesthetic agent could be dripped, the inhalation of which resulted in anaesthesia. He asked for another inhalational agent to be made available, the gas nitrous oxide, and was fortunate enough to be able to get some along with the appropriate apparatus.

Despite the passage of some 60 to 70 years between the discovery of anaesthesia and its use during the Great War, very little had changed. A demonstration of anaesthesia using ether took place in 1846 at the Massachusetts General Hospital just twelve months after Horace Wells had failed to produce a state of anaesthesia by using nitrous oxide at the same hospital.[2] The age of pain-free surgery had arrived and news quickly spread across the Atlantic to Great Britain and Europe. Keen to find other agents with the same effect James Young Simpson and friends in Edinburgh were experimenting after dinner one evening when they discovered that breathing chloroform rendered them

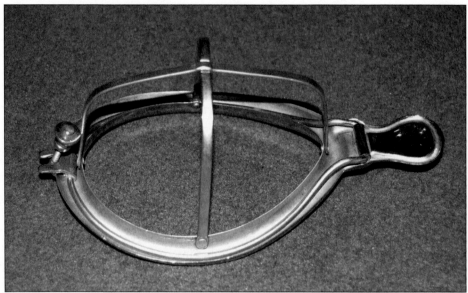

Figure 3.1 (a & b)   Schimmelbusch Mask, images showing the mask with/ without a piece of gauze, over which ether would be poured. (Reproduced by kind permission of the Association of Anaesthetists of Great Britain and Ireland)

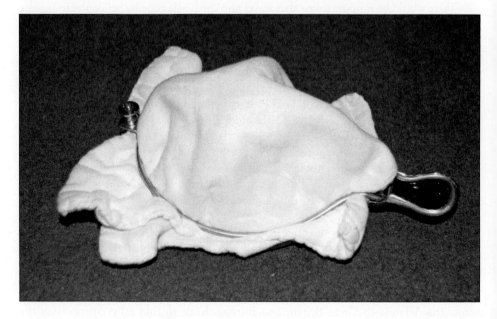

unconscious for a number of minutes. Chloroform acted more quickly than ether, but gradually reports of deaths from chloroform inhalation appeared. Fearing legal action in the event of death, Americans continued to use ether, but chloroform with rapid onset of anaesthesia, became popular in Great Britain. It was not until the early part of the 20th Century that scientific experimentation on animals revealed that the normal beating of the heart could decline into a quivering of the heart muscle known as ventricular fibrillation under the effects of chloroform.

These very early days of anaesthesia were dogged with arguments about exactly where the first anaesthetics had been given and who had given them, such was the desire to claim responsibility for the discovery. There were occasions when there was failure to produce a state under which surgery could be carried out (surgical anaesthesia) and there were complaints from some members of the medical profession that anaesthesia would be "bad" for patients. They regarded the pain of surgery as a "necessary evil" that kept the patient alive. However, such a welcome relief from suffering could not be suppressed and anaesthesia became an essential part of surgical practice.

However, when Britain went to war in the Crimea the old arguments surfaced once again. Despite the successful use of ether during the Mexican-American war in 1847 the Principal Medical Officer of the British Army, Sir John Hall, cautioned against its use in a memorandum published in the *Illustrated London News* in 1854:

> However barbarous it might appear the smart of the knife is a powerful stimulant and it is much better to hear a man bawl lustily than to see him sink silently into the grave.[3]

Fortunately his advice was largely ignored and chloroform was given for most operations. Perhaps doctors had been influenced by John Snow, who in 1847 advocated the use of anaesthesia for battle casualties:

> The pain endured by the bleeding soldier or sailor wounded in fighting battles of his country is deeply deplored by every feeling mind and a discovery which can prevent so much of it as depends on the operations necessary to save his life, must be hailed as a great blessing...[4]

Snow was a physician of great ability. Famed for his discovery of the spread of cholera through water he dedicated much of his life to the science of anaesthesia. He realized long before many others that good anaesthesia required close observation of the patient, a means of quantifying the dose given and a good bedside manner. Having invented a machine for delivering ether in known amounts which was later modified by another well known 19th Century anaesthetist, Joseph Thomas Clover, to give chloroform, he might well have been surprised to see ether being given from a drop bottle onto a piece of gauze held by a metal mask over the patient's face in the early days of the Great War.

Further experience was gained in military anaesthesia during the American Civil War and by the time the Boer War started in 1899, the British Army medical services were issued with 10 pounds of chloroform and 5 pounds of ether at every base hospital and doctors on horseback were given a bottle of chloroform in their saddlebag![5]

Ethyl chloride gained favour much later on than the other two agents. Its anaesthetic properties were first noticed in 1847 but it wasn't until 1895 that it came into general use when improvements in manufacture decreased impurities. Like chloroform it induces anaesthesia quickly but there was disagreement among physicians as to whether it was safer than other agents.

Various combinations of those four agents ether, chloroform, nitrous oxide and ethyl chloride had been advocated in order to make induction and maintenance of anaesthesia a safe and pleasant experience and they formed the backbone of inhalational anesthesia well beyond the end of the Great War. Induction of anaesthesia refers to the period between consciousness and the state of surgical anaesthesia which is defined as the state when it is possible to carry out surgery without the patient experiencing pain. Today, injections of drugs directly into a vein produce unconsciousness quickly and pleasantly but the inhalation of gases and vapours takes longer. In particular the use of ether on its own produces first a state of excitement during which the patient struggles before breathing becomes regular and surgical anaesthesia ensues. It takes considerable skill to produce a smooth induction, hence the desire to add other agents which speed up the process and make it more pleasant.

There was however, a form of anaesthesia available to surgeons which did not require the patient to be unconscious, that of local anaesthesia. Coca leaves were used in South America for their pain relieving (analgesic) properties and the active substance cocaine was isolated in 1859. Karl Koller, a German eye surgeon, was the first person to try out cocaine for its anaesthetic properties and in 1884 he used a direct application of it to carry out eye surgery. Hollow needles with syringes had been available since the 1850s and in 1892 Carl Ludwig Schleich infiltrated cocaine under the skin to "freeze" an area that could then be operated upon. Cocaine itself was poisonous but over the course of the next twenty years other local anaesthetic drugs were manufactured which could be used either under the skin or directly applied to a nerve to produce anaesthesia in the area supplied by that nerve. In 1891 the German physician Heinrich Quinke described the technique of lumbar puncture when a needle is inserted into the fluid which surrounds the spinal cord (cerebrospinal fluid).

Seven years later in 1898 one of his former students, August Bier, described the injection of small amounts of cocaine into the cerebrospinal fluid of six patients to produce abolition of sensation sufficient to allow surgery.[6] The ability of small amounts of local anaesthetic injected around the spinal cord to render large areas of the body insensitive to pain had been proven, and spinal anaesthesia was born. In order to reach a well-informed opinion, Bier decided that he should personally experience the technique and asked a colleague, Dr Hildebrandt, to carry out a spinal anaesthetic on himself. Inability to get a good fit between the syringe and needle resulted in a loss of local anaesthetic and the procedure was not successful. Hildebrandt then offered himself as a subject and the experiment successfully resulted in surgical anaesthesia, although both physicians suffered from terrible headaches.

Cocaine, however, failed to produce reliable results and the technique was abandoned until stovaine, another local anaesthetic, was discovered a few years later. It was so called because it was synthesized by Furneau, which is the French word for stove, and rapidly gained a place in the operating theatre. Several papers in the medical literature showed spinal anaesthesia to be a safe and reliable technique and Major Houghton of the RAMC (one of the first British Army anaesthetists) recorded its successful use on peace time army recruits in a series of papers carefully recording dosage, effect and side effects in all patients.[7] Usually, however, spinal anaesthesia fell under the jurisdiction of the surgeon and a separate anaesthetist was not involved. Many believed it to protect patients from the shock of surgery but in severely wounded battle casualties this was often not the case.

It should be noted that August Bier was not only famous for the introduction of spinal anaesthesia but was also responsible for introducing the distinctive steel helmet worn by German soldiers. Presumably after witnessing the disastrous effects of penetrating head wounds from shrapnel he realized that adequate protection was required.

The training of anaesthetists

But what of the training and experience of medical personnel whose duty included the giving of anaesthetics? Major Corfield, who was both a doctor and a barrister, had prior experience of the subject, having been employed as an anaesthetist at the Gordon Throat and Temperance Hospital, London and the Bristol General Hospital. At the outbreak of the war, such experience was the exception rather than the rule.

The idea that training in anaesthesia should be systematic and included in every medical student's curriculum was advocated in 1892 by Frederick Silk, assistant anaesthetist to Guy's Medical School.[8] Writing in *The Lancet* he argued that improvements in surgery required improvements in anaesthesia that would only be brought about by properly trained doctors devoting time and energy to the subject. Not only was equipment becoming more complicated but doctors were beginning to realise the importance of understanding the physiological effects of anaesthesia and surgery on the human body. In addition, Silk felt that the medical profession should do all in its powers to make it as safe a process as possible. The fact that having an anaesthetic was safer than a railway journey was not an excuse for the occasional death. Over the course of the next twenty years, specialist anaesthetists were appointed to many hospitals but even in 1901 Dudley Wilmot Buxton, anaesthetist at University College Hospital London, was still trying to get the teaching of anaesthesia included in the curriculum of every medical school.[9] A bill proposing that all general anaesthetics be given by medical personnel was put before Parliament in 1909 but it failed. Only in 1912 did the General Medical Council include anaesthetics as the last of 16 subjects to be included in the undergraduate curriculum of all medical schools.[10]

It is therefore understandable that most of the young men assigned the position of anaesthetist during the Great War had scant training and experience in the subject. They struggled to cope with the demand of two surgeons working between four or even six operating tables. During the Battle of The Somme, the Reverend Leonard Pearson found himself giving anaesthetics at Casualty Clearing Station No 44. Photographs and a scrap album of his were found in a rubbish skip and deposited at the Bodleian Library, Oxford. In Lyn Macdonald's book *The Roses of No Man's Land* he recounts his experience:

> I spent most of my time giving anaesthetics. I had no right to be doing this of course but we were so rushed … If they had had to wait their turn in the normal way, until the surgeon was able to perform the operation with another doctor giving the anaesthetic, it would have been too late for many of them. As it happened, many died.[11]

It is small wonder then that an approach was made to Geoffrey Marshall, a doctor serving on a hospital barge that was used to transport casualties who were too sick to go by train or road. Marshall described his time on the barge as most enchanting but the use of barges was sporadic and there were times of inactivity interspersed with a few days of desperate activity. In an interview in 1966 Marshall is quoted as saying:

A dreadful old man, who was the senior consultant, Sir Anthony Bowlby [see Chapter 2], drove up to my barge one day – lovely day – and said "Marshall we are having an awful lot of deaths in the forward hospitals from shock and you did a lot of work on the physiology of anaesthesia before the war so I want you to come along and see if you can do anything about these chaps.[12]

The development of anaesthesia during the Great War

"A dreadful old man" he might have been but Sir Anthony Bowlby had gained experience in the Boer War as well as the Great War and he knew exactly who to ask to sort out the problems of the large number of anaesthetic-related deaths. Marshall was a physician and respiratory physiologist who had worked at Guy's Hospital as a demonstrator in physiology, a recognized training ground for young physicians, and Bowlby remembered him from his pre-war days. The last thing Marshall wanted to be remembered as was an anaesthetist. However, in a carefully controlled study carried out at Casualty Clearing Station No 17 at Remy Siding near Ypres, he cemented the anaesthetist's role as peri-operative physician able to understand the physiology of shock and how the method of anaesthesia could be tailored to the condition of the patient with a resulting decrease in mortality.[13]

Patients arriving at casualty clearing stations often required immediate life-saving surgery but were suffering from the effects of shock and haemorrhage (blood loss).

When blood loss occurs, physiological changes take place which are designed to preserve the flow of blood to the most vital organs of the body and keep the person alive. First of all, small blood vessels in the skin constrict and then the blood flow to the kidneys is reduced. The heart rate increases and initially blood pressure is maintained. As the blood loss becomes more pronounced blood pressure falls and finally the patient becomes semi-conscious as the body fails to maintain flow to the most vital organ of all, the brain. Patients with blood loss are pale with a weak and rapid pulse. Many of the wounded had lain on the battlefield for some time and they were wet and cold, and in winter many suffered from bronchitis as well. Australian and Indian soldiers were particularly susceptible to the effects of the European winter. Hence Marshall said at the start of his paper:

A correct choice of anaesthetic is of the first importance: the patient's life will be as much imperiled by faulty judgment on the part of the anaesthetist as by a wrong decision on the part of the surgeon.

The methods of anaesthesia available to Marshall were:

1. Nitrous oxide and oxygen.
    Nitrous oxide differs from ether and chloroform in being a gas not a vapour and as such comes in pressurized metal cylinders. Metal was in short supply during the war as it was required for munitions and gaining a supply of nitrous oxide was difficult.
2. Ether and chloroform by the open method (i.e. a dripped onto a mask)
3. Ether and chloroform by Shipway's warm vapour apparatus.[14] The use of the open method allowed considerable loss of vapour into the operating theatre and loss of body heat from the patient. The evaporation of ether could result in the temperature of the inhaled vapour being 30-40° below that of the room. Shipway's apparatus allowed the patient to breathe warm vapour at a known concentration which was less irritant to the lungs and this decreased the incidence of post-operative bronchitis. Along with the addition of chloroform, it also improved the smoothness of induction.
4. Intravenous ether. Producing anaesthesia by injecting ether and also by instilling it per rectum (into the bowel) enjoyed a brief period of acceptance in the first twenty years of the 20th Century but it never really caught on, nor was it used to a large extent during the Great War.
5. Spinal anaesthesia with stovaine.
6. Local infiltration with novocaine. This was one of the local anaesthetics synthesised in 1905. It is known today as procaine and is still in use.

Nitrous oxide and oxygen

The commonest wounds were minor and required a quick anaesthetic with a rapid recovery so that the patient was fit for early evacuation by ambulance train. These patients were given nitrous oxide and oxygen and it suited short operations very well. Anyone who has inhaled entonox (50:50 nitrous oxide and oxygen) as carried by ambulances or on maternity wards will know that although it provides very good pain relief it rarely results in unconsciousness sufficient to allow surgery to proceed. It is no surprise that back in 1845 Horace Wells failed to demonstrate its use for anaesthetic purposes. The only way in which a state suitable for surgery can be produced is either by having a patient who already has a reduced level of consciousness due to blood loss or morphine administration or by giving 100% nitrous oxide. In the latter instance the patient is given nitrous oxide without oxygen and when asleep, sufficient air is allowed into the system so that the patient gets enough oxygen to prevent death from asphyxiation. Corfield described it as a compromise between consciousness and colour (a patient without sufficient oxygen would change from pink to blue), something which would be considered unethical today. When patients were already partly deadened to pain as a result of haemorrhage it would prove invaluable for a quick and definitive procedure such as a guillotine amputation. Marshall found that in patients close to death, a 'quick whiff' of nitrous oxide and oxygen would allow an arm or a leg to be amputated and blood vessels to be tied off to prevent further haemorrhage. Other anaesthetics would have killed the patient.

The disadvantage of nitrous oxide and oxygen alone was that while it produced analgesia for short procedures, it was of no use for prolonged operations requiring deeper levels of anaesthesia. These required ether and chloroform.

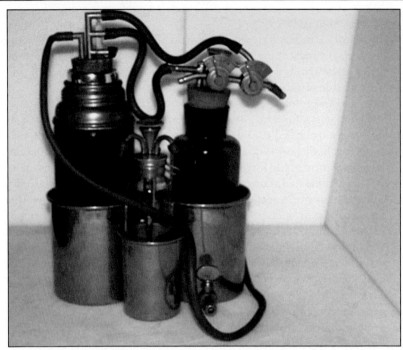

Figure 3.2 (a & b)   Shipway's Warm Ether Apparatus. The purpose of these bottles
is to warm the ether before it is administered to the patient, who otherwise may
become very cold. Shipway's apparatus was of particular use in longer operations
to help prevent the core temperature of the patient dropping. (Reproduced by kind
permission of the Association of Anaesthetists of Great Britain and Ireland)

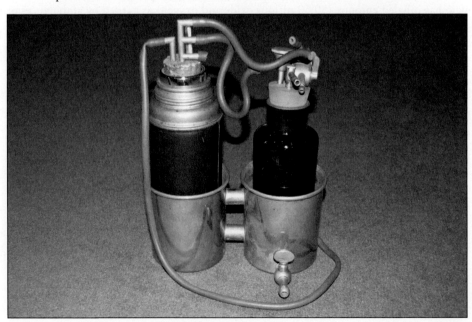

Ether and chloroform

Giving chloroform at the start of the induction and then proceeding with ether speeded up the time before the patient was ready for the surgeon's knife. Dripping these agents onto an open mask led to high levels of the vapours in the operating theatre and it must have been a very heavy and soporific atmosphere to work in. The advantages of Shipway's apparatus were such that one was issued to each hospital unit. Marshall felt it a huge improvement but Corfield was less impressed as he found it cumbersome and very tiring as there were hand bellows that required pumping.

Marshall's work on spinal anaesthesia

By the early 20th Century it was realized that the shock of surgery could be very harmful following on from the shock of being wounded. No longer did doctors believe that the stimulating experience of pain could be in any way beneficial. Spinal anaesthesia was thought to minimize the shock of operation and therefore ought to be used for wounds below the level of the umbilicus. Marshall found that if he used it at base hospitals when wounds were a few days old it proved a satisfactory method. It could also be used at casualty clearing stations if the wounds were not less than forty hours old.

However, when the wounds were more recent, spinal anaesthesia could be followed by profound drops in blood pressure. The radial pulse at the wrist might disappear completely and fatalities could result. He observed that it was loss of blood that made spinal anaesthesia particularly dangerous. He tried decreasing the dose of local anaesthetic but this just resulted in incomplete anaesthesia. He set about finding out which patients could be given spinal anaesthesia safely and which could not. He felt that neither the appearance of the patient nor the pulse and blood pressure were helpful in making this decision.

What was of use was the haemoglobin concentration in the blood. Blood consists of many different types of cells and haemoglobin, which gives the red cells their colour, is responsible for carrying oxygen around the body. When a patient bleeds and red cells are lost the haemoglobin falls. If the haemoglobin concentration was low in a recently wounded patient then this meant that they had lost a lot of blood and would collapse if given spinal anaesthesia. The normal range for haemoglobin is 97 to 120% and Marshall found that a safe level was above 100%.

The following chart looks at the pulse and blood pressure in a soldier with a shell splinter wound of the leg, who underwent surgery twenty-one hours after being wounded. The haemoglobin was 85% and the blood pressure fell to 81mms Hg. The patient died of gas gangrene 24 hours after the operation.

This collapse in blood pressure was not understood by Marshall. With the benefit of current knowledge, when a local anaesthetic is injected into the fluid around the spine it blocks not only the sensory nerves that carry the sensations of touch and pain to the brain and the motor fibres which allow the brain to send impulses to move the limb but also the fibres of the sympathetic nervous system. These sympathetic nerves innervate the small blood vessels in the body to alter their caliber in response to changes in blood volume and the outside temperature. When a person is shocked due to blood loss these small vessels constrict to direct blood to the brain and other essential organs in an attempt to preserve their function. Vaso-constriction caused by cold aggravates the problem. If that patient were to have a spinal anaesthetic so that the action of the nerves

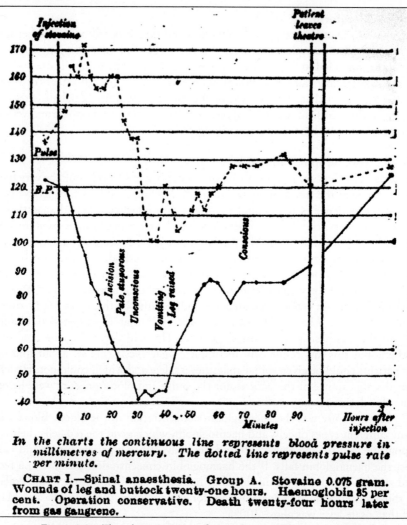

In the charts the continuous line represents blood pressure in millimetres of mercury. The dotted line represents pulse rate per minute.

CHART I.—Spinal anaesthesia. Group A. Stovaine 0.075 gram. Wounds of leg and buttock twenty-one hours. Haemoglobin 85 per cent. Operation conservative. Death twenty-four hours later from gas gangrene.

Figure 3.3   The administration of anaesthetics at the Front. (With permission from the *British Medical Journal* Publishing Group)

on the blood vessels is blocked, the effect is like pulling a rug from under someone's feet. This element of the compensatory mechanism that has been maintaining the blood pressure is withdrawn and the effect is dramatic. The peripheral blood vessels dilate uncontrollably. No amount of increase in the pulse rate will counteract the problem, and the blood pressure crashes. It is perhaps a testament to the fitness of youth that some men did survive this experience.

The problem of the seriously wounded soldier in a collapsed state

Having solved the problem of to whom not to give spinal anaesthesia Marshall turned his attention to the casualty with severe shock, the patient with a pale face and a very weak pulse. How was such a patient to be managed? He noted that these patients had a very cold skin and could be improved with hot water bottles (see Chapter 2). The blood pressure was taken regularly and if it was improving operation could be delayed for a short time, although too long a delay might result in gas gangrene setting in.

He warned that chloroform would result in death on the table and ether either by inhalation or intravenously would improve the patient initially and then result in profound collapse two hours later. Chloroform tended to depress the pumping of the heart resulting in death during surgery whereas ether stimulated it, resulting in an initial improvement which declined later. The only suitable anaesthetic in profoundly shocked patients was nitrous oxide and oxygen and although so light that there was occasional movement, there was no evidence of deterioration.

Shock due to haemorrhage occurred early on but septic shock took longer to develop. It might be due to infection of dead and damaged tissues that had been inadequately excised or to wounds of the abdomen which had resulted in bowel contents being spread into the peritoneum or bacteria being introduced with the offending weapon. Here the blood pressure is low but the pulse often full and bounding. We now know that toxins produced by bacteria act on the blood vessels to dilate them and on the heart to decrease the power of its pumping action. Although the pulse might not seem too fast and the blood pressure appear to be adequate, insufficient oxygen finds its way to the tissues and starting with the kidneys all the organs of the body fail. Marshall felt these patients were much more favorable subjects for spinal anaesthesia. Injection of stovaine around the spinal cord did not result in the same collapse as in haemorrhagic shock since the blood vessels were already dilated. The dramatic effect seen in the casualty with shock secondary to acute major blood loss did not happen. Ether could also be given without post-operative collapse, intravenous ether seemed to improve the patient's condition and nitrous oxide and oxygen could be used as well. Only chloroform was to be avoided as it had a direct depressant action on the heart.

Marshall's thoughts on anaesthesia for different types of wounds
Anaesthesia for severe limb wounds
Most of these patients were suffering from shock as a result of blood loss. They were cold and clammy, with pale faces and barely perceptible pulses. Marshall felt that many of their lives could be saved if correct procedures were followed. Morphine should be withheld as this would further depress the blood pressure. The only acceptable anaesthetic was nitrous oxide and oxygen, allowing the shattered limb to be quickly amputated. Anaesthesia might be so light that the patient would move when nerves were divided but the patient would be conscious five minutes after operation and able to "sit up and take nourishment".

Anaesthesia for penetrating head wounds
Marshall's opinion for head wounds was that local anaesthesia was far better than chloroform. Any general anaesthesia in a patient whose conscious level was impaired would have resulted in a depression of the patient's respirations and a rise in the carbon dioxide levels in the blood. This in turn would lead to the blood vessels of the brain dilating and the brain swelling, a condition referred to as cerebral oedema (See Chapter 9 for explanation of this). Without more modern agents and the ability to control the patient's ventilation any general anaesthetic would have been very dangerous. However if the casualty was completely awake, Marshall felt that if the

patient found cutting through the skull too upsetting, then warm ether could be recommended. As a mask would have got in the way of the surgeon he devised a way of passing a catheter down one of the patient's nostrils through which the anaesthetic vapour was passed.

Anaesthesia for Abdominal Wounds

Warm ether was of particular value, as temperature loss was a real problem when large amounts of the patient's intestines were exposed to the air. When the abdomen is opened, heat loss from exposed bowel is considerable and anything which counteracts a fall in body temperature is beneficial. Marshall found that when several feet of intestine were laid outside the abdominal cavity, the blood pressure fell. He suggested that surgeons should make large incisions and work within the abdomen. As casualties seemed to be able arrive at casualty clearing stations with several feet of intestine outside the abdominal cavity without any drop in blood pressure he attributed the deterioration in condition to heat loss from exposed blood vessels of the gut. If the casualty wasn't anaesthetized then the loss of heat was much less.

Ether itself would cause the blood pressure to rise but excessive manipulation of the bowel or pulling on the peritoneum which lines that abdominal cavity would result in a fall. The bowel and peritoneum are supplied by nerves from the sympathetic nervous system and stimulation of these nerves by pulling results in a slowing of the heart rate and fall in blood pressure. In other words the stimulation of the sympathetic nervous system by ether is counteracted by manipulation of the bowel. Bronchitis could be common after abdominal surgery as breathing and coughing are impaired due to the pain of the wound. Marshall found that he could decrease the incidence from 54% to 14.7% by using warm ether instead of open ether.

Operations on abdominal wounds could take a long time and it was important that surgeons proceeded quickly on a decisive course of action. Casualties might have holes in many parts of the intestine and these all had to be dealt with so that soiling of the peritoneal cavity was kept to a minimum. Just as it was important to excise dead tissue in a limb to prevent infection getting a hold so it was important to keep the peritoneal cavity free from intestinal contents. Once infection had set in it was difficult to combat. Even now septic shock from ruptured abdominal viscera may prove difficult to treat although support may be provided on an intensive care unit for every failing organ. When the operations took some time Marshall found that it was inadvisable to turn patients on their side to enable the surgeon to deal with a wound on the back.

The blood pressure in this situation fell markedly and it could be hours before the patient improved. Perhaps this was due to the patient being severely short of fluid. He stated that it was usual to give three pints of normal saline subcutaneously through a needle placed just under the skin during the operation but if the patient was shocked it would not be well absorbed as he showed in post-mortem studies. Three pints would be insufficient to replace the fluid that had evaporated from the surface of the intestines especially when combined with blood loss.

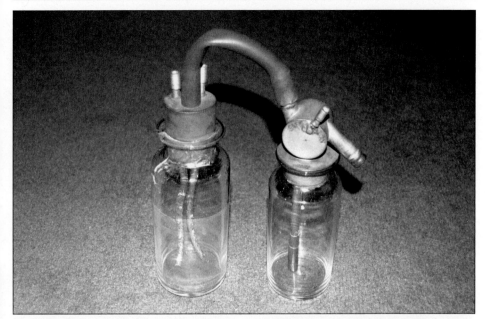

Figure 3.4 Marshall Gas/Oxygen/Ether Apparatus. Curved tubes deliver nitrous oxide and oxygen directly into the bubble bottle on the left. The bubbles of gas can easily be observed and the relative percentage of oxygen estimated. The gases then pass to the ether bottle on the right via a simple on/off valve. (Reproduced by kind permission of the Association of Anaesthetists of Great Britain and Ireland)

Anaesthesia for chest wounds

One operation in which chloroform proved superior to ether was when there was a penetrating chest wound. Ether in this situation provoked haemorrhage, perhaps because it had a tendency to raise the blood pressure.

As a result of Marshall's work, the place of nitrous oxide and oxygen became firmly established as a safe choice in difficult circumstances. Used in conjunction with ether for longer procedures an anaesthetic machine to regulate administration was required. Marshall designed such a machine. When home on leave he took his design to Coxeters, a manufacturer of anaesthetic equipment, who produced a machine for him which became the standard RAMC machine later on in the war. Marshall was encouraged to publish his work because "someone had borrowed their blocks".[15]

The "someone" in question was Captain Henry Boyle, who had by chance met an American doctor called James Tayloe Gwathmey in 1912 at the Seventeenth International Congress of Medicine in London. Before the war, in 1912, Gwathmey had developed an apparatus for giving nitrous oxide and oxygen which incorporated a device which could measure the flow of gases so that at a glance the relative proportions could be observed.[16]

Boyle acquired a Gwathmey machine when working in London. He adapted this, introducing reducing valves and used it on war casualties in London. Both Gwathmey and Marshall added bottles for ether or chloroform through which the gases were bubbled. These agents were introduced to enable Marshall to employ longer anaesthetics.

During the war chloroform was shown to lower the blood pressure whereas ether did not and if a small amount of ether was added to the nitrous oxide/oxygen mixture then the anaesthetic was still safe but could be used for more extensive surgery.[17]

However, it was Boyle who further developed the nitrous/oxide/ether machine and published his work on the new invention in February 1919. It was called a Boyle's Machine for many decades, the decline in the use of the term being a relatively recent phenomenon. Marshall did not really mind, because he had no wish to be remembered as an anaesthetist anyway.

Gwathmey went on to devise a method for giving nitrous oxide and ether to patients without the lungs collapsing during thoracic surgery. He delivered it through a mask which had an attachment containing an exit valve which had to be forced open before expired gases could escape. Thus the patient was breathing out against resistance and a continuous positive pressure was applied which kept the lungs expanded and allowed a lower percentage of oxygen to be given.[18]

Gwathmey also devised a simple method for giving analgesia to soldiers who required frequent wound dressings without removing them from their beds. He tried out a variety of mixtures deciding that a combination of paraldehyde, liquid paraffin and ether gave the best results. The smell and taste of paraldehyde was poorly tolerated but

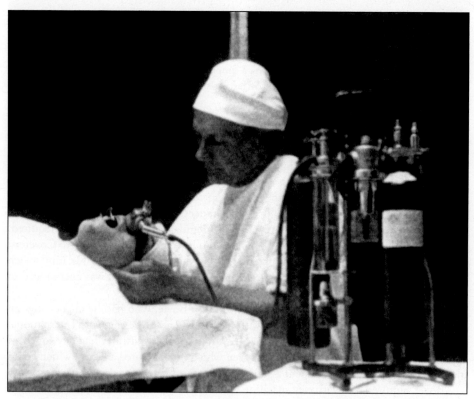

Figure 3.5   James Tayloe Gwathmey administering nitrous oxide/oxygen from his own apparatus. (from J.T. Gwathmey, *Anaesthesia*. New York: Appleton, 1914)

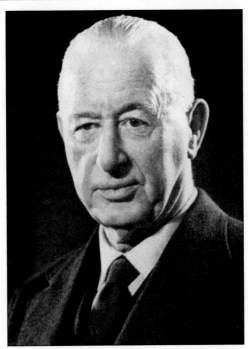

Figure 3.6   Sir Geoffrey Marshall. (Photograph originally published in K. Bryn Thomas, *The Development of Anaesthetic Apparatus*, 1975. Reproduced with permission of Wiley-Blackwell)

this was overcome by giving the soldiers a glass of port wine, an initial mouthful being followed by the ether mixture and then the remainder of the glass!

One of the hazards of general anaesthesia is the problem of operating on patients with a full stomach. This appears to have been given scant consideration during the Great War. An American anaesthetist called Flagg was one of the few to consider this problem in the emergency surgical patient.[19] In modern practice it is usual to fast people before surgery, so that there are no stomach contents that can be regurgitated or vomited, which could enter or obstruct the flow of air to the lungs. However, soldiers arriving at the casualty clearing stations cold and dehydrated were given a pint of hot tea (or coffee) whilst waiting for surgery. It warmed them up and helped to restore their blood volume and as it was liquid would hopefully not obstruct respiration if vomited. This might seem a strange practice to the present-day anaesthetist who would be concerned by the smallest amount of stomach contents entering the trachea (windpipe). The benefits might have outweighed the disadvantages but Flagg doubted this as he had observed that stomach movements ceased during anaesthesia and little would be absorbed. When wounds are suffered, gastric emptying is delayed and the stomach may remain full for many hours and for decades it has been accepted practice to perform maneuvers at induction which prevent regurgitation. This appears not to have been understood during the Great War as Major Corfield recalls one patient who brought up three bowls of bully beef and biscuit that he had consumed 28 hours earlier and been wounded two hours after it!

Largely as a result of Marshall's work, the need for a specialist anaesthetist as part of a surgical team was acknowledged.[20] Such team structure was haphazard to begin with in 1915, but as time went on, became more structured, so that by 1917 a surgical team with an anaesthetist was a well established group.

How Marshall managed to produce such high quality work with attention to detail in a casualty clearing station is remarkable, and careful charting of blood pressure and pulse rate during well given anaesthetics must have saved many thousands of lives. It is not clear how widespread the use of blood pressure measurement was in the hectic environment of a casualty clearing station. It is conjecture, but perhaps a finger on the pulse was the main monitor. Today it is unacceptable to use anything except 'minimal monitoring', that is an ECG recording heart beat, an automatic blood pressure measuring device, pulse oximetry (which indicates the amount of oxygen in the blood) and measurement of gases inhaled and expired including oxygen, carbon dioxide and anaesthetic vapours.

The use of a chart during anaesthesia to record blood pressure and pulse rate can be ascribed to an American Harvey Cushing who is best known for his work as a neurosurgeon.[21] He appreciated the importance of a meticulously given anaesthetic with routine blood pressure measurement. He had experienced a defining moment, when as a medical student in the 1890s, he gave his first anaesthetic to an elderly man. The patient vomited, inhaled and died. Cushing felt responsible. He was quickly reassured and told that such things happened frequently, and he should forget about it. He did not forget, and decided instead that he should train himself to be a better 'etherizer' and introduced charts to record pulse, respiration and temperature. He stated that careful anaesthesia and record taking:

> … was undoubtedly a step towards improvement in what had been a very casual administration of a dangerous drug.[22]

Initially, charts recorded pulse rate, respiration and temperature. The measurement of blood pressure by an inflatable cuff with a mercury column (sphygmomanometer) was described by an Italian, Riva Rocci, in 1896. On a visit to Switzerland in 1901 Harvey Cushing saw a simplified version of Riva Rocci's devise in use at the bedside at the Ospidale di St Matteo in Pavia. On returning to America the following year he introduced blood pressure measurement and a new anaesthesia chart into his clinical practice. The blood pressure was determined by palpating the pulse at the wrist and observing when it disappeared with the inflation of a cuff around the patient's upper arm.

In 1906 Korotkoff, a Russian doctor, described the changes in sound that were heard if a stethoscope was placed over the brachial artery at the elbow. In this way, both the systolic and diastolic blood pressures could be measured reflecting the pressure during contraction and relaxation of the heart. Marshall employed a Riva Rocci sphygmomanometer with stethoscope when he carried out his observations at Remy Siding.

Cushing therefore joins the ranks of men who realized the importance of anaesthesia as a subject even before the turn of the century. He served in the war from 1917 as a surgeon in chief at a base hospital in Boulogne where he took to work Gertrude Gerrard, a nurse anaesthetist who had worked with him in Boston. She was later decorated by the British Red Cross for her work at an advanced unit in Belgium. Nurse anaesthetists have a long history in the USA and are still used today. Their first training program was established in 1909, and when a surgeon by the name of Crile from the Lakeside Hospital, Cleveland, Ohio set sail for the American Hospital in Paris he took two nurse anaesthetists with him, Miss Agatha Hodgkins and Miss Mabel Littleton.[23]

Owing to a shortage of British anaesthetists the question of training British nurses was taken up by the DGMS in 1917.[24] A course was set up, and commenced in January 1918. It was open to all nursing sisters and VADs and lasted for three months, the first two months in selected base hospitals and the third month in a casualty clearing station. The nurses were taught to assess patients before surgery so that the correct choice of anaesthetic could be made, and they were taught how to manage an emergency. Two courses were held and 159 nurses trained although the use of VADs was not sanctioned and neither would the Australians allow their nurses to practice. The result appears to have been very successful but the withdrawal of experienced nurses from other duties was unfortunate.

The importance of the quality and training of personnel at casualty clearing stations became the concern of an American anaesthetist, Arthur Guedel, who was of the opinion that young medical officers could not become proficient and safe learning on the job. He set up training schools in Chaumont and Contrexville. He realized that they needed instruction in basic principles of airway control and depth of anaesthesia. He devised a chart which demonstrated the changes in the reaction of the pupils and certain reflexes under ether anaesthesia so that medical officers could recognize when they had achieved a suitable plane of anaesthesia.[25] To cement this training he became a well-known figure travelling between casualty clearing stations on a motorbike.

Text books of anaesthesia had been written from the 1890s but had to be rewritten after the war. Boyle and Hewer's *Practical Anaesthesia*, first published in 1907 and again in 1911, required an extra chapter on blood pressure and pulse reactions during anaesthesia when it was reprinted in 1923, presumably at least in part due to advances made during the Great War. It recommended regular charting of these parameters to detect changes from the patient's norm which would indicate the development of shock and result in prompt treatment with intravenous saline.[26]

Shock from the modern perspective

From a 21st Century perspective the areas of research which will be described appeared to be leading physicians down blind alleys and sidetracking them. The fundamental problem which nobody fully appreciated was that many wounded soldiers had lost massive amounts of blood. The clinical problem was aggravated by a lack of fluid intake both before being wounded and on the long transfer back to casualty clearing stations. Extreme cold also made things worse. If they continued to bleed either from a femoral fracture, if it was inadequately splinted, or internally from chest or abdominal wounds, then what might appear manageable at the beginning was life-threatening by the time they reached surgical help.

A healthy young man can lose up to 30% of his blood volume without a change in blood pressure and only a modest rise in pulse rate. He can compensate for even larger amounts of blood loss. He does this by constricting the blood flow to the skin and other organs. Deprived of blood flow and oxygen these tissues continue to function and survive by changing to what is called anaerobic (without oxygen) metabolism. The consequence of this is to produce an excess of acid. Cold makes matters worse. The flow of blood to the periphery is reduced to decrease heat loss and conserve core temperature. However, before measures were taken to keep casualties warm their core temperature must have fallen and we now know that cardiac output (the amount of blood pumped with every contraction of the heart muscle) falls directly with a decrease in body temperature.

When the compensatory mechanisms are inadequate for the blood loss the ability to preserve the blood pressure is lost and the shock worsens. These wounded soldiers needed fluid, blood, warming and early surgical intervention. Furthermore tissues deprived of oxygen provided an ideal environment for the bacteria responsible for gas gangrene to proliferate. These bacteria are classified as anaerobic as they flourish in an oxygen free environment.

The relationship between the amount of fluid in the vascular system and the alteration of the caliber of the blood vessels to compensate for the lack of fluid and blood is fundamental to understanding the mechanisms of shock. In order to direct blood to the vital organs of the body primarily the brain and heart, blood vessels constrict to reduce the blood flow to the skin and the kidneys. In this way the blood pressure is maintained. If the blood pressure falls much below 60mm Hg then the brain is no longer perfused and vital centres of the brain that maintain life cease to function. If a patient survives for any length of time with a very low blood pressure, it may be difficult to reverse, and kidney damage ensues. It should be noted that whenever a figure is given for blood pressure it refers to systolic pressure i.e. the pressure reached when the heart is contracting.

In retrospect it is frustrating to read about the attempts to understand shock when what the soldiers needed were massive amounts of intravenous fluids and pints of blood.

Understanding about shock and its causes before 1915

The different theories of shock are outlined below.

Crile's Kinetic Theory

Before the war Crile, an American surgeon, became interested in the nature and treatment of shock whilst working in Cleveland, Ohio where a large proportion of his practice was trauma cases due to industrial accidents. After serving in the Spanish-American War he returned to civilian practice in 1901 and developed the kinetic theory of shock. He believed that the brain became bombarded with stimuli from the wound and from the operation, and as a result of fear. It was proposed that the continuation of such stimulation led to exhaustion of the part of the brain that controls the peripheral blood vessels (vasomotor centre) with subsequent dilatation of vessels and a fall in blood pressure. He advocated that the painful stimuli should be abolished by the injection of local anaesthetic and that nitrous oxide be given to eliminate fear. He called this technique anoci-association. As he was using an appropriate anaesthetic along with pain relief that didn't worsen shock his technique had some value.

Yandell Henderson's acapnia theory

Another theory, the acapnia theory, was put forward by Yandell Henderson, an American physiologist. He suggested that the deep and rapid breathing seen after the infliction of a painful stimulus which results in a decrease of carbon dioxide in the blood results in a failure of the centre in the brain that is responsible for maintaining blood pressure. He claimed that when abdominal surgery was performed even more carbon dioxide was lost from the surface of the intestines which exacerbated the problem. In order to counteract this he suggested slow breathing or breathing through a long tube so that expired air was re-breathed. Furthermore warm saline saturated with carbon dioxide could be instilled into the abdominal cavity.

These are just two of the theories that were devised to explain the state of shock which could be defined as a "depression of all the vital functions of the body, the state being primarily induced by the infliction of injury on the body tissues and being characterized by a progressive fall of the blood pressure".[27]

During the Great War large numbers of patients suffering from wound shock were seen and their associated high death rate troubled doctors. If the survival rate was to improve then understanding of this condition had to advance. Marshall had solved the problem of which anaesthetics to use but the prevention and treatment of wound shock required the combined talents of a number of physicians and scientists.

The Medical Research Committee Investigative Committee on Shock during the Great War

In order to co-ordinate research and clinical observation on wound shock the Medical Research Committee (MRC) in 1917 appointed a Special Investigative Committee. This consisted of surgeons who were working at casualty clearing stations supported by physiologists in Britain carrying out research and laboratory doctors at base hospitals. In France a research group was organized in the First Army area. Professor Cannon, an American physiologist from Harvard and John Fraser, a Scottish surgeon who also did a lot of work on abdominal wounds (see Chapter 7), worked in the laboratory and surgical wards of a casualty clearing station in Béthune whilst Captain Ernest Cowell of the RAMC worked further forward.

Cowell established parameters for the normal limits of blood pressure found in fighting men by observing them when there was no active fighting.[28] [29] Knowing that the release of adrenaline in the body prepared the soldier for battle by increasing heart rate and blood pressure and releasing glucose from the body he wondered whether over a period of time this prolonged exposure to the effects of adrenaline might be harmful. He measured the blood pressure of men in the front line and found it to be raised compared to that of soldiers further back. During a full moon he measured the blood pressures of a garrison of a detached outpost in a part of the line that was exposed. He noted how their blood pressures became raised when danger increased and questioned whether outpouring of adrenaline contributed to the later development of shock if they were wounded.

He studied the onset of shock by making observations on casualties before they were evacuated to the casualty clearing stations. In early 1917, working at "Lone Farm" Advanced Dressing Station, he measured the blood pressure of casualties soon after wounding and observed what happened on the journey from the advanced dressing station to the casualty clearing station.

He was able to demonstrate to surgeons in the field how shock could develop and by now the terms primary and secondary shock were coming into common usage. Primary shock occurred when, after being wounded, a soldier's blood pressure would be low, but secondary shock didn't present until a few hours later. Some soldiers appeared in reasonable condition to begin with but after a journey back to the casualty clearing station with little attention paid to food, water and warmth the blood pressure might fall uncontrollably.

Looking back on this term in 1928 Cowell stated that several points stood out:

- The effect of the cold wasn't appreciated in the early months of the war,
- A correlation between the amount of shock and the extent of muscle injury was noted,
- The slowness of onset of shock was observed,
- Where the blood pressure was low and the patients survived it was beginning to look as if the low pressure predisposed to gas gangrene.

By the summer of 1917 Cowell worked at Casualty Clearing Station No 23 at Lozinghem, which received cases from around Loos. Here he was joined by Professor Cannon and together, at the suggestion of Professor Bayliss, another member of the Shock Committee, they looked at the effects of various intravenous solutions for improving blood pressure.[30]

Cowell's contribution to the investigation of shock was a very practical one and although a general surgeon in London during peacetime he became a senior army surgeon during the Second World War.

Cannon, however, had entered the war largely to research the problem of wound shock and he was a scientist. Realising that there was decreased circulation of blood and believing that it was pooling somewhere within the body, he was prompted to look at the use of a substance extracted from the pituitary gland of the brain (pituitrin) which if injected abdominally would constrict the vessels of the splanchnic bed and return the circulation to normal. Crile had already proposed that exhaustion of the vasomotor centre led to dilatation of blood vessels but it was a matter of which vessels the blood was hiding in. As the skin was pale in patients with shock he thought that the blood couldn't be here but must be in the huge area of blood vessels supplying the bowel (splanchnic circulation). Determined to investigate this at the front, when soldiers from the Battle for Hill 70 came into Casualty Clearing Station 23 he persuaded Cowell to let him inject pituitrin, however it did not work.

From autopsy studies Cannon learnt that there was no pooling of blood in the splanchnic circulation. In so doing, he effectively disproved the theory of splanchnic pooling as an explanation for shock. However, he was determined to solve the mystery of the missing blood and working with Fraser and Hooper in Béthune, Cannon then thought that pooling must occur in capillaries, tiny blood vessels connecting the arteries and veins.[31] He found that blood taken from capillaries was more concentrated than blood from larger veins. The greater the degree of shock the greater the discrepancy between the two figures

He concluded that blood was stagnating in the capillaries and that if this blood could be returned to the circulation then the blood pressure would improve. In other words, having disproved splanchnic pooling, he persisted in the mistaken belief that blood must be pooling somewhere else within the body, and he was determined to find out where.

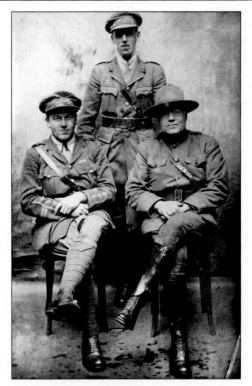

Figure 3.7

Photograph of Walter Cannon, John Fraser and A.N. Hooper, 1917. (Reproduced by kind permission of Harvard Medical Library in the Francis A. Countway Library of Medicine).

He was going from one blind alley (splanchnic pooling) to another (capillary pooling). The reality seems obvious to us now. The blood had been spilled onto the fields of France and Flanders.

Acidosis and shock – another misperception

Subsequently, Cannon turned his attention to measuring the amount of acid in the blood of shocked patients and he found it to be increased.[32] This is called acidosis or acidaemia. In cases of gas gangrene it appeared to be particularly severe and when operated upon it worsened still further. The acidosis was now thought to be a cause of shock and all that would be needed was baking soda! A method of giving sodium bicarbonate intravenously was devised and used with some success to improve the survival of shock.

In June 1918 Colonel Sir Almroth Wright wrote in *The Lancet* setting out to explain the acidosis seen in shock.[33] Work had already been done showing that muscles working without oxygen produced lactic acid and Wright concluded quite rightly that this was the same process as occurred in shock when arrest of the circulation cut off the supply of oxygen to the tissues and metabolism resulted in the production of acid.

As regards treatment of shock he paid particular attention to the warming of patients. Ideally he said prevention of heat loss was better than cure and the giving of hot drinks and application of warmth as early as possible was advisable. However once shock was established then too rapid resuscitation by warmth would convey large amounts of acid to the blood stream once the circulation was re-established. He suggested treating with sodium bicarbonate before resuscitation began and not subjecting the patient to anaesthesia and surgery before the blood alkalinity had returned to normal.

It seems to me that Almroth Wright, a laboratory physician, was beginning to understand the process. Firstly, he recognized that the acid blood was the result of a decrease in circulation to the tissues. In other words, acidosis was the result, and not the cause of shock. From this he concluded that trench foot and chilblains were also produced from the same process i.e. extreme cold decreased blood flow to the foot in such a way that metabolism changed to the anaerobic form and acid was produced in the tissues. He stated that:

The pathology of trench foot and anaesthesia would seem to lie poles apart, but in reality they would seem to have in common the factor of a shutting off of the circulation and the resultant cutting down of oxygen supply to the muscles.[34]

He recognized that prolonged and severe operations in cold operating theatres would be particularly likely to result in an acidosis and acknowledged Cannon's warning that it was very important not to superimpose an anaesthetic acidosis upon a wound acidosis. This was an important fact to have recognised not only during wartime but for future surgical practice. Long and difficult operations can only be carried out if the patient is kept warm and fluid and blood losses are replaced in a timely manner.

By the time Gray had written his book *The Early Treatment of War Wounds* in 1919, the priorities in the treatment of shock had been worked out.[35] Gray concluded that most cases of shock were due to haemorrhage and that the extent of blood loss was difficult to estimate and that the total amount lost was greater than generally supposed. In practical terms he stated:

Every effort should be made at the earliest opportunity to replenish the depleted fluid reserves of the wounded soldier by the administration of large amounts of fluid.

Fluid replacement therapy
As drinking water was limited at the front line, soldiers were already short of fluid, and when wounded any reserves were further depleted by perspiration. The preferred method of giving fluid was by mouth or by rectum, and for it to be preferably warm.

The recognition of the need to actively warm and rehydrate the wounded led to the introduction of resuscitation wards at casualty clearing stations. Special efforts were made to keep wounded men warm on the journey from the front. Blankets, hot water bottles, and better warming of advanced dressing stations all played their part. This reduced secondary shock and the period of resuscitation was shortened. A sister and orderlies acted under a special experienced medical officer who supervised the care of the wounded and prepared them for surgery. If oral and rectal fluids were not tolerated then intravenous fluids were required.

Professor W.M. Bayliss, who was a physiologist and a member of the Shock Committee, delivered a lecture to the Royal College of Physicians of London on 30 April

1918 on intravenous injections in wound shock.[36] He recognized that restoring the blood pressure so that oxygen could be delivered to the tissues was the single most important factor to reduce secondary shock. Although it would be thought that blood itself would be the best way to achieve this, he felt that it didn't show itself to be as superior to other solutions as might be expected. A dilute blood at high pressure was found to be more effective than normal blood under a low pressure. To some extent anaemia could be tolerated if the blood pressure was maintained.

Saline in Various Forms
The transfusion of normal saline or Ringer's solution (basically saline with a few other electrolytes) had been used for some years but as it leaked out of the blood vessels it provided only a transient improvement. The use of hypertonic saline, which is saline that is more concentrated than the surrounding tissues and should therefore hold the fluid within the blood vessels wasn't much better.

Gum
In order to achieve an increase in blood volume Bayliss introduced the use of Gum Arabica into clinical practice. A solution could be made of 6% or 3% in saline and the large molecules of galactose and arabinose present in gum were inert and stayed in the circulation. He found that it was useful in severe haemorrhage and in cases where haemorrhage and shock were not excessive but blood pressure fell after anaesthesia. In one case of gas gangrene where there was neither shock nor haemorrhage but a low blood pressure of 70mm Hg a transfusion of Gum Arabica restored the blood pressure. Gray was less impressed and felt that if the time interval between haemorrhage and the giving of Gum Arabica was prolonged then it was less effective. Therefore the use of this fluid was pushed forward to the field ambulances where it allowed a casualty to arrive at a casualty clearing station in a better condition where, if necessary, blood transfusion could be started.

Blood Transfusion
The introduction of blood transfusion during the Great War can rightly be ascribed to doctors from Canada and America where the subject had been given much more consideration in the first decade of the 20th Century than in Britain. However, the first person-to-person transfusions for acute haemorrhage were carried out in 1818 by James Blundell, a London obstetrician who had seen women dying of post-partum bleeding. Four of the ten transfusions that he carried out were successful, which is remarkable given that he didn't understand the presence of different blood groups or how to stop blood clotting on its route from one person to another. This meant that blood transfusion remained on rocky ground until 1900, when Landsteiner recognized the existence of three blood groups. The fourth group was recognized two years later in 1902. However the cross-matching of blood didn't become a practical proposition until almost a decade later when Moss, working at the John Hopkins University, developed a technique at the same time as Jansky, who was working independently in Bohemia.

Direct transfusion from donor to patient

George Washington Crile, who has already been mentioned in connection with his work on shock, was one of the earliest users of blood transfusion in the field of surgery.[37] His first transfusions were carried out without cross-matching or anti-coagulation (to stop the blood clotting) and he regarded it as an adjunct to the treatment of shock rather than a first line measure. He connected an artery in the donor's wrist to a vein on the inside of the patients elbow. By using a very short tube to connect the two he managed to overlap the two vessels and thus prevent clotting. A letter from Berkeley Moynihan, a surgeon in Leeds, appeared in *The Lancet* in June 1918, strongly rebuffing the idea that transfusion hadn't been used in Britain before the war. He had visited Crile in Cleveland, had learned the technique and used it to good effect.[38]

Blood transfusion during the Great War was first reported in the *British Medical Journal* in July 1916 by L. Bruce Robertson, a captain in the Canadian Army Medical Corps.[39] In cases of primary haemorrhage when initial wounding produced the blood loss, benefit would not be in doubt. However Robertson's first wartime transfusions were given at a base hospital in cases of secondary haemorrhage where infection had eroded into blood vessels resulting in major bleeding. Blood transfusion made the patient well enough to undergo further surgical intervention to stop bleeding, or boosted the patient's own condition, thus enabling him to combat the infection.

There were two problems with blood transfusion. The first was the possible introduction of infection from donor to patient, and it was important to establish as far as possible that the donor did not carry syphilis. Healthy donors could withstand the loss of 600 to 1000 ml of blood, which could be replaced by saline. There were also a few convalescent patients with minor fractures and sprains who were relatively healthy but unfit for duty who were ideal donors.

Rifleman Charlie Shepherd's experience as a donor is quoted in *The Roses of No Man's Land*. Finding himself in an American base hospital where a volunteer donor was requested, and seeing that most of the other casualties had both legs blown off, he offered his services. He was rolled into the operating theatre head to tail with the recipient and watched whilst his blood returned the colour to the face of the badly wounded soldier. This made him something of a hero and he was given champagne on his return to the ward. The best part was to be sent back to England for convalescence, when his own wound necessitated no more than two weeks out of the front line.

The second problem with blood transfusion was that of compatibility, where it was important that the donor and recipient blood when mixed together didn't result in destruction (haemolysis) or sticking together of the red blood cells. Establishment of the scientific basis of grouping and transfusing only compatible blood resolved this problem.[40]

Other factors that had to be overcome were how to prevent blood clotting whilst it travelled from donor to patient and how to measure the volume of blood transfused. The connection of a vein to a vein or an artery to a vein had the obvious disadvantage of not being able to observe and therefore measure the amount of blood that was transfusing. Initially this was overcome by using a syringe to extract blood from a cannula placed in the donor's vein, and then injecting it into a cannula in a vein in the recipient. Saline was injected through the cannulae after withdrawing or injecting blood to keep them patent. This process required two skilled operators and an orderly to run between them.

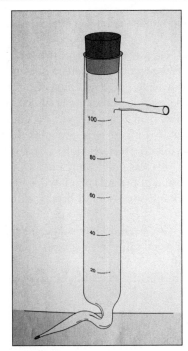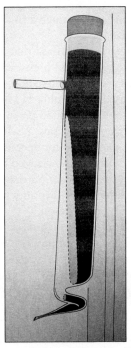

Figure 3.8 (a & b)   Diagramatic representations of Kimpton's Tubes (Gordon Stables, Department of Medical Illustration, University of Aberdeen)

Unger of New York devised a piece of equipment with stopcocks that allowed blood to be withdrawn from the donor and injected into the recipient without disconnecting. A saline flush was also incorporated which prevented the cannulae clotting up.[41]

Another ingenious method was Kimpton's tubes as shown in Figure 3.8.[42]

These consisted of a glass tube with a cannula drawn out at one end. This could be inserted into the donor's vein and placed in such a position that blood would run into it and then lain so that the blood would not escape. When inserted into the recipient's vein and held upright the blood would then enter the circulation. The tubes could be autoclaved for sterility and liquid paraffin was used to lubricate the inside of the tube and prevent blood from clotting.

Having successfully carried out blood transfusion in base hospitals, there was a desire to carry it forward to the casualty clearing stations and beyond, where primary haemorrhage was killing men. Saline infusions gave only a temporary improvement and Gum Arabica could be used with effect to tide casualties over if the haemorrhage was not too great, but for more seriously wounded soldiers it was insufficient. L. Bruce Robertson reported in 1917 his results of 36 transfusions in primary haemorrhage.[43] His results show that cases considered previously hopeless could be improved sufficiently to allow surgery to take place. Also, some patients who had undergone surgery and who then deteriorated due to the combined effect of wound and surgical haemorrhage could be saved by blood transfusion, which prevented them from sliding into irreversible shock. Blood was obviously a precious commodity and it was important to time the giving of a transfusion for maximum effect. Early transfusion would prevent the degenerative change seen if the exsanguinated situation (almost complete loss of blood) was allowed to persist.

By this stage it was realized that the best way of judging how much blood was lost was by measuring the blood pressure.[44] Haemoglobin measurements and blood counts didn't help, and the pulse rate could vary widely, although the danger of a rising pulse rate was recognized. If morphia had been given the pulse rate might be little over a 100 beats per minute. With a blood pressure less than 70mm Hg the patient was precarious and needed transfusion to save his life and if his pressure was less than 90 mm Hg he was not in a good state for operation. Blood pressures of less than 60mm Hg were rarely seen and it was acknowledged that this was only compatible with life for a short period. As shock without haemorrhage could also result in a low blood pressure it was important to realize that other anti-shock measures should be carried out at the same time as considering transfusion.

In his book *The Early Treatment of War Wounds* Gray suggested successive blood pressure readings while warmth, rest and rectal saline were given. If the pressure failed to rise then transfusion would be required.

The results of Robertson's 57 transfusions in cases of primary haemorrhage are summarized in Table 3.1.

Table 3.1

The results of Robertson's 57 transfusions in cases of primary haemorrhage

Effects of transfusion	Casualties
Life-saving (evacuated to base hospital in good condition)	36+
Immediately beneficial but died from shock	8
No benefit	4
Harmful (haemolysis)	2

+ 3 of these patients subsequently died from a combination of pneumonia, tetanus and sepsis.

The problem of donors in a casualty clearing station could be partially overcome by grouping all possible donors ahead of time and then having simple equipment available to type recipients. However the whole process of transfusion occupied two or three members of trained staff and in times of high numbers of casualties it was difficult to keep pace with the demand.

Stored Citrated Blood

The idea of having a bank of preserved blood available for these situations which could be administered by one medical officer offered a solution. Oswald Robertson of the US Army tested out this possibility at the casualty clearing stations of the British 3rd Army.[45] Rous and Turner, working at the Rockefeller Institute in New York, found that blood could be taken into a solution of dextrose and sodium citrate and preserved in the cold for several weeks. Robertson took volunteer donors from among the lightly wounded. Those with a history of malaria, trench fever or syphilis were excluded. The blood was collected and stored in heavy glass bottles called Winchester Bottles, which were kept in ice boxes until required.

Robertson carried out 22 transfusions in 20 individuals, 11 of whom were discharged to the base and nine died. All of them showed an improvement whether the blood had been stored for 3 or 26 days and the effect was as good as fresh blood. The transfusions were given in the resuscitation ward by one medical officer, thus leaving the operating room free for surgical procedures.

Blood was also transported in ambulance wagons over rough roads without suffering damage. Having introduced transfusion to casualty clearing stations there then came a desire to use it further forward in the field ambulances. Norman Guiou of the Canadian Army Medical Corps showed that it was possible to group patients in a field ambulance, find a suitable donor and transfuse them so that they could reach the casualty clearing station.[46] Clearly blood transfusions with either fresh or preserved blood could be carried out as far forward as the regimental aid post if the number of casualties was not overwhelming, and this ability to try to save even the desperately wounded had an important effect on the morale of the men. It should be noted that the amount of blood given, 1000ml at maximum, is small compared to the many litres which might be given to a road traffic victim in a modern emergency centre. Blood transfusion would allow a few lucky individuals to move from an unsalvageable situation to one which allowed life-saving surgery to be carried out.

Resuscitation teams

Towards the end of the war resuscitation teams were formed, which were able to advance as far forward as possible to treat the severely wounded. The first was probably established by Dr Holmes à Court of the 4th Australian Field Ambulance.[47] A shock centre had been established in early 1918 at No 3 British Casualty Clearing Station at Gezaincourt. As this was in easy reach of the Australian sector it may have been where Holmes a'Court conceived the idea of a field ambulance resuscitation team. They were ready for action at the Battle of Hamel on July 4 1918, which was a limited combined Australian and American offensive near Amiens. Such was their success that they were instituted as permanent establishments in each of the 5 Australian divisions. They consisted of two medical officers, one of whom was expert in rapid urgent surgery and blood transfusion while the other was experienced in anaesthesia, resuscitation and classification of blood donors. Supported by 4 others, 1 non-commissioned officer and 3 orderlies, they were attached to a main or advanced dressing station and had the use of a motor ambulance vehicle. On finding a casualty they would institute warming methods, infuse gum acacia, ligate any large bleeding vessels and amputate shattered limbs. This enabled the wounded to reach casualty clearing stations in a much better state than they would otherwise have been and saved many limbs by the early removal of tourniquets.

℘

This account of the practice of anaesthesia and resuscitation starts well before the Great War. The anaesthetic agents used during the war were the same ones as had been used before. It was the pioneering work of Geoffrey Marshall and others that led to a better understanding of the applicability of the various agents to the seriously wounded. As a result of this work, there was great improvement in survival. It also became clear

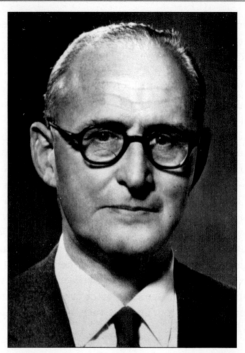

Figure 3.9   Sir Ivan Magill. (Photograph published in K. Bryn Thomas, *The Development of Anaesthetic Apparatus*, 1975. Reproduced with permission of Wiley-Blackwell)

that there was a definite need for specialist anaesthetists in military service whose role extended to preparing the wounded for surgery pre-operatively.

These pioneering individuals not only brought the benefits of improved understanding of the use of agents leading to safer anaesthesia, but also the need for a scientific basis of practice, development of equipment and proper training of anaesthetists. They were responsible for making the specialty what it is today. The influence of the Great War on practice continued beyond 1918 and led to one of the most important anaesthetic developments of the 20th Century, introduced by one of the most able anaesthetists of the time, Sir Ivan Magill.[48]

Magill worked with the plastic surgeon Harold Gillies at the Queen's Hospital for Facial and Jaw injuries at Sidcup in Kent. Born in Northern Ireland he qualified from Belfast in 1913 when he was issued with a certificate confirming that he had in his training administered one anaesthetic. During the war he joined the Royal Army Medical Corps as a captain and acted as medical officer to the Irish Guards at the Battle of Loos in September 1915. He also worked in a base hospital near Rouen. After the war he worked originally in Barnet before moving to work with Gillies at Sidcup. The anaesthetics were very challenging. It wasn't possible to hold a face mask on the patient because of where the surgeon was operating, and the patients often required many operations.

When Magill joined the hospital the usual method of giving ether was through the back passage but this resulted in inadequate anaesthesia at the beginning of surgery progressing to unnecessary depth during surgery and a prolonged recovery. Magill introduced the use of tubes which could be passed into the windpipe through the nose through which ether from Shipway's warm ether apparatus was passed. The ether was insufflated into the windpipe by a motorized pump that drove air through the ether. However it had to come back out of the patient when he exhaled and any obstruction in the throat or mouth would prevent this happening, leading to laboured breathing and increased haemorrhage. Harold Gillies once remarked:

> Maggi – you seem to get this anaesthetic into the patient alright, don't you think you could devise a method of getting it out again so I am not anaesthetized?[49]

The answer came in one particular case when the patient's breathing became so laboured that it was necessary for Magill to put another tube down the patient's other nostril to allow the gases to escape. The back of the throat was then packed with gauze. This eventually led to Magill developing a single endotracheal tube which was passed into the windpipe from the nose and allowed to and fro breathing. At first his invention was treated with scepticism but by the 1970s most anaesthetics were given through an endotracheal tube. Necessity is the mother of invention, and the difficulties anaesthetizing facio-maxillary wounds led directly to the invention of one of the most important pieces of anaesthetic equipment still in use today.[50] [51]

It is unfortunate that it required the large number of casualties of the Great War to launch advances in the practice of anaesthesia. The agents available had hardly changed, but the training of anaesthetists, development of equipment, the preparation of the patient for surgery and post-operative care were revolutionized. The mystery of wound shock began to be unravelled and the lessons learnt applied to civilian practice, enabling more complicated and extensive surgery to be carried out than could have been imagined before 1914.

Above all the advance of anaesthesia owes everything to the clear thinking men and women who felt the subject worthy of their full attention both in peacetime and in war.

Notes

1   Corfield, C., "Six months experience at a C.C.S. on the Somme", *Practitioner* 1917; 24: pp.251-254.

2   Snow, S.J., *Blessed Days of Anaesthesia*. New York: Oxford University Press, 1978.

3   Connor, H., "The use of chloroform by British Army surgeons during the Crimean War", *Medical History* 1998; 42: pp.161-193.

4   Snow, J., "On the inhalation of vapour of ether in surgical operations", *The Lancet* 1847; 50: pp.551-554.

5   Metcalfe, N.H., "Military influence upon the development of anaesthesia from the American Civil War (1861-1865) to the outbreak of the First World War", *Anaesthesia* 2005; 60: pp.1213-1217.

6   Wulf, H.F.W., "The centennial of spinal anaesthesia", *Anaesthesiology* 1998; 89, No 2: pp.500-506.

7   Houghton, J.W.H. & C.G. Spencer, "Spinal anaelgesia with notes of fifty cases", *Journal of the Royal Army Medical Corps* 1905; 4: pp.447-449.

8   Silk, J.F.W., "Anaesthetics a necessary part of the curriculum", *The Lancet* 1892; 139: pp.1178-1180.

9   Buxton, D.W., "On the advisability of the inclusion of the study of anaesthetics as a compulsory subject in the medical curriculum", *British Medical Journal* 1901; 1: pp.1007-1009.

10 General Medical Council, *British Medical Journal* 1912; 2: pp.536-538.

11 Macdonald, L., *The Roses of No Man's Land*. London: Papermac, 1984.

12 Evans B., "A doctor in the Great War – an interview with Sir Geoffrey Marshall", *British Medical Journal* 1982; 285: pp.1780-1783.

13 Marshall G., "Anaesthetics at a casualty clearing station", *Proceedings of the Royal Society of Medicine* 1917; 10: pp.17-36.

14 Shipway, F.E., "The advantages of warm anaesthetic vapours and an apparatus for their administration", *The Lancet* 1916; 1: pp.70-74.

15 Metcalfe, N.H., "The effect of the First World War (1914-1918) on the development of British anaesthesia", *European Journal of Anaesthesiology* 2007; 24: pp.649-657.

16 Thomas, K.B., *The Development of Anaesthetic Apparatus*. Oxford: Blackwell Scientific Publications, 1975.

17 Marshall, Geoffrey, "Two Types of Portable Gas-Oxygen Apparatus", *Proceedings of the Royal Society of Medicine* 1920 (Section Anaestheology); 13: pp.16-19.

18 Gwathmey, J.T., *Anaesthesia*. London: Churchill, 1925, 2nd ed.

19 Flagg, P.J., "Anaesthesia in Europe on the Western Battle Front", *International Clincs* 1918; 3: pp.210-228.

20 MacPherson, W.G. (ed.), *History of the Great War based on Official Documents. Medical Services. General History*. London: HMSO, 1924, Volume 2, pp.44-45.

21 Hirsch, N.P., "Harvey Cushing: his contribution to anaesthesia", *Anaesthesia and Analgesia* 1986; 65: 288-293

22 Beecher, H.K., "The first anaesthesia records (Codman, Cushing)", *Surgery, Gynaecology & Obstetrics* 1940; 71: pp.689-693.

23 Bennet, J.A., "War of Ideas", *Proceedings of the History of Anaesthesia Society* 1994; 15: pp.59-64.

24 MacPherson, *op.cit.*, Volume 2, pp.165-166.

25 Guedel, A.E., "Third Stage Ether: A sub-classification regarding the significance of the position and movements of the eyeball", *American Journal of Surgery* 1920; 34: pp.53-57.

26 Boyle, H.E.G. & C.L. Hewer, *Practical Anaesthetics*. London: Hodder & Stoughton, 1923, 3rd ed.

27 Fraser J., "Operation shock", *British Journal of Surgery* 1923; 11: pp.410-425.

28 Cowell, E.M., "The initiation of wound shock", *Journal of the American Medical Association* 1918; 70: pp.607-610.

29 Cowell, E.M., "The pathology and treatment of traumatic wound shock", *Journal of the Royal Army Medical Corps* 1928: 51; pp.81-102.

30 Benison, S., A.C. Barger & E.L. Wolfe, "Walter B. Cannon and the mystery of shock: A study of Anglo-American co-operation in World War I", *Medical History* 1991; 35: pp.217-249.

31 Cannon, W.B., J. Fraser & A.N. Hooper, "Some alterations in distribution and character of blood in shock and haemorrhage", *Journal of the American Medical Association* 1918; 70: pp.526-531.

32 Cannon, W.B., "Acidosis in cases of shock, haemorrhage and gas infection", *Journal of the American Medical Association* 1918; 708: pp.531-535.

33 Wright, A.E. & L. Colebrook, *The Lancet* 1 1918; 191: pp.763-765.

34 *Ibid.*

35 Gray, Col. H.M.W., *The Early Treatment of War Wounds*. London: Henry Frowde, 1919.

36 Bayliss, W.M., "Intravenous injection in wound shock", *British Medical Journal* 1918; 1: pp.553-556.

37 Boulton, T.B., "The role of George Washington Crile in the development of anaesthesia", *Proceedings of the History of Anaesthesia Society* 1991; 9B: pp.54-59.

38 Moynihan, B., "The operation of blood transfusion – letter to the editor", *The Lancet* 1918; 191: p.826.

39 Robertson, L. Bruce, "The transfusion of whole blood", *British Medical Journal* 1916; 2: pp.38-40.

40 Moss, W.L., "A simplified version for determining the iso-agglutinin group in the selection of donors for blood transfusion", *Journal of the American Medical Association* 1917; 68: p.1905.

41 Unger, L.J., "A new method of syringe transfusion", *Journal of the American Medical Association* 1915; 64: pp.582-584.

42 Kimpton, A.R. & J.H. Brown, "A new and simple method of transfusion", *Journal of the American Medical Association* 1913; 61: pp.117-118.

43 Robertson, L.B. & C. Gordon Watson, "Further observations on the results of blood transfusion in war surgery", *British Medical Journal* 1917; 2: pp.679-683.

44 Robertson, L.B., "Blood transfusion in war surgery", *The Lancet* 1918; 191: pp.759-762.

45 Robertson, O.H., "Transfusion with preserved red blood cells", *British Medical Journal* 1918; 1: pp.691-695.

46 Guiou, N.M., "Blood transfusion in a field ambulance", *British Medical Journal* 1918; 1: pp.695-696.

47 Westhorpe, R., "The introduction of a mobile resuscitation service – 1918", in: Fink, B.R., L.E. Morris & C.R. Stephen (eds.), *The History of Anaesthesia: Third International Symposium* Illinois: Wood Library, Museum of Anesthesiology, 1992: pp.435-438.

48 McLachlan, G., "Sir Ivan Magill KCVO, DSc, MB, ChB, BAO, FRCS, FFARCS (Hon), FFARCSI (Hon), DA, (1888-1986)", *Ulster Medical Journal*, 2008; 77(3): pp.146-152.

49 Pallister, W.K., "Sir Ivan Whiteside Magill (1888-1986)", in: Atkinson, R.S. & T.B. Boulton (eds.) *The History of Anaesthesia; Proceedings of the Second International Symposium*. London: Royal Society of Medicine, 1989: pp.605-609.

50 Rowbotham, S., "Ivan Magill", *British Journal of Anaesthesia* 1951; 23(1): pp.49-55.

51 Rowbotham, E.S. & I. Magill, "Anaesthetics in the plastic surgery of the face and jaw", *Proceedings of the Royal Society of Medicine* 1921; 14: pp.19- 27.

4

Pathology during the Great War

Robin Reid

Introduction

Pathology may be defined as the study and diagnosis of disease. The word pathology is from Greek πάθος, *pathos*, "feeling, suffering"; and -λογία, *-logia* "the study of".

Although not a frontline service directly dealing with the wounded being brought into the various medical facilities, it should not be thought that "pathology", which is an encompassing term for laboratory medicine concerned with the cause and effect of disease, did not make a significant contribution to the British and Allied war effort.

Many extremely distinguished doctors worked in this area of medicine, and their contribution to the understanding of a variety of conditions which affected soldiers, both wounds and disease, will be highlighted within the relevant sections of this chapter. Some topics will be discussed in detail, and an attempt will be made to put them into perspective from nearly one hundred years later. It was only by understanding the mechanisms of damage to cells and tissues, as well as the body's response to injury and disease, that there could be the scientific development needed to understand and treat the wounds and illnesses that occurred during the Great War.

Fighting conditions experienced by the British Army during the Great War differed from those encountered in any previous conflict in which they had been involved. Since the Battle of Waterloo in 1815, a number of small colonial wars had been fought, mainly in Asia and Africa. However, only the Crimean War and the Second Boer War could be considered to be on the scale of major conflicts, although neither approached the magnitude of events between 1914 and 1918. Lessons had been learned from the Crimean War (1853-1856) and the Second Boer War (1899-1902) about the risk to troops of infectious diseases and the necessity of good hygiene (see Chapter 1). This knowledge was supplemented by observations of what occurred during the American Civil War (1861-65) and the Russo-Japanese War (1904-05). Arguably much more could, and should, have been learned from these conflicts. For example, this particularly applies to the management of abdominal wounds sustained by the Russians in the Russo-Japanese War, as will be discussed in Chapter 7.

Pathology in 1914 was at a fairly early stage of its development, both as a science and as a branch of medicine. Rudolf Virchow was a German doctor who is considered to be the father of histopathology, which is the study of disease at a cellular level. Virchow initially described the concept in 1854, and had died in 1902, just a few years before the start of the Great War.

Of particular importance for the development of surgery was the introduction of anti-septic surgery. This really started in 1867 when it was introduced by Joseph Lister, Professor of Surgery at the University of Glasgow. Anti-sepsis reduced the risk of patients developing infections after undergoing surgery although the reasons why this worked were not fully understood. The first micro-organism, a bacterium, was only identified in 1876 when Robert Koch, another leading German doctor who had studied under Virchow, demonstrated the bacteria which caused the disease anthrax. Koch was subsequently awarded the Nobel Prize for Medicine for his work in 1910. Further developments in the study and identification of bacteria led to specific ways of seeing bacteria under the microscope by staining them with special chemicals. Two keys methods of doing this were by means of the "acid fast" and Gram's stains, which were introduced in 1882 and 1884, respectively.

It is important to remember that although bacteria had now been identified as the cause of infections, antibiotics to kill them would not be available for many years to come. However, innovative doctors and scientists tried using a variety of chemicals which were administrated to patients to kill bacteria, usually without success. Notable exceptions were the developments of Atoxyl to treat sleeping sickness and Salvarsan to treat syphilis. Salvarsan was developed in 1909 by Paul Ehrlich, who was born in East Prussia (now partly Poland, partly Russia). It was the first really successful chemical treatment for syphilis, and a chemical that did not damage the patient! After being introduced into clinical practice in 1910, it became one of the most commonly prescribed drugs in the world until it was replaced by penicillin more than 30 years later. Ehrlich, too, was awarded a Nobel Prize for his contribution to medicine.

Surgical histopathology and Crown Prince Frederick of Germany

Surgical histopathology became established in the 1880s. There was one very famous example illustrating the early difficulties encountered using histopathological diagnosis. In January 1887, the Crown Prince Frederick of Germany, who was married to Victoria, the eldest daughter of Queen Victoria, became persistently hoarse, and a small lump was removed from his vocal cords. A cancer was suspected by his German doctors, and Dr Ernst von Bergmann was involved in his treatment. Originally Bergmann was from what is now Latvia and had been professor of surgery in Dorpat and Würzburg before moving to Berlin in 1882. Von Bergmann played a key role in the advance of surgery by introducing the sterilisation of surgical instruments.

He recommended to the Crown Prince that surgery was necessary to remove the affected area of the vocal cords and this would be a major undertaking. Therefore, before proceeding with the surgery, it was decided that a further opinion should be sought from Dr Morell MacKenzie, a British doctor who was regarded as "the greatest living authority on diseases of the throat". MacKenzie had studied in Paris, Vienna and Budapest where significant and rapid advances were being made in many branches of medicine, and he had acquired great experience. His practice was at the London Hospital.

Summoned to Berlin in May 1887, Mackenzie insisted that unless the growth could be proved (by taking a sample of tissue called a biopsy) to be cancer, then the radical and extensive surgery proposed should be cancelled. A biopsy was taken from the Crown Prince's larynx, and was examined by Dr Virchow, who was then Director of the Pathological Institute of Berlin. Virchow pronounced the growth to be benign, but he was incorrect in his diagnosis. It was in fact malignant, as the Crown Prince's subsequent clinical progress confirmed. The tumour gradually grew, and obstructed his airway until he was unable to breathe properly.

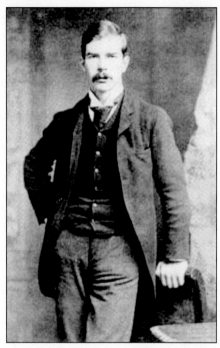

Figure 4.1   Sir Almroth Wright. (Wikimedia Commons)

It became necessary to perform a tracheotomy (making a cut in the neck directly into the trachea or windpipe) and a silver tracheotomy tube was inserted into his trachea so that he could breathe. This was of course a palliative measure, and his cancer relentlessly and, painfully, progressed, finally resulting in the death of Frederick who had by then become Emperor Frederick III of Germany, albeit only for a short-lived reign. This medical error may well have been an important contributory factor in the background to the Great War, because it alienated Frederick's son Wilhelm, who became Kaiser Wilhelm II on his father's death, and helped fuel mounting Prussian antagonism towards Britain.[1]

The study of pathology in the army

It is worth noting that the Royal Army Medical Corps was only formed in 1898; this is discussed in some detail in Chapter 1. Prior to this, in 1860, the Army Medical School had been established, although the study of bacteria – bacteriology – was only included in the curriculum in the 1890s. This delay reflects what was happening simultaneously in the general curricula that were being offered to medical students in the medical schools of the British universities at that time.[2] Under the leadership of Almroth Wright, Professor of Pathology from 1892 to 1900, the Army Medical School was established at the leading edge of research in bacteriology and hygiene.

Wright was born in 1861, and graduated from Trinity College Dublin in 1883. He was appointed Professor of Pathology at the Army Medical School, Netley in 1892 and rapidly took an interest in typhoid, and in particular the possibility of developing a bactericidal antibody directed against the bacterium which causes typhoid, salmonella typhi, by injecting heat-killed bacteria into the body as a vaccine, to stimulate the body to make antibodies against this bacterium, thus enabling it to destroy it should there be subsequent exposure. This followed the example set by Louis Pasteur to protect against the bacterium responsible for causing anthrax. Although trials were successful, his proposal to inoculate all soldiers with the vaccine who were going to be travelling to South Africa for the Second Boer War was rejected and only 4% of soldiers were protected in this way. In the three years of the war, there were 57,000 recorded cases of typhoid and this resulted in 9,000 deaths.

Further studies demonstrated the worth of inoculation against typhoid so that in the Great War every soldier was encouraged to be protected against the disease. As a result, only 20,000 cases and 1,191 deaths were seen in this much larger conflict. Wright had moved to St Mary's Hospital, London, as Professor of Pathology and Bacteriology, a position he held until 1946, the year before his death at the age of 85. After the outbreak of the Great War, he established a laboratory in the Casino at Boulogne and took particular interest in wound infections, receiving help from another famous doctor, Alexander Fleming.

Alexander Fleming was born in Darvel, Ayrshire in 1881 and studied medicine at St Mary's Hospital, London, graduating in 1906. He became assistant bacteriologist to Almroth Wright and served in the RAMC. He demonstrated that antiseptics were counter-productive in treating deep-seated anaerobic infections and he is best remembered for his work after the Great War – the serendipitous discovery of the antibiotic penicillin in 1928 which was the basis for his Nobel Prize, awarded in 1945.

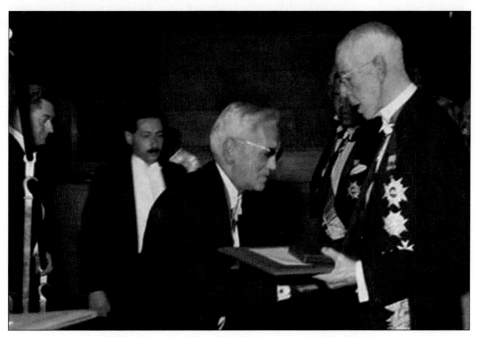

Figure 4.2   Sir Alexander Fleming receiving the Nobel
Prize for medicine. (Wikimedia Commons)

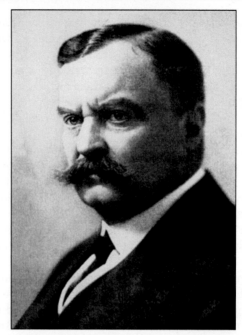

Figure 4.3   Sir David Bruce. (Wikimedia Commons)

A leading protagonist in the development of this scientific basis for medicine was David Bruce, an Australian by birth but who graduated from the University of Edinburgh in 1881. He made major contributions to the understanding of tropical diseases and was commandant of the Army Medical College during the Great War. His name lives on in the disease Brucellosis (a disease which chiefly affects cattle, but can cause undulant fever in humans) and in Trypanosoma brucei, (the cause of sleeping sickness).

Pathology during the Great War

Practical application of these disciplines in the British Army lagged behind that of the French and German armies. When speaking in 1914 Sir William Osler, a Canadian who had been Professor of Medicine at the University of Oxford since 1905, observed that in the Second Boer War, the "microbe killed more than the bullet".[3] Indeed he was correct because in that conflict, 14,048 soldiers died of disease, compared with about half that number – 7,994 – who were either killed in action or died of wounds.[4] This happened because soldiers had not been immunised against typhoid, despite the excellent work of Almroth Wright.

Pathology in the period of the Great War was a medical specialty which encompassed several different areas of laboratory medical specialties. Nowadays, doctors who focus on laboratory medicine work in their own highly specialised areas for the benefit of patients, for example, histopathology (the study of tissues removed from the body which are examined microscopically to allow a disease to be diagnosed), microbiology (the study of microorganisms such as bacteria, fungi and viruses which cause disease), biochemistry (the study of the various chemicals which are in the blood and the different body tissues) and haematology (which is the study of the cells in the blood stream and the bone marrow where they are produced). The doctors and staff working in pathology during the Great War had a broad overview of laboratory medicine, in the same way that surgeons were "general", and able to turn their hands to any procedure. Specialisation had yet to develop at that point in time.

Laboratories were involved in diverse areas, especially microbiology, which was concerned both with the identification of bacteria responsible for wound infections, (such a major problem during the Great War), as well as trying to ensure the maintenance of good (or as best as was possible) general health in soldiers. They did this through prevention and diagnosis of the normal range of infections to which large numbers of young men, who were kept in fairly close contact, would be liable to develop, for example, measles and tuberculosis. In 1914, tuberculosis was a disease responsible for killing great numbers of people, and was rightly feared. But what about measles, which today is generally regarded as of little importance, although it may have the most serious of consequences? When men of the 51st (Highland) Division, went to Bedford near London to complete their training before embarking for the Western Front, there was an outbreak of measles. There were 529 cases of measles, and 65 men died of the disease, a mortality of 10.8%, which may well be surprising to the reader. The epidemic was more deadly in the case of men from the more northern parts of Scotland, and from the Western Isles, according to the Official History of the 51st Division.[5]

There was a high prevalence of venereal (sexually transmitted) diseases, with official statistics recording a total of 416,891 cases of venereal disease in all theatres of war between 1914 and 1918.[6] From August 1914 to December 1918, there were 153,531 admissions to hospitals in France as a result of soldiers contracting sexually transmitted infections. Prevention of venereal disease was thought to be best achieved by "moral persuasion". What exactly does that mean? The official policy was to encourage men to spend their recreational hours engaged in wholesome pursuits in "places of healthy amusement" and so they would be better placed to resist "temptation". For example, skittle alleys, organised sports, libraries and gyms were provided for the men as an alternative to sexual activity. The prevention of venereal diseases was generally regarded as much a moral issue as it was a medical one. There was a variety of health guides available for the soldiers, which encouraged virtues such as "cleanliness, moderation, pure air and self control". If men were diagnosed with a venereal disease, their pay was stopped and leave was withheld for 12 months, and for the first two years of the war the patient's family were informed of the fact that their relative had a venereal disease. Furthermore, there were random checks made where men would have to lower their trousers and be inspected for signs of these diseases – in front of their superiors. This was called a "dangle parade" but will not be discussed further here!

There was extensive debate about how to reduce the increasing numbers of soldiers who were contracting venereal diseases, for example, licensing and medical checks of those who worked in brothels, putting soldiers through a chemical decontamination process after they had visited brothels or even giving each soldier six "preventive outfits" (chemicals to use on themselves with the intention of destroying the causative bacteria) when they went on leave. Furthermore, these should only be supplied to "those who deliberately set out to gratify their sexual desires".[7] There was certainly a great need to overcome prejudice and to apply the scientific basis of medicine to help in the prevention of venereal disease rather than by some of the methods that were employed!

A number of apparently newly-identified disease entities were recognised during the Great War, and their patho-physiology investigated, and as far as possible defined. The reader is referred to the *History of the Great War based on Official Documents, Medical Services, Pathology* edited by Major Sir W.G. MacPherson and others, and published in 1923.[8] Alexander Fleming, Robert Muir and Almroth Wright were amongst the contributors to this volume. Robert Muir was Professor of Pathology at the University of Glasgow, and was a Lieutenant-Colonel in charge of the pathological and bacteriological work at the 3rd and 4th Scottish General Hospitals during the Great War. Later, he went on to write a textbook of pathology, which became of such importance that it is still available in updated format in the 21st Century for the current generation of pathologists and medical students to use.

Organisation of pathology services

The experiences of the British Army in the Second Boer War, notably the significant number of deaths from enteric fevers (typhoid fever and paratyphoid fever), influenced thinking in the RAMC, especially in terms of sanitation and the supply of pure water to the troops. A recommendation was made by the Sanitary Advisory Board that all troops should receive anti-typhoid inoculations, but this was not followed by the Army Council.

In 1908 it became apparent that only six posts were available to officers qualified as specialists in microbiology, although 31 such were qualified in this field. Although the Sanitary Advisory Board recommended that all hospitals with more than 100 beds should appoint a clinical pathologist, no attempt was made to increase the number of army appointments. Unsurprisingly, the existing resources in the army for the provision of pathology services were inadequate for the scale of war which rapidly developed between 1914 and 1916, and most civilian laboratories sent the bulk of their staff to serve in the army.

In 1914, the post of Advisor in Pathology to the Director-General of Medical Services, British Forces in France, was established. The first incumbent was Sir William Leishman, a graduate of the University of Glasgow, who had previously identified the causal organism of Kala-Azar (Leishmaniasis), which is a tropical disease caused by a microscopic parasite called a protozoan, and is transmitted by the bite of sandflies.

By the outbreak of the Great War, the Royal Army Medical College had recognised the importance of providing microbiological support to the armed forces at home and abroad, particularly in tropical areas of the Empire, through junior and senior courses in pathology. On completion of the latter three-month course, officers might choose a further three-month course covering all areas of microbiology, resulting in registration as a specialist in microbiology. Only around 50 men worked in the laboratories at home and abroad, with a smaller number held in the reserve.

Although large numbers of casualties with serious wound infections, including tetanus and gas gangrene, were noted in the initial phases of the war where there was a great mobility of troops, it was impossible to develop proper microbiology services at this stage. As trench warfare became established, and the movement of troops and their units reduced, it became possible to set up laboratories in relationship to the medical facilities. These were mobile laboratories, the first being a bacteriology laboratory which reached France in October 1914. This was followed by a hygiene laboratory the following month,

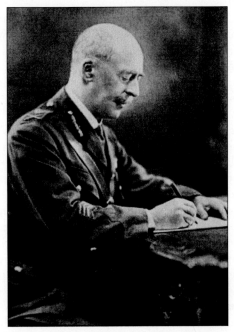

Figure 4.4   William Leishman. (Wikimedia Commons)

and by 1915, each army was allocated two bacteriology laboratories, and one hygiene facility. Static hospital laboratories were established, initially at No. 2 and No. 4 General Hospitals at Le Havre and Versailles, respectively. Eventually, three types of laboratory were established.

Mobile bacteriology units

These were truly mobile and could support the forward area, particularly the casualty clearing stations. This mobile capacity was of great value during the retreat during the German Spring Offensives of 1918, and Allied advances in the autumn offensives during the final one hundred days of the war (see Chapter 1). Mobile units were equipped to a level which would allow them to function autonomously. They carried autoclaves (machines using steam under pressure for sterilising surgical instruments), incubators (for growing bacteria on special plates and allowing their identification) and centrifuges. Twenty-five such laboratories were supplied, and eighteen were allocated to the Western Front, seven being divided between Salonika, Egypt and East Africa. Their work lay largely in the routine diagnosis of patients with suspected enteric fevers (typhoid and para-typhoid fevers), dysentery, diphtheria and meningitis. Sputum and urine examination and blood counts were carried out, and autopsies (post-mortem examinations) were also required.

The requirement for microbiology services related to wounds clearly varied depending on how busy the casualty clearing stations were, being obviously much greater during periods of heavy fighting.

Post-mortem studies were of great importance in helping to understand the effects brought about by different wounds and how these resulted in the death of a soldier. This is well illustrated in Chapter 7, which deals with abdominal wounds, and will be fully explained in that part of the book. Post-mortem studies performed on soldiers dying from abdominal wounds revealed that haemorrhage (bleeding) was the main cause of death, usually occurring soon after the wound had been inflicted. In contrast, infection caused deaths a few days after the wound had been sustained. This new knowledge impacted on treatment, leading directly to early operative intervention in these patients, with considerable improvement in prognosis.

Hospital laboratories

These were key parts of all general hospitals of 520 beds and over, and each had a single microbiologist. The duties of this laboratory were similar to those of the mobile unit, but the balance shifted towards the management of soldiers with severe wound infections. While it was suggested that economies of scale might be achieved by concentrating services in large general hospital bases, the benefits of close liaison amongst the patient, the responsible clinician and the microbiologist were considered to mitigate against such centralisation. However, a central mortuary and autopsy facility was established at Étaples. It is interesting to note that there are similar debates regarding centralisation of services in many areas within the National Health Service at the present time.

Research Laboratories

No thought had been given initially to the provision of central research laboratories, which could be freed from the burden of day-to-day routine analyses of samples so that they might advance understanding and help in the development of new treatments. Colonel Sir Almroth Wright in effect established the first research laboratory at No 13 General Hospital, which was located in Boulogne. Assisted by colleagues from St Mary's Hospital London, including Alexander Fleming, he made significant contributions, for example to wound healing and to the understanding of gas gangrene. Wright's major contribution to the understanding of shock has already been discussed at length in Chapter 3. This clearly illustrates the great importance of research laboratories in helping to understand the causes of clinical problems and by so doing, helping to find solutions and improve treatment.

Whilst this was happening, hospitals in the UK required pathological expertise to cope with the needs of men undergoing military training and the increasing flow of men who had been wounded and were returning home to the UK. General military hospitals were often established in, or close to, existing civilian hospitals and medical schools, and utilised their laboratories services. Staff members from civilian hospitals were often commissioned into the RAMC or the Territorials.

The microbiology and pathology of wounds

The principles of wound healing, effectively the production of granulation tissue (discussed in chapters 2 and 6), fracture callus (the body's healing process for fractured bones) and epithelial regeneration (healing of skin), were already known before the outbreak of the war, and no major advances in these areas were made. From a pathological standpoint, wounds were classified by pathologists during the Great War as falling into one of four categories

- Wounds where tissue had been avulsed, and carried away, for example the ripping away of an arm or leg, usually by a large irregular metal fragment of exploding shell casing,
- Perforating and fracturing wounds, where a projectile had struck bone and fragmented it, these fragments either leaving through an exit wound or if not, forming irregular cavities within the tissues (see Chapter 6 for the example of compound fracture of the femur),
- Sutured amputation wounds, with collection of pus deep to the flaps of skin which had been stitched back together,
- Implunging wounds caused by nearly spent pieces of shrapnel ball, bullet or shell casing having enough residual energy to penetrate the skin.

Regardless of this classification, and in contrast to the experience of surgeons dealing with the wounded in the Second Boer War of 1899 to 1902 which had been fought on the hot dry battlefields of South Africa, it became clear early in the war fought on the arable soil of the Western Front, that almost every type of wound sustained in the manured fields of France and Flanders could became infected.

Bacteriology and Pathology of Specific Wound Infections
Streptococcal infections
Infections with the bacteria streptococcus were very common and led to diffuse infection and inflammation of the tissues called cellulitis. This is a rapidly spreading infection through the skin and subcutaneous tissue adjacent to the site of a penetrating wound. The skin of the entire limb may become red, indurated, and feel very hot to the touch. The infection may spread to the lymph nodes, and to the bloodstream (septicaemia) with fatal consequences.

The poet Rupert Brooke sailed with the British Mediterranean Expeditionary Force on 28 February 1915, but developed septicaemia from an infected mosquito bite. He died on 23 April 1915 in a French hospital ship moored in a bay off the island of Skyros in the Aegean on his way to Gallipoli. He lies buried "in some corner of a foreign field that is forever England". There were no antibiotics in 1915 but had there been, Brooke and many others who developed septicaemia may well have survived.

Gas Gangrene
There were numerous cases of gas gangrene, an infection characterised by spreading necrosis (death) of tissue with the production of gas. Gas gangrene was seen frequently in the early months of the war, and indeed occurred in around 10% of the wounded. It presented with two distinct clinical patterns. The first pattern was seen when the infection spread in the subcutaneous plane (under the skin) with the formation of gas and fluid-filled bullae (loose, baggy, fluid filled blisters in the skin). The second pattern of presentation involved deep infection within skeletal muscle, the limb becoming cold and hard and death following invariably, unless the limb was amputated immediately with complete removal of all involved tissue. The buttocks, calves and hamstrings were particularly common sites for gangrene, the trunk being seldom affected. The surgical prevention of gas gangrene, and its treatment once established, is discussed in detail in Chapters 2 and 6.

The pathology of gas gangrene was investigated urgently as this was a major clinical problem.[9] Impairment of the blood supply to muscle resulted in a deficiency or absence of oxygen in the tissues, which was an ideal milieu for the growth of bacteria, which only thrive in the absence of oxygen (anaerobic bacteria). These bacteria produced toxins which in turn caused further muscle damage culminating in the death of muscle. The tissues affected rapidly became very oedematous with the accumulation of fluid within them, later to be followed by the death (coagulative necrosis) of the muscle fibres.

Coagulative necrosis is a term used to describe death of cells which has been caused by loss of their blood supply. It is characterised by a "ghostly" appearance of the cells under the microscope, and reflects death of the cells due to absence of oxygen. In time, the bacteria invade and grow within these necrotic fibres. Culture of many of these anaerobic organisms outside the body (in vitro) was difficult, although not for Clostridium welchii, one of the principal organisms responsible for gas gangrene. Consequently, laboratory diagnosis was carried out by inoculation of an emulsion of necrotic muscle and oedema fluid into animals previously treated with specific anti-toxins. The clinical state of the animal and histological examination of its tissues gave information as to the likely causative bacterium of the infection.

A move to early surgery with radical wound excision led to a dramatic reduction of these overwhelming and lethal infections, so that only 1% of wounded developed this complication by 1918. Also, by 1918 an anti-toxin against Clostridium perfringens (another bacterium causing gas gangrene) was used, but with limited success. It became clear that this was at best an aid to surgical therapy, and not a substitute for it.

Almost 100 years later, gas gangrene remains a problem in civilian and military medicine to this day.[10]

Tetanus

Significant advances were made in the understanding of the pathology of tetanus. Like the organisms responsible for gas gangrene, the bacteria causing tetanus are anaerobic. There was a problem growing and identifying these bacteria in the laboratory, given that they only grew in the absence of oxygen. Anaerobic culture was made simpler however, by the finding that oxygen need not be excluded if fragments of meat were added to the culture medium, forming a "meat broth". Several subtypes of Clostridium tetani were identified, but all appeared to produce the same toxin, which could be neutralised by the same anti-toxin. It became clear that Clostridium tetani could be isolated from many wounds in patients who did not suffer from tetanus, and that the disease might follow many months after the wound had been sustained due to germination of spores. Spores are produced as part of the bacterium's life cycle where it can exist and survive in an almost inert state for long periods of time before it begins to grow and multiply. This resurgence in activity, growth and multiplication of the bacterium can be provoked by further tissue damage, be it mechanical, chemical or due to co-infection, especially with other anaerobic bacteria. As has already been discussed in Chapter 2 this explains why many cases of tetanus occurred long after the casualties returned to the UK.

Most importantly, routine administration of tetanus antitoxin (serum from an animal infected with the disease, and therefore by anti-tetanus toxin antibodies) to the wounded resulted in a great reduction in the incidence of tetanus, to approximately one-sixth of that seen early in the war. In addition, the mortality of those who developed the disease despite prophylaxis was greatly reduced.

Other important pathological conditions seen during the Great War

A number of clinical entities were "discovered" during the Great War, and some of the more important ones are discussed in the following paragraphs. While these examples go into detailed histopathology, of principal interest to the specialist pathologist, it should be appreciated that pathology research laboratories responded vigorously to these new entities, and did so "despite there being a war on" in order to help the war effort by understanding disease and helping to point the way towards finding solutions to problems.

Trench Fever and the the Body Louse

In the spring of 1915 in Flanders, the first patients affected by this disease were described by Graham[11] with a more complete clinical account by Hunt and Rankin following shortly thereafter.[12] The term was coined by soldiers themselves and although it was not confined to those serving in the trenches, that is where it first appeared. Clinically, the soldiers with the disease were characterised by a fever lasting 5 to 7 days, often followed by a single short relapse after which the soldier was fit to return to duty. Subsequently, some patients were noted to suffer from a shorter period of fever but with more frequent and severe relapses that resulted in a longer period of incapacity.[13] In addition, those affected complained of headaches, skin rashes, experienced pain in their bones and there was often enlargement of the spleen (splenomegaly). There were no deaths from this condition and therefore no autopsies were carried out, other than in those who had been affected by the disease but were dying of other causes, usually severe wounds. The disease occurred widely within France, affecting French and German soldiers and referred to as "fièvre des tranchées" and "febris Wolhynica" and appears to have been transferred to the Salonika Front in the autumn of 1915. Overall, almost one million soldiers appear to have been affected during the war.

From the outset an infective cause was considered likely, perhaps related to enteric fevers. Standard bacteriological techniques were employed, to try and track down the causative organism. These tests included culture agglutination techniques, which were negative, and initial haematological examinations showed only leucocytosis (an increase in the number of white blood cells to combat infection). In 1916 His and colleagues described dumb-bell shaped bodies some 1-2 microns in length lying free or within the red blood cells, especially during episodes when the patient had a fever. These dumb-bell shaped bodies resembled similar bodies described in Rocky Mountain Spotted Fever and in Typhus Fever.

An important pathologist who was keen to understand and learn more about disease was John McNee, who was born near Glasgow in 1887. He graduated from Glasgow University in 1909 and as Major McNee of the RAMC, served as assistant advisor in pathology to the 1st Army before later returning to Glasgow as Professor of Practice of Medicine. Experimental pathology was carried out by McNee and his colleagues initially by inoculation of experimental animals, but, as it became clear that there was no threat to life attempts were then made to transmit the disease to volunteers, which were successful.[14] Transfer of whole blood from patients to volunteers by the intravenous or subcutaneous route resulted in the development of the disease.

The mechanism of transmission in the trenches was explored further by Hunt and McNee, and as the disease continued during the winter of 1915-16, flies were exculpated.

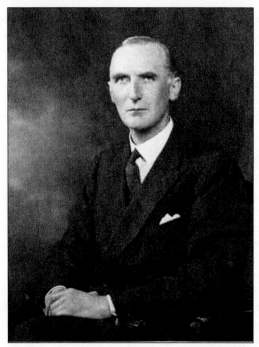

Figure 4.5   Sir John McNee. (With permission of the University
of Glasgow Archive Services GB0248 UP1/357/1)

Circumstantial evidence suggested the body louse, pediculus corporis, was the vector
and this was confirmed by a series of British and American experiments during 1917 and
1918. Additionally, the microscopic bodies described on blood films were demonstrated
within the faeces of lice by Topfer in 1916.

Subsequently, the infective agent was identified as Rickettsia Quintana (so called
because of the periodicity of the fever of 5 days), and now reclassified as Bartonella
Quintana. It may be of interest to note that "urban trench fever" is found in the homeless
in the present time[15] and, perhaps, more so to those interested in military history of the
Napoleonic Wars, within La Grande Armée.[16] The common factor, of course, linking
the trenches of France and Flanders with the homeless of today, is the body louse. The
histological features include perivascular lymphocytic infiltrates, and granulomatous
inflammation within lymph nodes, akin to those seen in cat-scratch fever.[17]

A standard pastime of troops in the trenches was to rid themselves of lice whenever
they could. Lice were frequently referred to as "chats" and men would gather in groups to
de-louse themselves (ie 'to chat'). One favoured method of eradicating lice was to quickly
run a lit candle along the seams of clothing, where lice would typically converge.

Trench Nephritis
This disease first appeared in early 1915, especially affecting troops in the trenches[18], and
reaching a maximum of 100 per 100,000 troops in December 1916. It was noted that
officers were seldom affected and cases in civilians in areas of high prevalence were not
identified. German, Austrian and then French soldiers were also subject to this disorder,

which was not seen in the trenches of Gallipoli. It was the most important renal (kidney) disorder of the war and accounted for 5% of medical admissions.

Previously healthy soldiers rapidly became unwell with proteinuria (the presence of protein in the urine, and indicative of kidney damage), facial oedema (swelling of the face), often fever and dyspnoea (breathlessness), headache and sore throat. Examination of the urine confirmed the proteinuria and also revealed haematuria (blood in urine) and the presence of urinary casts. Urinary casts are cylindrical structures produced by the kidney and are present in the urine in certain disease states.

While most patients recovered rapidly some developed recurrences and progressed to subacute nephritis and a significant number died; many of those who died were subjected to post-mortem examination. Dunn and McNee described the renal lesions in 35 fatal cases, all dying within 2 weeks of onset.[19] Unsurprisingly, the main abnormality was glomerular.

A glomerulus is a capillary tuft that performs the first step in filtering blood to form urine. The glomeruli were enlarged and hypercellular, with enlargement and proliferation of endothelial cells with fibrin thrombi. There was a mild infiltration of polymorphonuclear leucocytes and lymphocytes. Crescents were seldom seen in the acute phase. The initiating event in all glomerular crescents is the development of a physical gap, or hole, in the glomerular capillary wall. The presence of crescents in glomeruli is a histologic marker of severe injury. The appearances were therefore those of an acute glomerulonephritis, or active inflammation of the glomeruli. Secondary changes were found in the lungs with oedema, and formation of diffuse alveolar damage (damage to the air sacs in the lung), and a non-specific response to damage to the alveolar walls. The appearances, for example, were noted to be similar to those seen in chlorine gas inhalation. Unfortunately of course, pathologists had an opportunity to study the effects of exposure to chlorine gas, which was first employed by the Germans on the Western Front on 22 April 1915, during the Second Battle of Ypres.

In later stages, glomerular sclerosis with crescent formation was seen, with secondary changes of atrophy and dilatation of the renal tubules and fibrosis and lymphocytic infiltration of the interstitium. While these histological details will really only be of interest to pathologists, they serve to illustrate that research laboratories were able to devote time to understanding the behaviour of a "new disease", and could do so while there were enormous clinical pressures being exerted elsewhere in the service.

It was very important to have surgeons and anaesthetists working on the never-ending numbers of wounded. It was equally important to have pathologists working in the relatively protected environment of research laboratories, trying to help resolve new clinical problems as they cropped up.

Unfortunately, as often happens in medicine, the aetiology of trench nephritis has never been established with conviction, although a post-infective cause seems most likely.[20] Interestingly, a similar form of nephritis appears to have affected soldiers in the American Civil War.

Leptospirosis (Weil's disease)

Two outbreaks of fever and jaundice which occurred during the Great War were shown to be due to infection by the spirochaete, Leptospira icterohaemorrhagica (a particular type of bacterium). Although sporadic cases occurred in 1915 and later in the war, the first main epidemic occurred near Ypres in the summer of 1916, and the other in the British Army in Italy. In Japan in 1916 it became clear that the spirochaete was responsible and that the common rat was the animal host, the organism being excreted in the urine. From an accidental laboratory transmission, the incubation period was shown to be 6 to 8 days, and the clinical features were of fever, malaise, myalgia (muscle pain), conjunctivitis and headache, followed by jaundice.

In the Flanders outbreak, fewer than 10% of patients who were infected died. In those, autopsy showed severe jaundice, haemorrhage within viscera (abdominal organs) and serous membranes and consistent changes within the kidneys of acute tubular necrosis (reflecting acute kidney failure) and acute interstitial nephritis, an inflammation of the kidney. The liver changes were variable, in some there being marked centrilobular necrosis which is a particular pattern of cell death, with lack of cohesion of the liver cells and white blood cell infiltration, while in others there was little abnormal.

Again, while the detailed histopathology may only be of interest to medical readers, the wider issue here is that a potentially fatal cause of infective jaundice was identified and analysed by laboratory studies. As a result of this important research, Captain Philip Gosse was appointed to the post of "Rat Officer" to the British 2nd Army, with a remit to draw up schemes for the catching and destruction of rats. Schools of sanitation ran "rat classes", and there were "rat lectures", all designed to help rid the trenches of the vermin, thus reducing the probability of contracting a potentially fatal disease.

Blood transfusion

Although Landsteiner described what became known as the ABO blood groups and their incompatibilities in 1900, in general, blood transfusion was seldom used in civilian practice before 1914. Its major impact came in the last two years of the war, and the contribution of two military doctors, one Canadian and one American, was very significant.[21]

The first, Lawrence Bruce Robertson, a surgeon who served in the Canadian Corps of the British 3rd Army from 1915 to 1917, described blood transfusion of non-crossmatched blood directly from donor to recipient, albeit by a syringe–cannula technique rather than direct artery to vein contact.[22] Although death could occur as a result of acute haemolysis where the red blood cells were broken down, the effects were strikingly beneficial to those who did not have a transfusion reaction. The limitations of direct transfusion in a war zone are obvious, and his namesake, the American Oswald Hope Robertson, introduced the use of previously stored citrated (to prevent clotting) blood during the Battle of Cambrai in 1917.[23] Initially, only Group O blood was used (at that time classified as Group 4) and was given in a casualty clearing station. Of the 20 transfused patients, all of whom were expected to die, 11 survived. By 1918, transfusions were administered closer to the front than casualty clearing stations, including in a field ambulance.[24]

Spanish Influenza

It is often correctly stated that more people died in the influenza pandemic of 1918 to1919 than in the Great War itself. Estimates of the number of deaths that occurred worldwide vary at between 50 and 100 million. It was called Spanish 'Flu because Spain was a non-belligerent nation, and being a neutral country, had no reason to exert censorship on the truth by concealing the numbers of its citizens who had succumbed to the disease. It was no more common in Spain than elsewhere. Nor did it have its origin in Spain. Indeed, the pandemic probably had its origin in the conflict, possibly at the British military base at Étaples, where 100,000 men mixed with pigs, ducks and geese may have been the source.[25] There was little doubt at the time that the sporadic cases of purulent bronchitis and bronchopneumonia described in the winters of 1916 to 1918 reflected the same process as some aspects of the influenza pandemic.

Hammond and colleagues described a series of fatal cases of purulent bronchitis in February and early March 1917, this accounting for 71 out of 156 consecutive autopsies.[26] The changes were most marked in the smaller bronchi which were filled with pus, and whose epithelium, initially intact, was shed and replaced by inflamed granulation tissue. In some, but not all patients, the inflammatory process had spread to adjacent lung parenchyma giving bronchopneumonia. The influenza bacillus (Haemophilus influenzae) could be identified on gram-staining, but this of course was not the primary causative agent. Similar findings were reported from Aldershot, from Canadian troops at Boulogne and from American recruits in camps in Texas and Iowa in the winter of 1917 to 1918. Notably, an infiltrate of mononuclear cells, especially small lymphocytes, occurred within the bronchial wall. In time, it was shown by Abrahams and colleagues, who had reported the Aldershot cases, that the changes of purulent bronchitis were identical to the post-mortem findings in fatal cases of influenza.[27]

These contemporary descriptions of the pathological findings of influenza are only a small part of the story. They are a description of post-mortem findings of patients who died as a result of bacterial infections of the bronchi and lungs, which were secondary phenomena, and were complications of the primary viral illness. The viral cause was not isolated until 1933.

There were two waves in the 1918 Spanish Influenza pandemic, the first in the spring, and the second in the autumn. This in itself is unusual, most influenza outbreaks occurring in the winter months. The spring outbreak followed the expected course, causing complications in the very young, immunologically immature, and in the very old, immunologically compromised. Secondary purulent bronchitis and broncho-pneumonia were responsible for deaths in these two groups, and the contemporary pathological descriptions outlined above apply to victims of this wave. Young, fit individuals usually dealt with the disease without difficulty.

The second autumn wave was much deadlier, the virus having mutated to a lethal form. This time, it behaved in a very different way, affecting particularly strong, fit , young individuals causing a significant mortality in that young adult group. It also killed them very quickly, with descriptions of soldiers being well one day, and dying the next, drowning in their own secretions. It may well have represented a strong immune response to the virus, the very strength and vigour of the response ironically causing release of inflammatory mediators in what may be described as a "cytokine storm" resulting in pulmonary oedema and death. Post-mortem studies revealed a "wet lung" sometimes with haemorrhagic appearances. This may be described as an adult respiratory distress syndrome described elsewhere in this book.

The spread of this deadly mutant was assisted by the circumstances of the war. In civilian life, those who get very sick stay at home, isolating themselves. During the Great War, those who became very sick were sent on crowded trains to even more crowded general hospitals, concentrating the deadlier virus in these locations, and thus facilitating its spread amongst the troops, and carried to all parts of the world from that dense reservoir of deadly virus.

It is particularly ironic, given the terrible wounds inflicted by high explosive shells and bullets, in what was an appalling illustration of the destructive effects of industrial warfare, that it should be a disease that carried off more people worldwide than all the ordnance that belligerent nations could hurl at each other.

Conclusion

In conclusion, pathology services during the Great War made a very important contribution to the war effort. They did so firstly in the day-to-day service provided by mobile and hospital laboratories. Of particular importance, an understanding of the pathology of abdominal wounding led to improved management of these patients, with better chances of survival. Secondly, pathology research laboratory facilities gave brilliant scientific minds an opportunity to develop new ideas, and make original contributions to the clinical problems encountered during four years of conflict. Young Alexander Fleming, working in Colonel Sir Almroth Wright's research unit at No13 General Hospital in Boulogne, would go on in later years to make a major impact on management of wounds in the Second World War. He would discover penicillin.

Notes

1   McInnis, W.D., W. Egan & J.B. Oust. "The management of carcinoma of the larynx in a prominent patient, or did Morell Mackenzie really cause World War I?", *American Journal of Surgery* 1976; 132: pp.515-22.

2   Atenstaedt, R.L., "The development of bacteriology, sanitation science and allied research in the British Army 1850-1918: equipping the RAMC for War", *Journal of the Royal Army Medical Corps*, 2010; 156: pp.154-8.

3   Cushing, H., *The Life of Sir William Osler* Volume 2. Oxford: Oxford University Press, 1925, pp.427-428.

4   Mitchell, T.J. & G.M. Smith, *History of the Great War based on Official Documents. Medical Services. Casualties and Medical Statistics.* London: HMSO, 1931, p.270.

5   Bewsher, F.W., *The History of the 51st (Highland) Division.* Edinburgh: Blackwood, 1921, pp.4-5.

6   Mitchell & Smith, *op.cit,* p.74.

7   *Ibid,* p.78.

8   MacPherson, W.G., S.L. Cummins & W.B. Leishman (eds.), *History of the Great War based on Official Documents. Medical Services. Pathology.* London: HMSO, 1923.

9   McNee, J.W. & J.S. Dunn, "The method of spread of gas gangrene into living muscle", *British Medical Journal* 1917; 1: pp.727–729.

10 Titball, R.W., "Gas gangrene: an open and closed case", *Microbiology* 2005; 151: pp.2821–2828.

11 Graham, J.H.P., "A note on a relapsing febrile illness of unknown origin", *The Lancet* 1915; ii: pp.703-4.

12 Hunt, G.H. & A.C. Rankin, "Intermittent fever of obscure origin occurring among British soldiers in France. The so-called "trench fever"", *The Lancet* 1915; ii: pp.1133-6.

13 McNee, J.W., A. Renshaw & E.H. Brunt, "Trench Fever", *British Medical Journal* 1916; 1: pp.225-234.

14 *Ibid.*

15 Foucault, C., K. Barrau, P. Brouqui & D. Raoult, "Bartonella quintana bacteraemia among homeless people", *Clinical Infectious Diseases* 2002; 35: pp.684-9.

16 Raoult, D., O. Dutour, L. Houhamdi, R. Jankauskas, P.E. Fournier, Y. Ardagna et al. "Evidence for louse-transmitted diseases in soldiers of Napoleon's Grand Army in Vilnius", *Journal of Infectious Diseases* 2006; 193: pp.112-20.

17 Maurin, M. & D. Raoult, "Bartonella (Rochalimaea) quintana infections", *Clinical Microbiology Reviews* 1996; 9: pp.273-92.

18 Raw, N., "Trench nephritis. A record of five cases", *British Medical Journal* 1915 ; 2: p.468.

19 Dunn, J.S. & J.W. McNee, "A contribution to the study of war nephritis", *British Medical Journal* 1917; 2: pp.745-51.

20 Atenstaedt, R.L., "The medical response to trench nephritis in World War One", *Kidney International* 2006; 70: pp.635–640.

21 Stansbury, L.G. & J.R. Hess, "Blood Transfusion in World War I: The Roles of Lawrence Bruce Robertson and Oswald Hope Robertson in the 'Most Important Medical Advance of the War'", *Transfusion Medicine Reviews* 2009; 23: pp.232-236.

22 Robertson, L.B., "The transfusion of whole blood. A suggestion for its more frequent employment in war surgery", *British Medical Journal* 1916; 2: pp.38-40.

23 Robertson, O.H., "Transfusion with preserved red blood cells", *British Medical Journal* 1918; 1: pp.691-695.

24 Guiou, N.M., "Blood transfusion in a field ambulance", *British Medical Journal* 1918; 1: pp.695-696.

25 Oxford, J.S., R. Lambkin, A. Sefton A., "A hypothesis: the conjunction of soldiers, gas, pigs, ducks, geese and horses in Northern France during the Great War provided the conditions for the emergence of the "Spanish" Influenza pandemic of 1918-1919", *Vaccine* 2005; 23: pp.940–945.

26 Hammond, J.A.R., W. Rolland & T.H.G. Shore, "Purulent Bronchitis: a Study of Cases Occurring amongst the British Troops at a Base in France", *The Lancet* 1917; 2: pp.41–45.

27 Abrahams, A., N. Hallows & H. French, "A further investigation into Influenza Pneumococcal and Influenza Streptococcal Septicaemia: Epidemic Influenza Pneumonia of highly fatal type and its relation to Purulent Bronchitis", *The Lancet* 1919; 1: pp.1–9.

5

X-Rays during the Great War

Alexander MacDonald

Introduction

Having an X-ray taken in the present day is a common experience for many patients throughout the world, for a variety of reasons. After a short, or indeed perhaps long, wait in a warm waiting area, the patient is taken into the X-ray room and positioned so that the affected part of their body which is to be X-rayed is placed comfortably between a large and heavy X-ray tube, and an X-ray film inside a cassette (similar to a standard photographic film), or perhaps nowadays a digital system. There is a small opening in the metal tube casing of the X-ray machine, which is narrowed right down so that almost the entire X-ray beam is delivered accurately to the patient's affected part.

When the radiographer, who is the person trained to take the X-ray, has sought protection by moving behind a protective lead glass window to avoid being exposed to radiation, the X-ray is taken. The kilo-voltage, which determines the penetrative quality of the energy of the X-ray beam, is adjusted along with the milli-amperage, which is the quantity of energy to be delivered in this beam. When the radiographer presses the button to take the X-ray, the energised tube sends X-rays through the selected part of the patient for a mere fraction of a second and the image is recorded on film or digitally. Finally, the exposed film is processed through a machine which produces a final image in just a few minutes. In the years 1914-1918 during the Great War it was all very different.

The discovery of X-rays

When Professor Wilhelm Conrad Roentgen discovered X-rays in 1895, he was studying a Crookes tube.[1] This was a bulbous glass cylinder from which the air had been evacuated using a strong vacuum pump, and into which had been fused two wires, one at each end so as to investigate what happened when a high voltage was generated between the two wires.

One wire, called the cathode, was connected to the negative pole of a battery, and the other, the anode, to the positive pole. Like some of his contemporaries, he was studying "rays" that were being emitted from the cathode when a high voltage was applied between the wires. These cathode rays were later discovered to be electrons. Roentgen's genius was to recognise that very odd rays were actually being emitted from the opposite, anode end of the tube. These rays were of such penetrating quality that they blackened a chemically treated plate (coated with barium platinocyanide) on his bench, even when a thick sheet of cardboard was interposed between the device and the plate. He called these X-rays, for want of a better term, and his first piece of research on these newly discovered rays was to determine what different materials they were able to penetrate. He even involved his wife in his research. When he put her hand between the tube and the plate, he could distinguish the bones from the soft tissues in her hand, which immediately suggested to

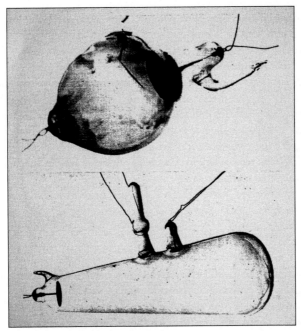

Figure 5.1   Top – original Crookes Tube; bottom – pear-shaped tube used
by Professor Roentgen. (From E.H. Burrows, *Pioneers and Early Years: A
History of British Radiology.* St Anne, Alderney, Channel Islands: Colophon,
1986, appears courtesy of the British Institute of Radiology)

him the remarkable medical potential of his discovery. Within a matter of weeks, he had
determined most of the basic properties of this astounding new form of electro-magnetic
energy. He disseminated his findings throughout the scientific world, by sending a copy
of his first research paper, "On a New Kind of Rays" in December 1895 to friends and
colleagues whom he knew to be working in the same field, and were working, in the
main, in Europe and North America. He was awarded the first Nobel Prize for Physics
in 1901 because of this most important work in discovering X-rays.

Early development

Roentgen's new discovery was immediately embraced by some members of the medical
and scientific communities, who began to set up "Electrical" departments. One of these
was Dr James Mackenzie Davidson, from Aberdeen, about whom much will be said later.[2]
Within the first decade of worldwide research on X-rays following their discovery, the
fundamental principles of radiography (the process of taking X-rays) and radiology (the
interpretation of the images obtained) were established. One of Mackenzie Davidson's
seminal contributions to radiography and radiology was to devise a technique for the
localisation of foreign, metallic material which was lying deep within the human body.

This technique was used extensively in a variety of different ways during the Great
War, given that so many wounds were caused by penetrating fragments of shrapnel, shell
casing, or bullet. Mackenzie Davidson's technique was only superseded when specialised
scans such as CT and MRI scans were introduced within the last 30 years and which

allow very high quality, high definition images to be taken in different planes and taking "cuts" through the body at different levels.

After their discovery, what we now know as X-rays were called roentgen rays by everyone except Roentgen himself. However in 1915, such was the antipathy in the UK to all things German that the term X-ray was substituted permanently and has been used in the UK ever since. It was the same antipathy that led King George V to change his family name from Saxe-Coburg and Gotha to the House of Windsor in 1917!

The original Crookes tube was subsequently adapted for X-ray emission only, modified to produce more X-ray energy. Some limited success was achieved in directing the emission of X-rays to a particular area of interest, which in this early primitive equipment was scattered in many different directions.

At the outbreak of the Great War, an X-ray machine was still very recognisable as a vacuum Crookes tube!

Dangers of X-rays

Roentgen himself had recognised that, since the X-rays were emitted in all directions, not only was this inefficient, but everybody and everything in the vicinity was being irradiated. Dangers associated with this widespread and uncontrolled spread of X-rays were not fully understood at this time nor even for some years subsequently. Roentgen died as a result of cancer of the intestine although it was unlikely that this was related to radiation exposure. His assistant, however, eventually did die as a direct consequence of over-exposure to radiation. Some effort at protection was made, but not all workers took the risk of exposure to X-rays seriously, protection was varied in terms of quality and efficacy, and was completely unregulated.

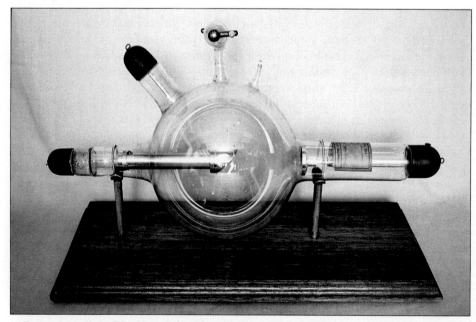

Figure 5.2   Great War X-ray tube. The cathode, now a small dish, is on the right, and the anode, now angled, is close to it on the left. (Courtesy of the Museum of Technology, London)

After a few years, the health of many early workers suffered. The hands of these individuals were particularly affected as they were exposed whilst the affected part of a patient was manipulated under a beam of X-rays to obtain the best possible image. This was especially so in casualty clearing stations and base hospitals during the Great War. The need to provide a useful image for surgeons to understand as much as possible about the wound the casualty had sustained, overrode any protective measures for patient and worker.

The deaths of some of those who used X-rays in the early years following their discovery and initial applications to clinical practice is commemorated on a memorial stone to 'X-Ray Martyrs' which was erected in 1936 in St. George's Hospital, Hamburg. A few of those with radiation damage to their hands (causing ulceration, deformities and cancers) from exposure to X-rays which had been taken during the Great War were still working in the National Health Service in the United Kingdom until the late 1950s.[3] The respected doyen of French radiology at that time, Dr. Ledoux-Lebard, estimated that by 1920, over 100 people who had worked with X-rays had lost their lives due to radiation.[4]

X-rays in warfare

The first reported use of X-rays during warfare was in the Abyssinian War of 1896, when an Italian doctor was able to show fractures and retained bullets in two soldiers who had been wounded. This was only a few months after Roentgen's discovery and illustrated how quickly it was introduced into clinical practice, albeit it in an early form.[5] The first use of X-rays by the British was recorded in subsequent hostilities in the Greco-Turkish War of 1897. This was also called the Thirty Day War and took place against a background of growing concern by Greece over conditions of the Greek Christian majority who were living in Crete under Turkish domination. Relationships between Christians and their Muslim rulers had been deteriorating steadily. This was a conflict between the Kingdom of Greece and the Ottoman Empire. Germany and Great Britain took sides and Germany sent a German Red Cross X-ray apparatus and accompanying physician to Constantinople to support the Turks. While the British Red Cross were reluctant to help, British pioneers, including Francis Charles Abbott, a surgeon from St Thomas's Hospital in London, who was in charge of the medical team, voluntarily travelled to Greece and established the advanced basic military hospitals that were to provide the earliest facilities with military radiology.[6] The British team had their X-ray machine located in Athens.

Experience was also gained in the Tirah Campaign of 1897, which was a conflict located on the North-West Frontier of India between India and Afghanistan, the War in the Sudan in 1898, the Spanish-American War, and, importantly, in the Boer War between 1899 and 1902.

X-rays during the Great War

The advantages of X-rays to the surgeon managing patients who had been subjected to trauma were obvious. This undoubtedly accelerated any improvements in X-ray equipment, but the fragile X-ray tube remained an overriding and ongoing problem, so that, despite better generators, multiple batteries and improved transformers to provide electrical power, the tubes could easily be overloaded and overheated. They could only be used for an hour or so at a time. This was clearly inadequate when there was a sudden increase in the numbers of wounded following a major battle. The answer was to have two or three tubes per medical unit, if they were available, so that they could be rested in rotation – unlike the technicians who were working the equipment!

Meanwhile, there was a major advance in tube technology, namely the Coolidge heated cathode tube, invented by William Coolidge in 1913 and manufactured in the USA.[7] This produced much more X-ray energy. Its development was made possible by other innovations, including the use of tungsten (which increases the intensity of the X-rays and previously was thought to be unworkable), and other harder metals in the manufacture of the anode and cathode. A form of intrinsic cooling was also introduced. A limited supply of Coolidge tubes, unfortunately, did not become available to the British Army until sometime after the USA had entered the war in April 1917. Some of the old Crookes' type tubes were still being used into the 1920s.

Another practical improvement was the introduction of cellulose-based film to replace the fragile and cumbersome glass plates. Interestingly, the glass that was used originally came only from Belgium and Germany, not an ideal source in the circumstances which prevailed between the years 1914 and 1918!

For the first two to three years of the war, while ancillary developments improved the quality of the images produced by X-ray apparatus, tube limitations necessitated X-ray exposure times of minutes rather than the fractions of a second needed by the equipment in modern X-ray departments. Today's radiologists looking at reproductions of X-rays taken during the Great War would comment how poor the penetrative quality of the image was. They would also express some astonishment, given the circumstances under which they had been taken, at how useful the images were, especially when used to locate the presence of foreign bodies such as pieces of metal, bullets etc. Along with all the other problems, it has to be remembered that the ingenious X-ray 'mobile unit' workers also had to process their films or X-ray plates on which the image had been taken in X-ray vans, using developing, fixing, and washing baths (similar to the process of developing and printing a camera film before the age of digital photography) that could be packed into what was a very limited space.

Applications of X-rays during the Great War
Foreign bodies

The actual use of X-rays in the Great War was mainly in the demonstration of foreign bodies such as bullets and shell fragments, which were localised using a "Mackenzie Davidson" technique, if possible, before the essential early wound excision. Sir James McKenzie Davidson, who pioneered this approach, was a surgeon who graduated from the University of Aberdeen and worked in Aberdeen, and who specialised in the eye. He became interested in X-rays and actually visited Roentgen in Würzburg before leaving Aberdeen to move to London in 1909 to take charge of the Roentgen Ray departments at the Royal London Ophthalmic and Charing Cross Hospitals. He described in his seminal research paper how taking two X-ray images at different angles would allow the accurate localisation of a foreign body by taking measurements from a series of fixed positions on the surface of the body. His technique was originally described for locating foreign bodies in the eye and his original foreign body eye localiser is still in the Marischal College Museum in Aberdeen. Too old for a commission during the

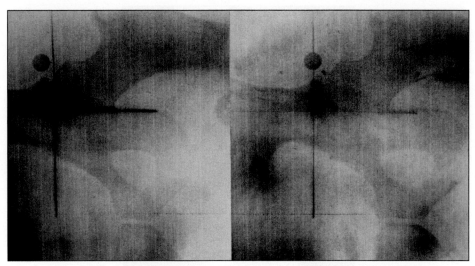

Figure 5.3   Localising technique of J. MacKenzie Davidson. The cross wires are on the skin at the point of entry, and the tube shift is 10cms. A poor quality image, but of great historical value. (Courtesy of the *British Medical Journal*)

Great War, McKenzie Davidson, nevertheless, was in overall charge of radiology in the hospitals in Great Britain for most of the Great War.

Fractures

X-rays were not routinely used in "closed" fractures because they were not used in civilian practice at that time. A "closed" fracture is one where the bone is broken, and the overlying skin is undamaged. Such fractures would be common in civilian injuries, but uncommon in war wounds. Indeed, it would be many years before orthopaedic surgeons would use X-rays routinely to help in the management of fractures. Most fractures in a war setting of course were "open" or "compound" where the skin was penetrated by a piece of shrapnel or bullet piercing the skin before striking and shattering the underlying bone. An X-ray would have been desirable before proceeding with radical wound excision, so that the surgeon would be aware of the approximate location(s), and the number, of fragments of shrapnel or bullet. Wound excision is discussed in detail in Chapters 2 and 6.

Role of X-rays in diagnosing infection

Not all foreign material which predisposed to life-threatening infection could be seen on an X-ray film. For instance, the soldier's clothing, if dragged into the wound by a missile, was not dense enough to show up. However, the presence of a metallic foreign body would alert the surgeon to the possibility that fragments of clothing might also have been dragged in to the wound by the missile, and could be lying in the proximity of the metallic fragment. One grotesque feature of battlefield wounds was that the foreign body could be soft tissue or bone from fallen comrades, killed or maimed by the same shell.

The demonstration of gas gangrene on an X-ray film was possible three or four days after the introduction of the bacteria responsible. One of the clinical features of gas gangrene is that the bacteria produce gas, which then forms bubbles within the body tissues. Such gas is relatively easy to detect by X-ray, because of the extremely low X-ray density of air or gas when compared with the body's tissues. Unfortunately by the time

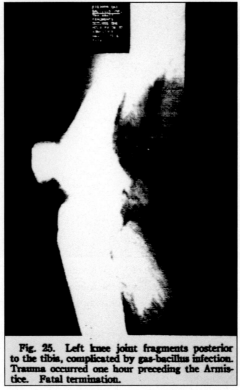

Fig. 25. Left knee joint fragments posterior
to the tibia, complicated by gas-bacillus infection.
Trauma occurred one hour preceding the Armistice. Fatal termination.

Figure 5.4   X-ray of gas gangrene, behind shattered lower thigh bone (femur).
The metallic fragment and gas within the muscle of the leg are shown. Of very
grainy quality, this image reflects the inherently poor clarity of imaging available
at the time. (Courtesy of the Radiological Society of North America)

this was demonstrable on X-ray, it was often too late to save the patient's limb or life
because the infection had progressed to such an extent that amputation of the affected
limb or death of the patient was inevitable (see Chapter 6 for more details).

X-ray screening

Unfortunately, an essential part of battlefield radiography was the use of X-ray screening,
using a glass plate which was coated with chemicals fluorescent to X-rays. This screening
allowed a limb to be held in the optimum position for a film to be exposed, and was also
an integral part of metal localisation. Since the screening might take many seconds, or
minutes, the resultant irradiation of both patient and technician was considerable.

Chest X-rays

Since the chest contains a high proportion of air, which is normally only in the lungs,
the amount of beam penetration is not large, but the long exposures required, because of
the low tube output must have been a major problem, and for the wounded service men,
must have required a great deal of stoicism. Any blurring of the X-ray image cause by
breathing movements or because of pain and discomfort would have made interpretation
of the X-ray image very difficult. The detection of blood or other fluid within the chest

cavity (see Chapter 8) requires a horizontal tube position to demonstrate fluid levels, and this was not always possible.

Chest X-rays were in widespread use in the UK in 1914 and were used for routine screening of army recruits in an attempt to detect tuberculosis of the lung, which was extremely common and resulted in many deaths at this time. Tuberculosis was the major killer disease at the time of the Great War, and the very mention of tuberculosis caused fear in much the same way as cancer does today.

Abdominal X-rays

Taking an X-ray of the abdomen required long exposure times to obtain a good image and as in the case of chest X-rays, patient movement, and any movement of the intestine which was certainly not controllable, also compromised abdominal films by blurring the images. However, if the abdominal X-ray was mainly used to locate a metallic foreign body then this was still possible as finer detail was not required.

Skull X-rays

Patient movement was also a potential problem of skull X-rays, because of the difficulty of immobilising a semi-conscious patient. When localisation of a foreign body that had penetrated the skull was required, this was possible and relatively straightforward because front and side views only required half-rotation of the head for the two most useful X-ray films to be taken.

The use of X-ray equipment during the war

Records show that the extent to which X-ray equipment was used in France and Belgium varied considerably. In 1941 an American radiologist Dr Ernst wrote a fascinating reminiscence of his experiences during the Great War.[8] Ernst came to France in April 1917 with Base Hospital 21 from Washington, after the USA had entered the war. This hospital took over the running of British General Hospital No. 12 at Rouen. As discussed in Chapter 2, when the United States entered the war, its Government sanctioned the dispatch of personnel for the staffing of six base hospitals to work as complete US units, on British lines of communication. Each of these units had 23 medical officers, 50 nursing sisters, and a complete establishment of NCOs and men. Each unit would fly the flag of the United States, and personnel would be paid by the US Government. This arrangement permitted the freeing up of British personnel so that they could carry out other duties.[9] On his arrival, Dr Ernst found that there was one X-ray tube of the old type, and electricity to power this was supplied by eight wet storage batteries, charged by a small one cylinder petrol engine. This produced maximum X-ray strength of only 2 milli-amps, and a very low screening current of only half of this. Glass X-ray plates were still in use and had not yet been replaced by film-type ones. The throughput of patients that he recorded during his time was remarkable. Base Hospital 21 produced more X-ray film than all the British hospitals put together. This is partly explained by a difference in the British and United States organisation of how the casualties were managed and the systems and processes that they had in place to facilitate this.

The wounded soldier in a United States-run base hospital was admitted via the X-ray department, and X-ray films taken readily, and perhaps more routinely. In hospitals run by British medical services, the casualty was usually first admitted to a ward for clinical assessment, and was only taken to the X-ray department if the medical team thought that this was required after clinical examination. French base hospitals were located

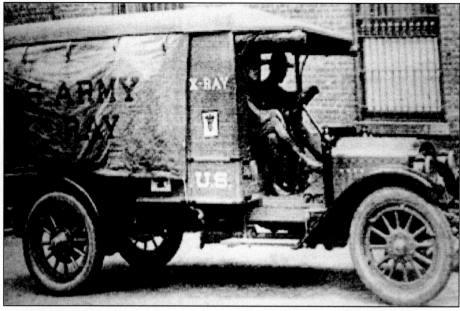

Figure 5.5   USA Army X-ray van. (Courtesy of the American College of Radiology)

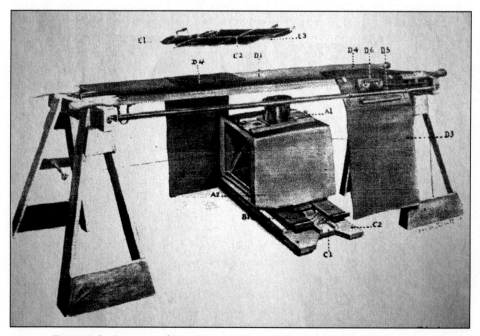

Figure 5.6   Diagram of Base Hospital X-ray table, under-table tube, and over-
table screen. (Courtesy of the Radiological Society of North America)

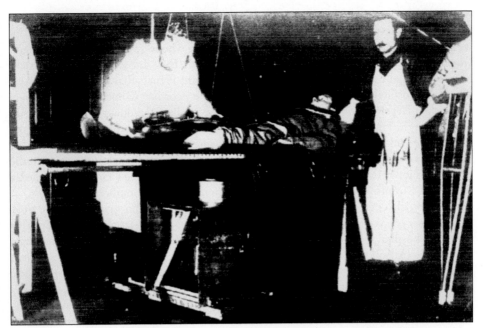

Figure 5.7   This is a similar table to that in Figure 5.6 and is in use with a casualty having an X-ray being taken. The poor quality of the photograph is contemporary, however as possibly the only image in existence showing a table of this type in actual use during the War it is of great historical value. (Courtesy of the Radiological Society of North America).

mostly in and around Paris, and could be reached from the front in about 12 hours. Their protocols for casualty management and flow through the hospitals were similar to those used by the British medical units.[10]

The evacuation pathway of casualties, as detailed in Chapter 2, meant that the wounded were taken from the regimental aid posts, through collecting or relay posts, to the field ambulance level. There were often facilities at main dressing stations, but if not, then a mobile van could be called up if required urgently.

These vehicles were sometimes converted cars, whilst others were caravan-type cabins, pulled by a tractor. Although called Mobile X-ray Units, "moveable" might be a better description, because it required a considerable period of time to set them up, arrange the stretcher table, connect the X-ray tube, and organise the processing facilities for the X-ray films. Static, slightly more sophisticated machines were usually located at the casualty clearing stations, and of course, in the base hospitals and not in more forward medical units.

X-Ray Personnel

As the Great War continued, the need for trained doctors who were skilled in the interpretation of X-ray films (radiologists) became apparent, and eventually many were recruited. Equally important were the 'assistants', who did most of the actual work required to obtain an X-ray image.

Amongst the doctors working as radiologists was a women working in an all-women volunteer hospital unit from Great Britain. Initially, women had not been allowed to work with the RAMC in the war, but there were some who were determined to help and would not be put off by this attitude shown to them. They did so by joining a variety of international organisations, such as the British and French Red Cross and Scottish Women's Hospitals (SWH) for foreign service. The Scottish Women's Hospitals were established largely through the efforts of Dr Elsie Inglis, a graduate of the University of Edinburgh. Her association with the campaign for women's suffrage resulted in the War Office and British Red Cross declining her offer of help, and financial support for her hospitals came from women's suffrage organisations. The French did not share the prejudice shown by British authorities, and the Scottish Women's Hospitals opened a hospital at Royaumont Abbey near Paris a few months after the outbreak of the war.

A Scottish doctor who worked here was Agnes Savill, who graduated MA from St Andrew's University before going on to study medicine at Glasgow University. This voluntary hospital made a major contribution to the management of casualties, having a total of 600 beds. It treated French soldiers, and Savill was given an X-ray car by a French general, General Le Bon. Savill published a paper on gas gangrene in 1917 where she described the X-ray appearances of gas gangrene[11], but returned to her original speciality of dermatology after the war, enjoying a long and distinguished career, both in medicine and in literature. She edited a textbook of medicine written by her late husband, and also had an interest in military history, authoring a book about Alexander the Great.

The first male specialist radiologist in the British Army came from Aberdeen. His name was Dalziel B. McGrigor.[12] He qualified in medicine at the University of Aberdeen in 1907 and then joined the RAMC in the same year. His initial training in radiology was in the Indian X-ray Institute, during his time of service in India. On return he was appointed to be specialist in charge of the X-ray and electro-medical units at the Queen Alexandra Military Hospital, Millbank; he was also a lecturer at the Royal Army Medical College. During the Great War he served in France, leading No 1 Field X-ray Section with the Indian Expeditionary Force. He subsequently became interested in localisation of foreign bodies within the eye and his localising 'spectacles' were to be found in X-ray departments in the UK into the 1950s.[13]

The X-ray workers in those days were not much interested in terminology, and the terms "radiographer" and "radiologist" were very loosely used, certainly until the end of the war. This confusion is evident in the early reports and papers from that time, which makes the term "X-ray worker" useful. The responsibility for taking the X-rays in the British Army was sometimes with a qualified radiographer. Following the experience of the Boer War, the British Army opened what was probably the world's first radiographer training school in Southampton in 1903.[14] However, in the field, any willing and interested soldier could be recruited on the spot, and asked to "carry on" after having received minimal training. Apparently a remarkable number of these individuals remained in the occupation of radiography after their return to civilian life. At the beginning of the war there were a few fully accredited medical doctors who specialised in radiology and would now be called radiologists. Most of those acting as such during the war were doctors pressed into service, usually because they had an interest in the relatively new technique. Quite a number went on to full radiology training after the war, while others reverted to their original interests.

As the war went on, all branches of the medical profession came under severe pressure. Just as there was a general shortage of medical manpower by 1917, so there was also a shortage of radiologists. In Chapter 6, the shortage of orthopaedic surgeons is discussed, as a result of surgeons in training being sent to fill vacant positions in forward medical units – someone had to do this, but it could also be interpreted as callous disregard for experienced medical manpower, in a way not unlike the lot of the "fighting soldier" at the hands of some of the generals.[15] The situation improved when the United States entered the war, bringing with them a number of doctors, including fully trained radiologists, to staff British general hospitals, thus alleviating the shortages in the British Army brought about by three years of relentless conflict.

Provision of X-rays by other combatant nations
At the outset of hostilities in 1914, the British Army was well equipped to deal with the demands of radiology and this, in part at least, was because of experience gained during the Boer War.

Unfortunately, the French Army was not so well prepared in this respect. In fact the French High Command seemed at first indifferent to the need for radiology.[16]

An important figure in championing the potential importance of X-rays in the clinical management of the wounded was Marie Curie. She was born in Warsaw, Poland, but had to leave Poland to secure an education, and after a period of financial hardship was able to enter the Sorbonne in Paris to study and complete a Masters degree in Physics and Maths. This was quickly followed by a doctorate in 1903. She was the first woman in France to achieve this distinction. Curie's scientific work was of the highest quality and she obtained two Nobel Prizes, the first for Physics in 1903, and the second for Chemistry in 1911.

At the outbreak of the Great War, Curie was very concerned about the lack of X-ray facilities available to the French Army. There were X-ray facilities in larger hospitals but not in the field hospitals where they were clearly needed. It is reported that in order to give something back to the country of her adoption, she took a personal interest in France's contribution to this war, even offering to donate her two Nobel Gold Medals and the money she had received from the Nobel Prizes. She undertook a short course in anatomy and radiography, and began training young women including her own daughter, Irene (who also won a Nobel Prize for Chemistry), to be radiographers. Using her position as the pre-eminent French scientist, she begged and borrowed money and cars from her well-off friends and then persuaded car-body shops to turn them into X-ray vans! For the actual X-ray equipment, she went around hospitals and private clinics, wherever X-ray machines were under-used, and somehow obtained them to equip the vans for use in the war.

Beginning in 1914, she sent out over 20 mobile units and permanent units equipped with trained technicians to take X-rays to provide an X-ray service for wounded French soldiers. The first van was staffed by herself and her daughter. Probably the presence of these brave women also helped the morale of the soldiers. The vans were called *petite Curies* by the combatants. Madame Curie also helped increase X-ray facilities in the base hospitals when they began receive the wounded from the forward areas. She opened, and ran, a training school for X-ray workers from the United States, possibly in her spare time. Over two hundred individuals qualified from her academy[17] and consequently by

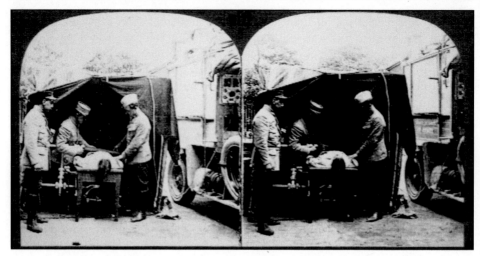

Figure 5.8   French X-ray van in action. Viewing the X-ray screen in daylight
is puzzling, but may be for the photograph only; this is to give a three-
dimensional stereoscopic image of the scene. (Adrian Thomas)

the end of the war, the French medical service had an X-ray division comparable with
that of other combatant nations.

By the time the United States entered the war, their industry was already making
the improved Coolidge tubes. With fewer raw material restrictions than Great Britain,
they had researched and manufactured better screens which enhanced the image. They
used films instead of glass plates, and introduced Potter Bucky diaphragms, an advance
which cleaned up the final picture, but which required a more powerful unit than
the old X-ray tube. They were able to take advantage of the pathways of evacuation,
already established by the French, British and Belgian medical services. They did
not have the 'benefit' of the Boer War experience, but the short ten-week Spanish-
American War in 1898 had demonstrated the need for X-rays.[18] The American Roentgen
Society realised the significance of the need for trained staff and established schools of
military roentgenology.[19] A close working relationship developed between surgeons and
radiologists as they realised the value of working together. American military radiologists
were also well informed of their British colleagues' work and problems in Flanders.

Captured German X-ray units were found to be very similar to those used by their
opponents.[20] The German Army medical service was equipped with both static and
moveable X-ray machines, the latter used mainly in the Balkans and the Eastern Front,
where battlefronts moved frequently. The X-ray units on the Western front were situated
in the German Base Hospitals.

In conclusion, improvements in men and machinery were accelerated by the Great
War, but most of the significant advances were made before 1914. While the majority of
X-ray workers did their job out of range of shot and shell, they did suffer casualties, and
many received high doses of radiation. This cohort of men and women gave their health,
wittingly or not, to the cause they believed in. Along with the millions of others who
fell, they should also be remembered for their contributions to the care of the wounded
in this war.

Acknowledgement
Much of the background for this chapter makes use of the detailed work of the late E.H. Burrows and the research of Adrian M.K. Thomas, who also gave generous advice.

Notes

1   Burrows, E.H., *Pioneers and Early Years: A History of British Radiology*. St Anne, Alderney, Channel Islands: Colophon, 1986, p.1.

2   Anonymous, "MacKenzie-Davidson, J.", *British Medical Journal* 1919: 1: p.468.

3   Personal observation.

4   Rolleston, H., "On the effects of radiations on patients and radiologists – the Mackenzie Davidson Lecture", *Radiology* 1928; 10: pp.165-166.

5   Thomas, M.K., "The first 50 years of military radiology, 1895-1945", *European Journal of Radiology* 1945; 63: p.2.

6   Ramoutsaki, I.A., E.N. Giannacos & G.N. Livaadas, "The birth of battlefield radiology: the Greco-Turkish War of 1897", *Radiographics* 2001; 21: pp.263-266.

7   Knox, R., "Discussion on experiments and experiences with the Coolidge tube", *Proceedings of the Royal Society of Medicine* 1916; 9 (Electro-Therapy section): pp.98-142.

8   Ernst, E.C., "Reminiscences of roentgenology during the last war, 1917-1919", *Radiology* 1941; 3: pp.421-438.

9   MacPherson, W.G. (ed.), *History of the Great War based on Official Documents. Medical Services. General History*. London: HMSO, 1923, Volume 2, pp.98-101.

10 *Harvard Graduates' Magazine* September 1915 Volume 24, No 93, p.3.

11 Savill, A., "X-ray appearances in gas gangrene", *British Medical Journal* 1917; 1: p.15.

12 McGrigor, D.B., "Radiology (In Arduis Fidelis), 1898-1948", *Journal of the Royal Army Medical Corps* 1948; 90: pp.334-338.

13 Personal observation.

14 Burrows, *op.cit.*, pp.218-219.

15 Clark, A., *The Donkeys*, London: Pimlico, 1991.

16 Quinn, S., *Madame Curie, A Life*. London: Heinemann, 1995.

17 Blair, J.G.S., "Marie Curie's other role", *Journal of the Royal Army Medical Corps* 2005; 151: pp.117-118.

18 Cirillo, V.J., "The Spanish-American War and military radiology", *American Journal of Roentgenology* 2000; 74: pp.1233-1239.

19 Rosenberger, A., W. Fuchs, O.B. Adler, J. Braun, U. Kleinhaus, D. Goldsher, A. Engel, M. Pery, J.K. Kaftori, "Radiology of War", *Acta Radiologica Supplement* 1986; 367: pp.1-82.

20 Thomas, *op.cit.*, pp.214-219.

6

Developments in orthopaedic surgery

Thomas R Scotland

To mark the seventieth birthday of the surgeon Sir Robert Jones, some of his former colleagues presented him with a volume of original essays on various topics relating to orthopaedic surgery. They did so as a mark of respect for his contribution to the emerging specialty of orthopaedic surgery over the years. His good friend, and renowned surgeon, Lord Moynihan from Leeds, addressed Jones in the preface to the work. In it Moynihan wrote:

> At the head of the Orthopaedic Department at the War Office (during the Great War), Robert Jones found his destined place. He became the guide, the counsellor, the example to a large band of workers who really assimilated his teaching, and were able to practise it on a scale hitherto unimaginable. The genius of Owen Thomas, the skill of Robert Jones, found their highest expression in treatment of wounded. The methods of these two, previously little known, and rarely practised, except by such old friends such as Harold Stiles, Henry Gray, and Lynn-Thomas, now became the inheritance and enjoyment of all who cared to seek acquaintance with them.[1]

These five men – Jones, Stiles, Gray, Lynn-Thomas and Moynihan himself – were largely responsible for the development and establishment of orthopaedic surgery during the Great War, and their contribution to the surgical war effort will be examined. However, one must go a generation further back from this new dawn of specialisation in surgery, precipitated by the Great War, and reflect on the work of Welsh practitioner, Hugh Owen Thomas, the uncle by marriage of Robert Jones.

Thomas was a Welsh medical practitioner descended from a long line of bonesetters. Thomas made a conscious effort to break with the family "bone-setting" tradition, preferring to gain a recognised medical qualification. He went to medical school at Edinburgh University and University College London, graduating in medicine in 1857. He went on to study surgery in Paris before returning to Liverpool. Initially, he went into practice with his father, but the two soon parted company, and Thomas set up on his own. He became established in 11 Nelson Street, where he continued in practice for the rest of his life.[2] His patients were the poor, the crippled and the destitute from the area around the docklands of Liverpool. Many suffered from tuberculosis, and frequently showed evidence of joint damage caused by tuberculosis, a condition rarely seen by orthopaedic surgeons today as it is now relatively simply treated by antibiotics whilst in its early stages in the lungs.

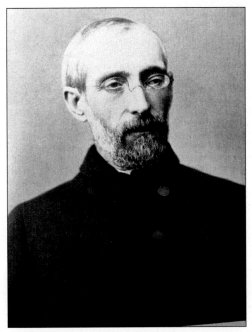

Figure 6.1   Hugh Owen Thomas (1834-1891). (Private collection)

Thomas was a strong advocate of absolute rest for the treatment of joint damage secondary to tuberculosis. He had a workshop on his premises, where he invented and manufactured a wide variety of splints, including one designed for complete immobilisation of the knee joint. It so happened that the Thomas Knee Splint (see Chapter 2) was also ideally suited for the effective immobilisation of fractures of the thigh bone (femur). Little did Thomas know when he was hard at work in the slums of Liverpool that his splint would one day revolutionise the management of the wounded soldier with a fractured femur on the Western Front during the Great War, and make one of the most significant contributions to the advance of orthopaedic surgery in the 20th Century.

Thomas was a very innovative practitioner, but he didn't really fit into the medical establishment, and he never held a hospital appointment. He started work very early in the morning, and finished late every evening. He conducted a free clinic for the poor every Sunday. He never took a holiday. He published his work, but was in the habit of not appending his own academic qualifications to his writing, and consequently many thought that he, like his ancestors, was an unqualified "bonesetter".[3]

In 1857, he published his first book on *Diseases of the Hip, Knee and Ankle Joint*, in which he described his splints which were destined to become famous round the world, and are still in use today. He remained a recluse throughout his career and he worked in isolation. Had it not been for Robert Jones, his nephew, his work might never have survived him. Thomas died in 1891, at the age of fifty-seven years.

Robert Jones was born on 28 June 1857, and went to live with his uncle from the age of sixteen onwards. He admired the work of his uncle, and grew up to be greatly influenced by him. Jones studied medicine at Liverpool University, and graduated in

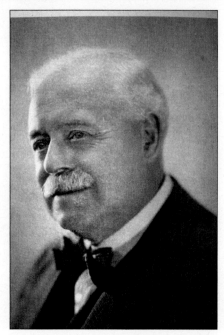

Figure 6. 2   Sir Robert Jones (1857-1933). (Private collection)

1878, afterwards proceeding to gain the qualification of Fellow of the Royal College of Surgeons of Edinburgh. He worked with his uncle in Nelson Street, becoming his assistant, thereby receiving a unique education in orthopaedics, at a time when the specialty as such did not exist. All surgeons were really "general" surgeons, who were able to turn their hand to any and every procedure. It would be some time, and it has to be said, against much opposition from the surgical establishment in London, who were "general" surgeons in the broadest sense (and opposed to specialisation) before orthopaedic surgery would emerge as a specialty in its own right.

Unlike his uncle who was quiet and reserved, Jones was friendly, outgoing and gregarious. He was appointed surgeon-superintendent to the Manchester Ship Canal which was begun in 1887 and completed in 1894. Around 20,000 workmen were employed on its construction, and Jones treated more than 3,000 injuries in strategically built hospitals close to the construction sites. He had to deal with over 200 major injuries during this time. [4] No doubt, he employed his uncle's knee splint for the treatment of fractures of the femur, his ever-growing clinical experience establishing him as a leading authority in the management of fractures. This experience would stand him in good stead during the years 1914 to 1918.

He was appointed to the position of Honorary Surgeon to the Southern General Hospital in Liverpool in 1889, and it was during his time here that Agnes Hunt, who had a little hospital for crippled children in the village of Baschurch near Oswestry, first brought patients to Jones for consultation. Soon, he paid visits to Baschurch, and began doing regular Sunday clinics there, which he continued doing until the outbreak of the war, becoming consulting surgeon to the hospital in 1904. [5] Today, the Robert Jones and Agnes Hunt Hospital in Oswestry is a world famous orthopaedic unit.

While orthopaedic surgery did not exist as a surgical specialty, Jones was to all intents and purposes developing expertise in the surgical management of the problems of bones and joints, a fact acknowledged by numbers of American orthopaedic surgeons who crossed the Atlantic to the port of Liverpool, and spent time watching Jones at work in his clinics and operating theatre. He was a skilful surgeon, who displayed economy of movement, and had very big operating lists during which he operated on many patients. Such was his dexterity that visiting surgeons from the United States were unanimous in their appreciation of his work.[6] Unlike this country, the medical profession in the United States had already recognised that orthopaedics was a distinct specialty, having formed and established an American Orthopaedic Association.

Jones' association with surgeons from North America was to prove of great importance when the United States declared war on Germany in April 1917. One of the first things they did was to send orthopaedic surgeons to train and work with Jones in the United Kingdom. This was to prove invaluable, since by 1917, Jones was developing major orthopaedic centres all round the United Kingdom. These were short-staffed, partly because of his expanding service, and partly because he was always under constant threat of having surgeons under his instruction being taken away to fill posts in advanced medical units on the Western Front.

During the Great War, Jones primarily focussed on the late problems of wounds affecting the musculoskeletal system. By the very nature of this work, he frequently had to deal with problems associated with complications secondary to poor initial management, frequently with associated major wound infection. Jones, however, was instrumental in solving one of the most serious acute clinical problems on the Western Front, namely the compound gunshot fracture of the femur (thigh bone), which had a documented mortality of around 80% in 1914 and 1915. He solved the problem with the help and support of his good friend and colleague, Henry Gray.[7] [8]

Henry Gray was born in Aberdeen in 1870, the son of an Aberdeen wholesale provision merchant. After going to Merchiston Castle School in Edinburgh, he returned to Aberdeen to join his father's business. After two years, he enrolled in the Faculty of Medicine, University of Aberdeen and graduated in 1895. He went on to pursue a career in surgery, and became a Fellow of the Royal College of Surgeons of Edinburgh. He travelled abroad before taking up post as assistant surgeon to the Aberdeen Royal Infirmary in 1899. In 1904 he became surgeon to Aberdeen Royal Infirmary, and is credited with bringing aseptic surgery to Aberdeen. On a national level he was responsible with Sir Henry Barker for introducing local anaesthesia to surgery in Britain.[9]

Like Jones, Gray was a general surgeon. His operating lists would include a caesarean section (then a very rare procedure), drainage of an acutely infected mastoid (a bone just behind the ear which could become infected with pus leading to serious complications), a cerebral decompression (a brain operation), a hysterectomy (removal of womb), a total cystectomy (removal of urinary bladder), and the joining together of two ends of a fractured bone using a metal plate and screws. Many abdominal cases were done under spinal anaesthesia, and hernias and operations on the limbs were performed under local anaesthesia.[10]

Gray was an original member of the Moynihan Provincial Surgeons' Club[11], begun by renowned Leeds surgeon Sir Berkeley Moynihan. This was an important group of surgeons, because hitherto there had been a belief (held mainly in London)

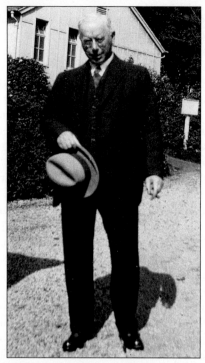

Figure 6. 3   Sir Henry Gray (1870-1938). (Dr Iain Levack)

that development in surgery only came from the capital, and certainly not from the far North! The reality was that surgical development was every bit as likely in provincial units, as in the well established prestigious institutions in London.

At the outbreak of the war in 1914, Gray at first joined a Red Cross unit. Then, after a brief return to the United Kingdom, he went back to France, where he spent three and a half years from November 1914 until June 1918. Part of this time was spent as Consulting Surgeon to a group of base hospitals in Rouen, and partly as Consulting Surgeon to the British 3rd Army.[12] Gray's responsibility to the 3rd Army was to ensure that the standard of surgical work was as high as possible. Indeed, the quality of Gray's work over three and a half years of concentrated experience in France earned him the award of C.B. in 1916, the C.M.G. in 1918, and the K.B.E. in 1919. He was mentioned in despatches five times.[13] In 1924, the University of Aberdeen bestowed the honorary degree of LLD for his outstanding contributions to surgery.[14]

It may be said that Robert Jones and Henry Gray complemented each other. While Jones spent most of his war in the United Kingdom, establishing Military Orthopaedic Services in the UK, Gray spent three and a half years in France, dealing with acute surgical problems in the forward surgical units. It was Gray who documented the high mortality from the compound gunshot fracture of the femur, quoting a mortality of 80% in 1914 and 1915.[15][16] He encouraged Jones to employ the Thomas Splint for treating these fractures.[17] If Robert Jones introduced the Thomas Splint, then it was Henry Gray who helped to bring about its widespread acceptance on the Western Front.

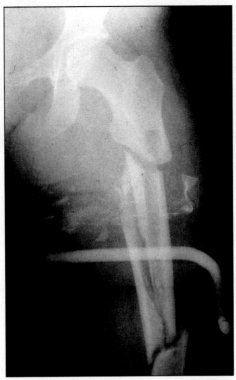

Figure 6. 4   Fracture of the femur (thigh bone). This is a high-energy civilian injury as opposed to a war wound. The fracture is in several bits (comminuted). One cannot say from the radiograph if the fracture is compound (skin broken). All war wounds involving a fracture of the femur were compound, allowing entry of bacteria which caused infection. (Author's photograph)

The clinical problem confronting them was indeed a serious and potentially lethal one. A compound fracture is a broken bone where the skin has been punctured, potentially allowing a route for bacteria to gain access to the fracture site and cause a very deep-seated infection. Compound fractures of the femur were particularly serious because of the large amount of muscle damaged at the time of the fracture, and the loss of at least a couple of pints of blood into the thigh. The huge area of the wound with many possible recesses was predisposed to foreign bodies lying undetected within its depths. Pieces of shrapnel and contaminated clothing, lying within an area of damaged muscle, created the ideal setting for establishment of major infection.

If the muscle had been so badly damaged that there were areas deprived of a blood supply, then the bacteria responsible for gas gangrene had an opportunity to thrive. Such bacteria can only live when there is no oxygen in the tissues. They are called "anaerobic", which means they can only survive in the absence of oxygen. Wounds caused by bullets or fragments of shrapnel from an exploding shell were always compound. As well as direct damage to the body's tissues from irregular pieces of shrapnel derived from exploding shells and fragments of clothing and other debris carried into the innermost depths of the wound, the shock wave from a penetrating missile also caused destruction of adjacent

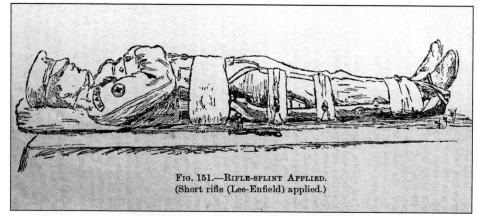

Fig. 151.—Rifle-splint Applied.
(Short rifle (Lee-Enfield) applied.)

Figure 6. 5   The Rifle Splint, based on the Liston Splint. A Lee-Enfield Rifle was bound to the affected limb and to the pelvis and abdomen. It did not effectively immobilise the fracture. This illustration is taken from *Royal Army Medical Corps Handbook* of 1911.

muscle, creating an ideal environment for anaerobic infection. Very importantly, the soil from the agricultural areas in France and Flanders where the battles were fought had been enriched with manure, a ready source of potentially deadly organisms.

When the British Army went to war in 1914, it did so with a variety of inadequate splints for treating fractures of the femur. Most were based on the principle of the Liston Splint. Liston had been a famous man, and part of the establishment in the early to mid 19th Century. His splint, however, was ineffective. It did not immobilise the fracture adequately. The only splint mentioned in the Royal Army Medical Corps handbook, published in 1911, was the Rifle Splint, based on the Liston Splint, as shown in Figure 6.5.[18]

A Lee Enfield Rifle was tied to the patient's trunk, thigh, and leg, and while its aim was to stabilise the fracture, it was simply inadequate for the purpose. It allowed the bone ends in the thigh at the fracture site to move and grind against each other, causing great pain and further, excessive blood loss. In contrast, the Thomas Splint was effective in immobilising the fracture. The thigh was well supported, and traction applied to the leg and fixed to the bottom of the splint maintained the fracture in a reduced position. It was easier to apply in a battlefield situation, and once fitted, the patient could be transferred effectively back down the line to the appropriate casualty clearing station in relative comfort. In the illustration here, skin traction has been employed as it was during the Great War. An adhesive bandage, fixed to the skin with glue, was attached to the leg from mid-thigh level to just above the ankle. Traction was then applied and cords from the skin traction apparatus tied round the bottom of the Thomas Splint.

Thomas, however, had been an eccentric provincial surgeon, and unlike Liston, was not an accepted establishment figure. So the British Army took the Liston Splint to war in 1914, not the more effective Thomas Splint.

Robert Jones described the fractured femur as the "tragedy of the war".[19] This was partly because so many soldiers died unnecessarily, and partly because poor splinting caused late problems for the casualties who survived. Many had significant overlap of the bone ends with shortening of up to 5 inches. Fractures then went on to unite in

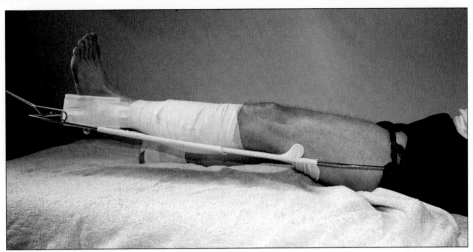

Figure 6. 6   Thomas Splint. A patient with fracture of the femur in a Thomas Splint using skin traction; a firm pull is applied and cords are tied round the bottom of the splint. In this way, traction maintains the fracture in a reduced position. (Author's photograph)

this grossly shortened position. Mal-union is a term used to define fractures which heal with significant shortening or angulation, and this could have been prevented by proper splinting in the first place.[20]

When soldiers with badly splinted fractures arrived back at casualty clearing stations, they frequently arrived in a state of shock, due to excessive blood loss and pain.[21] These men required radical surgery to save their limbs and lives. Wound excision has been dealt with in general terms in Chapter 2, and the method for dealing with a compound fracture of the femur was no different in principle. Entry and exit wounds would have to be extended widely, removing all dead skin and fat. The damaged muscle would then have to be carefully directly inspected and all devitalised muscle removed by cutting it away, frequently in huge amounts, until all dead muscle had been removed. It was essential that only healthy muscle tissue be left behind. This was judged by a fresh appearance to the muscle and the fact that it was able to bleed. The bone ends of the femur at the fracture site would then have to be pulled out of the wound and be inspected directly. Any loose fragments of bone with no blood supply would have to be removed along with fragments of clothing and general battlefield filth. If any dead muscle had been left behind at the completion of surgery, then the operation would have been inadequate, and the likely outcome would have been loss of limb or life, from the effects of gas gangrene which would develop and become apparent a day or two later.

Infection of the greatest severity took hold very quickly, and this is something surgeons today perhaps find difficult to appreciate, working in the aseptic environment of the modern operating theatre. Major infection clearly caught surgeons by surprise in 1914, prompting urgent policy changes, referred to in Chapter 2, when Sir Anthony Bowlby declared that wound excision would have to be carried out before the patient was sent back to base, and before gas gangrene had a chance to become established.[22]

Wounded soldiers arriving at casualty clearing stations with a weak pulse, and low blood pressure secondary to excess blood loss due to inadequately splinted fractures would be unlikely to survive the major procedure just described, thus explaining the very high mortality from this wound. The challenge which confronted Jones, and in particular, Gray who was working in the forward areas on the Western Front, was to reduce this high mortality.

They did this by ensuring that the Thomas Splint would be used to transfer patients with compound femoral fractures to a designated casualty clearing station, and so arrive in good clinical condition thanks to adequate splinting of the fracture.

It has been suggested that Dakin's Solution (see Chapter 2), administered through a series of irrigation tubes to kill bacteria was a major contributory factor in reducing the high mortality from the compound fracture of the femur, and not the Thomas Splint.[23] While Dakin's Solution may have been useful in cleaning up infected wounds, it was no substitute for surgery. No antiseptic solution would make any difference to the outcome unless the patient had first undergone successful radical wound excision.

As a direct result of arriving at casualty clearing stations in good clinical condition patients were able to undergo necessary limb and life-saving surgery with a greater chance of survival than ever before. This can be illustrated by Gray's experience of casualties at the Battle of Arras in April 1917, when in a six week period 1,009 soldiers were admitted with a compound femoral fracture.[24] The Thomas Splint was used exclusively at Arras, and all regimental medical officers were taught how to apply it. They, in turn, instructed their stretcher-bearers in its application and use. Prior to the Battle of Arras the majority of patients had arrived at clearing stations in a shocked state in a variety of splints. With the exception of the Thomas Splint, all were ineffective. Gray quoted a mortality rate in the casualty clearing station of over 50% for these shocked casualties. Using the Thomas Splint exclusively, all but 5% of patients arrived back at the casualty clearing stations in good clinical condition, and could proceed safely to radical wound excision. The mortality rate was 15.6%, a reduction of more than 30%. Although there are no available figures, it may also be assumed that fewer soldiers died before they reached the casualty clearing station thanks to effective splinting. This represents a major improvement in survival.[25]

Before the widespread use of the Thomas Splint, there had been a school of thought that all compound fractures of the femur should be treated by amputation of the limb. This was based on work done by Marshall (see Chapter 3) at Casualty Clearing Station number 17 at Remy Siding, near Ypres. Marshall had noted that shocked patients needing an amputation stood a better chance of survival using a short anaesthetic of nitrous oxide and oxygen, and then quickly "whipping off the leg".[26] Chloroform, ether, or spinal anaesthesia tended to be associated with a potentially fatal fall in blood pressure (see Chapter 3).[27] By extrapolation, if all shocked patients with a compound fractured femur had a "whiff of gas and a quick amputation" then more might survive than the 20% before the Thomas Splint found favour. Fortunately, thanks to the Thomas Splint, those who favoured immediate amputation for all cases of compound femoral fractures never had to put their hypothesis into practice.

The amputation rate for Gray's series of casualties was only 17.2%. Many of these patients would have had major nerve or blood vessel wounds, or wounds which were infected beyond any hope of recovery, making amputation the better, if not the only option.[28] It should be pointed out that reconstruction of major arteries was not yet a possibility during the Great War and the repair of a vessel by directly suturing one end to the other was only rarely feasible. Gray also made the observation that of those who died, many had lain out in No Man's Land for a prolonged period and were beyond help, whatever measures had been employed.[29]

During a battle, the incidence of compound fracture of the femur was one case per fifty to sixty admissions. The incidence during a military advance was greater than during defensive trench warfare. When the wounded arrived at the casualty clearing station, they were immediately prepared for theatre, and were anaesthetised. Field dressings were taken off to expose the wound[30] and they underwent wound excision. Gray insisted that no patient was ever sent back to base hospital without first having surgery. Occasionally, a wound might appear so innocuous as to make it seem that the patient could safely wait for definitive surgery at the base, but the damage was always worse than it appeared, and to leave such a wound could well have fatal consequences.[31]

It was vital that surgery was undertaken by surgeons most experienced in dealing with this type of wound, and so there were clearing stations for dealing specifically with compound fractures of the femur. Such facilities were usually situated further forward at a range of around 10,000 yards from the front line, so that patients could get there more quickly. During Third Ypres, for example, which began on 31 July 1917, casualty clearing stations at Brandhoek were designated to take chest wounds, abdominal wounds, and patients with compound femoral fractures which all required early surgery.[32]

After wound excision, primary closure of the wound (stitching the skin back together) was possible in selected cases allowing more rapid recovery.[33] Such a course of action, however, would only have been safe if performed early, within twelve hours, by the most experienced surgeons exercising sound clinical judgement as to when it was, or was not safe, to employ primary closure. Delayed primary closure was used if there was doubt about complete removal of devitalised tissue. Secondary closure and healing by secondary intention were the conservative options available for established major infection. Amputation was the fall back surgical position for major infection. The accompanying table summarises the different ways of dealing with the wounds of soldiers with compound fractures of the femur.

Table 6.1
Possible ways of managing compound wounds of the femur

Different ways of dealing with wounds	Description	Comments
1 Primary Closure	After wound excision of recently inflicted wound with no sign of infection, wound closed and skin sutured	Rapid wound healing provided wound excision complete; high price to pay for inadequate wound excision
2 Delayed Primary Closure	After wound excision, in recently inflicted wound; not sure about completeness of procedure; saline pack and second look 2-3 days later; if clean, wound closed.	Safer option than 1. Wound excision at CCS and delayed primary suture at base hospital 2-3 days later.

Different ways of dealing with wounds	Description	Comments
3 Secondary Suture	Wound severely infected at first surgery due to delay. After surgery, various antiseptics till wound clean. Once healthy granulation tissue formed, wound sutured at 2-3 weeks.	Could be considered a very satisfactory outcome in an infected wound, if wound heals after secondary suture without further complications.
4 Healing by Secondary Intention	Wound so infected that it never cleans up enough to suture. It granulates and very slowly and gradually fills up from its depths. Even then, uncertain outcome. Infected non-union of fracture likely outcome.	Prolonged period in hospital; likely ongoing problems with infection; doubtful if fracture would ever unite; option 5 would crop up in discussions as a way out of a hopeless situation for limb.
5 Amputation	Best option in severely mangled limb with major vessel or nerve involvement; amputation straight away always better than doing one weeks later due to complication of other regime(s).	If things went badly wrong with options 1-4, then option 5 would be indicated.

Delayed primary closure of fractures of the femur during periods of severe pressure was employed by Gray. After wound excision in the casualty clearing station hypertonic saline packs were inserted[34], and the wounded sent back to designated general hospitals with a saline dressing (see Chapter 2). Patients would then be taken back to theatre, anaesthetised and the wound inspected. Usually, after a couple of days the wounds were clean enough so that they could safely be closed. When there had been delay in getting the patients to the casualty clearing stations, wounds would almost certainly have been grossly infected, and would have to be left for many days until healthy granulation tissue had formed, and then closed by secondary suture. Such wounds would also have been suitable for irrigation with antiseptic solution to help clean them up, but as already stated in Chapter 2, irrigation was as well as, and not instead of, wound excision.

The various antiseptic solutions and their method of application, described in Chapter 2 were more often employed at base hospitals, where these treatments were more appropriate than at the casualty clearing stations, where there was high turnover and limited scope to use the more complicated techniques involved.[35] This treatment involved "too much paraphernalia and attention."[36]

In particularly severely infected cases, wound healing by secondary intention would have to be employed (see Chapter 2). This would take weeks, if not months. Under such circumstances, the chances of such a fracture progressing to union would be impaired, so that amputation might be required late on. Psychologically, it is very bad for a patient to endure a prolonged course of conservative treatment, only to eventually need an amputation. It is much better to have an early amputation, get the wound healed, and then positively embark on rehabilitation by fitting an artificial limb. It requires the most experienced surgeon to make the most appropriate treatment plan for any wounded soldier to ensure the best outcome for any individual.

Part of the tragedy of the femoral fracture referred to by Jones was the appalling loss of position of fractures in soldiers coming home to the United Kingdom after inadequate splinting. Gross shortening and deformity frequently occurred amongst survivors, making the patient a cripple for the rest of his life.[37] Jones pointed out that it was not uncommon to see patients with four or five inches of shortening of the femur due to poor initial management. To help overcome this problem, and to ensure that these cases were looked after by surgeons who knew what they were doing, all cases of fractured femur were looked after in designated base hospitals, and were retained in France for four to six weeks.[38]

This would have ensured that fractures had progressed sufficiently towards union to make them "sticky". By that is meant that one could apply one's hands to the patient's thigh, and attempts to "wiggle the fracture" would reveal that it was no longer moving. It would be at low risk of shortening or becoming angulated, and consequently safe for transfer to the United Kingdom without loss of position. The patient could then continue in traction in the Thomas Splint until hopefully his fracture would go on to bony union some weeks later. During the Battle of the Somme in 1916, there were 3,173 cases of fractured femur in base hospitals in France (see Chapter 2). They were distributed as shown in Table 6. 2.

Table 6.2
Distribution of compound fractures of the femur in base hospitals in France during the Battle of the Somme

Hospital location	Number
Rouen	1,023
Étaples	762
Boulogne	743
Abbeville	318
Le Havre	134
Le Tréport	75
St Omer	62
Calais	56

This policy did create problems. The large accumulation of casualties meant beds were blocked, with resultant congestion of hospital accommodation. Specialised medical officers, nursing sisters and other ranks had to be retained, and were thus unavailable for duties elsewhere. The immobile nature of Thomas Splints and fracture apparatus put patients at risk from air raids. During the German offensives in the spring of 1918, it became necessary to lift restrictions on transfer of patients with femoral fractures to the United Kingdom.[39]

There is no doubt that Henry Gray was a much respected figure and regarded as an authority in surgery for the treatment of war wounds in the forward areas. Reference has already been made to the observations of Carberry, writing in *The History of The New*

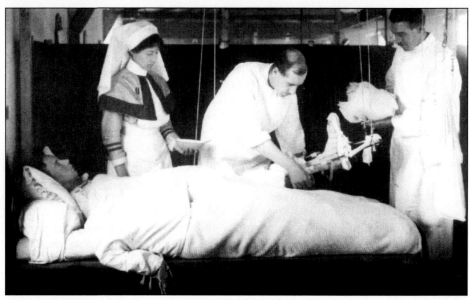

Figure 6.7   A Thomas Splint at a base hospital. (Imperial War Museum Q33472)

Zealand Medical Services in The Great War[40], where he documented that Gray had been noted for his work on the treatment of compound gunshot wounds (of the femur), and that his book, *The Early Treatment of War Wounds* epitomised the advancing knowledge of the period.[41]

Gray's memoranda, issued by the British 3rd Army in 1917, formed the basis of front line surgical practice of all British armies. New Zealand medical officers, working in the forward areas, had all been given the opportunity to attend Gray's regular series of lectures on dealing with surgical problems in the forward areas, giving treatment of shock and splinting of fractures as examples.[42]

There was, however, one dissenting voice, speaking out against the overwhelming body of opinion relating to the severity of the compound gunshot femoral fracture. Following the publication of Gray's book *The Early Treatment of War Wounds* in 1919, which was based on a series of scientific papers written by Gray and published during the war, Sir Anthony Bowlby attempted to discredit the evidence for the high mortality of the gunshot fracture of the femur in the early years of the war, declaring it to have been significantly less than the quoted figure of 80%. In a letter published in the *British Medical Journal* in January 1919, he stated it to have been only 16% at casualty clearing stations in 1915.[43]

In a very sharp response, Gray issued a strongly worded letter in the *British Medical Journal*, criticising the very inaccurate and misleading figures Bowlby had employed in arriving at his mortality figure of 16%.[44] Gray suggested that Bowlby's figures had been based on numbers documented in notoriously inaccurate 1915 admission books at casualty clearing stations. He pointed out that the diagnoses entered in these books were frequently inaccurate, especially during battle periods. For example, the admission and discharge books at three casualty clearing stations used by Bowlby only recorded 141 cases of gunshot wounds of the femur.[45] There were 23 deaths, giving a mortality of 16%. However, this was a far smaller number of gunshot wounds of the femur than would have been expected to have occurred during that period. The accepted incidence of compound femoral fractures was 1 per 50 to 60 admissions. Bowlby should have had an additional 500 cases on which to base his mortality assessment.

Gray went on to say that in cases of multiple wounds admitted to casualty clearing stations the fractured femur was often not even mentioned, and some other component of the patient's multiple injuries was documented in the record. The diagnosis in the casualty clearing station record was usually copied straight from the rudimentary field card which had been filled out under stressful conditions, and was usually illegible and inaccurate. Gray concluded that Bowlby's figures were completely skewed, and were based on inaccurate data, derived from a group of patients whose sole wound was a fractured femur, and he had probably missed 500 cases which should have been included. Gray, in contrast, had based his assessment on a careful study of all cases when he arrived at a mortality figure of 80%.

Gray went on to severely criticise Bowlby, perturbed that he was trying to play down the severity of the compound femoral fracture, which was acknowledged to be one of the gravest of wounds. Gray continued with the following:

Had his remarks gone unchallenged, then those who had not given serious consideration to the matter would receive a wrong impression of the appalling seriousness of this injury, especially in the early years of the war.[46]

Gray went on to say that it was a pity that Bowlby had attempted to diminish appreciation of the excellent progress in the handling of such cases:

Speaking generally, the enormous improvement in treatment and consequently results is one of the brightest records of the medical service.[47]

In an address to the American College of Surgeons in 1920, Bowlby contradicted himself, by stating that during the German Spring Offensive of 1918, French soldiers, with inadequately splinted fractures, had arrived in British casualty clearing stations in a state of shock, and many of them had died, while British casualties, with effectively splinted fractures, arriving at the same casualty clearing stations, were in much better clinical condition and had done much better.[48] It is not clear what Bowlby was trying to achieve in his correspondence with the *British Medical Journal*, when he challenged the existing evidence for the high mortality of compound fractures of the femur.

Perhaps the relationship between Bowlby and Gray was a difficult one, as this exchange of correspondence in the *British Medical Journal* might suggest. Both were clearly key people in their field, determined, driven and single-minded, in order to succeed. They would have had to display great determination and conviction as pioneering surgeons, dealing with appalling wounds. Gray was a general surgeon with an emerging expertise in front line, hands on, orthopaedic military surgery, while Bowlby was perhaps a product of the surgical establishment. This may have been a source of friction between the two men. What is certain is that both men were doing their best to establish policies to deal with the dreadful wounds from the trenches of France and Flanders.

Reference has been made in Chapter 1 to the fact that data collected was not always accurate. Given the circumstances they worked under, dealing with vast numbers of casualties, this is hardly surprising. There were so many patients to treat under the most trying of conditions. Even today, in carefully controlled clinical trials, data collection has to be given careful attention and even now, errors and omissions occur.

Gray published his work extensively during the war. He was instrumental in developing hypertonic saline dressings[49], as already mentioned. He wrote about gun-shot wounds of the knee joint.[50] [51] The outcome of wounds of the knee joint in the early part of the war was disastrous, and was frequently association with loss of limb or life. According to Gray:

> At the record of a healed stiff joint one felt almost inclined to cheer, while the story of movement following an operation sounded like a fairy tale.[52]

Improvement in the treatment of knee wounds was due to early surgery, and the thoroughness of the procedure. The principle of treating wounds of the knee joint was exactly the same as for other wounds. Early surgery with wound excision was of paramount importance, and primary closure was essential to save the joint and retain movement. Once infection was established, then virulent infection usually resulted in disintegration of the joint and breakdown of the patient's general resistance, so that amputation was the only way to save the patient's life.

Patients were transferred promptly to a casualty clearing station in a Thomas Splint, and foreign bodies, bullets or fragments of shrapnel, were localised using X-rays. For radical limb-sparing conservative surgery, great experience was required to adequately excise the wound and yet still be able to close the joint, if not completely, then by stitching the synovial lining of the joint, thus excluding it from the "outside world" and the risk of infection. X-ray localisation of foreign bodies greatly helped in their removal. Patients whose wounds were associated with major fractures or vessel damage were best treated by immediate amputation. For others, radical wound excision and primary closure brought good results.

> Now, what were fairy tales are commonplace, and great is the satisfaction to those who were out in the dark days of surgery.

Gray discussed the treatment of infected gunshot wounds[53], gunshot wounds of the head[54], and gunshot wounds of the spinal cord[55]. Surgical treatment of head injuries will be discussed in a later chapter, although once again, the principle of early excision of devitalised tissue is the same. Gray was a protagonist of treatment of gunshot wounds by excision and primary closure[56], and he wrote a paper on removal of a bullet from a soldier's heart under local anaesthetic[57], which illustrates that he, like all others at the time, was a surgeon in the most general sense with wide ranging skills and an expansive knowledge and understanding of the problems he faced. He had very definite views about prevention and treatment of gas gangrene[58], which came down in the end to radical removal of all devitalised tissue. If there was no dead muscle left, then the patient would not develop gangrene. By the same token, if the patient had gangrene, then he could only be saved by excision of all dead tissue.

Gray was highly rated by his peers and like-minded contemporaries. John Lynn-Thomas from Cardiff was Consulting Surgeon and Deputy Inspector of Military Orthopaedics, Western Command, having been appointed to this position by Robert Jones. Publishing his remarks on a simple modification of the "guillotine" or" flapless" method of amputation of a limb, he acknowledged Gray's major contribution to the management of septic wounds of the limbs, and where amputation was necessary, he commented on Gray's method of packing amputation stumps with gauze soaked in hypertonic saline or Dakin's sodium hypochlorite solution.[59]

Lynn-Thomas was also strongly linked to Robert Jones in his ideology. He published an appreciation of Hugh Owen Thomas in the *British Medical Journal*, and in particular the use of the Thomas Splint in military surgery, reinforcing, if any reinforcement were required, the essential role it had come to play in military orthopaedics.[60] Lynn-Thomas concluded that with the Thomas Splint, the fractured femur could be restored to perfect length and alignment. He also made reference to the failure of contemporaries to acknowledge Thomas and again highlighted the quality of the work outside of the capital:

> ... in dealing with the professional blindness of the old London school to advancements made in the Provinces.

It is sad to reflect, that had the medical establishment given Thomas his due recognition, then the British Army would have used the Thomas Splint from the outset of the Great War, and many lives, particularly in 1914 and 1915, would have been saved.

Crippled soldiers

In 1914, Robert Jones was fifty-seven years old. He joined up at once as a captain in the Reserve, and was attached to the 1st Western General Hospital. He was soon promoted to the rank of Major and as part of his responsibilities he inspected the hospitals of Western Command. He drew attention to large numbers of soldiers, with late orthopaedic problems, who would require prolonged treatment in specialised orthopaedic units.[61] They had often been passed from one hospital to another in order to free up beds, and had not been provided with the necessary continuity of care to ensure the best possible outcome from their wounds. As a result, hospitals were full to overflowing with crippled soldiers, neither fit for military duty, nor for discharge back into civilian life.

At the conclusion of his inspection, Jones wrote a damning report, which soon reached Sir Alfred Keogh, Director-General of Army Medical Services. As a result, Jones was asked to open an experimental orthopaedic unit in Alder Hey, Liverpool, in the spring of 1915. He was allocated two hundred and fifty beds, which soon expanded to five hundred and sixty.[62]

Sir Alfred Keogh had been very involved with Richard Haldane in the military reforms in 1906-1908, during which time he had worked closely with Haldane to improve efficiency of military medical care. Now, in Keogh, Jones found a very supportive ally when he was given the opportunity to help eliminate military wastage by improving management of late orthopaedic problems. The aim was to concentrate under one roof, a medical staff trained in orthopaedic surgery, and supplied with the necessary equipment to be able to provide for all stages of treatment allowing restoration of function. In

March 1916, Jones opened the first orthopaedic centre on the site of the Hammersmith Workhouse in Shepherd's Bush, London. This was made easier by a grant from the British Red Cross. In opening this centre, he was not only treating wounds inflicted by the Germans, but was also having to take on the establishment of powerful general surgeons, who did not always look favourably on specialisation and stated:

> We find a specialist for the treatment of fractured jaws; another for fractures of the thigh; and strange inconsistency, we meet with a third department, that of orthopaedics—for which a special course of a few months in some instances suffices to qualify—claiming almost the whole field of the surgery of injuries.[63]

During the development of orthopaedic services, Jones sought advice from, and welcomed the input of his colleagues Henry Gray and John Lynn-Thomas. They concluded that the most diplomatic solution would be to set up a clearing house scheme, which would perhaps minimise existing friction with the general surgical establishment and Jones wrote:

> The collection of orthopaedic cases presents a difficult problem, details of which will require considerable thought. I have had long conversations with Gray and Lynn-Thomas, and we agree that a clearing house scheme offers perhaps the least objection, and would not invite friction amongst the members of the staffs. A clear definition of the scope covered by the term "orthopaedics" should be supplied to the CO of each general hospital in the Command, making him responsible for evacuation of orthopaedic cases from his hospital and its auxiliaries into a clearing house, to which should be attached a good surgeon of orthopaedic training.[64]

It certainly required considerable tact, since Jones was effectively declaring that general hospitals were not competent to handle a large percentage of the wounded soldiers. As far as Jones was concerned, orthopaedic cases required supervision in a specially designated orthopaedic military hospital. Treatment required administration by men of special experience and knowledge, able to provide cohesion between all aspects of care. The unit was required to be able to deal with more complex cases from all over the country.[65]

In opening his first orthopaedic centre in Shepherd's Bush, Jones was seeking a demonstration institution in London which might convert sceptical or frankly hostile opinion from establishment figures.[66] At around the same time that Jones opened the first orthopaedic centre at Shepherd's Bush in London, he was made Director of Military Orthopaedics, at the instigation of Sir Alfred Keogh. In this matter, Jones had to overcome much opposition from the general surgical establishment. Sir Berkley Moynihan played a pivotal role in securing this appointment for Jones.[67]

The start of the war found Moynihan (1865-1936) attached to the 2nd Northern General Hospital of the territorial RAMC in Leeds. In November 1914 he was commissioned temporary Colonel to the Army Medical Service and left for France in December 1914. Moynihan's visit lasted until March 1915, at the conclusion of which he was called upon by Sir Alfred Keogh. In providing Keogh with a summary of his visit to the medical services on the Western Front, Moynihan expressed the view that the

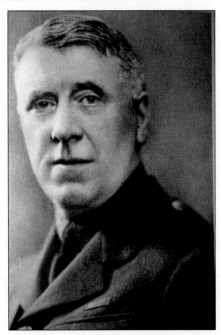

Figure 6. 8   Sir Berkeley Moynihan (1865-1936). (Private collection)

treatment of compound fractures in France was deplorable, and that the country would soon be "flooded by men doomed to deformity and crippling".[68]

Keogh realised that Moynihan wanted Robert Jones to be appointed Director of Military Orthopaedics. Keogh responded by saying that if he appointed Jones the London surgeons would have his head on a charger, to which Moynihan retorted that if Jones were not appointed, then he, Moynihan would resign. So Jones became Director of Military Orthopaedics. The story of Moynihan's influence in Military orthopaedics does not end there with the appointment of Robert Jones. The success of Alder Hey and Shepherd's Bush Orthopaedic Centre aroused opposition which was both powerful and bitter. The segregation of a wide range of wounds, under army council regulations, to be treated by a relatively small group of young and unknown surgeons selected by Robert Jones was anathema to a number of senior general surgeons in the United Kingdom.[69]

As well as installing Jones in his position as Director of Military Orthopaedics, Moynihan was also powerful enough to ensure that Jones kept his job. A formal objection to Jones' appointment was lodged with the President of the Royal College of Surgeons of England. The Council of the College at first seemed ready to rescind the appointment of Jones. Delivering the Eleventh Moynihan Lecture in Leeds on 25 May, 1961, orthopaedic surgeon Sir Harry Platt described how Moynihan, supported by Lynn-Thomas and Ernest Hey Groves:

> ... used all the eloquence at his command to dissuade the Council from taking a disastrous action. The College acted wisely.[70]

Jones remained Director of Military Orthopaedics.

Moynihan's admiration and affection for Jones remained unshaken through the years of the war and beyond. He used to refer to him as "Grandpa".[71] Moynihan's powerful and unswerving support allowed Jones to develop his orthopaedic centres while keeping opposition at bay. By the end of the war, Moynihan had been promoted to the rank of Major-General and was a powerful figure indeed. He had been chairman of the Army Medical Advisory Board since 1916, and President of the Council of Consultants 1916-1919.[72] In this role he was responsible for advising on retention and distribution of medical officers in the United Kingdom, and economy in the administration of hospitals. He was responsible for selection of electro-medical apparatus and for deciding on patterns of surgical instruments and appliances. His remit also included establishing measures for prevention and treatment of tetanus, and prevention and control of dysentery. He was responsible for selection, inspection and testing of x- ray equipment, and training of orderlies in their use. He was also responsible for pathological work undertaken in the army generally.[73]

Before the war, Moynihan had been responsible for creating the Provincial Surgeons' Club. Its objective was to bring like-minded men together to advance their surgical skills.[74] Among the founding members were John Lynn-Thomas, Henry Gray, Harold Stiles and Robert Jones.[75] [76] The Provincial Surgeons' Club had sent a clear message to the surgical establishment in London indicating that it was perfectly possible for surgical innovation and development to take place in the provinces. Most of the members of the Provincial Surgeons' Club became involved with Jones during the war.

Jones' appointment to the position of Director of Military Orthopaedics coincided with a breakdown of medical services in Mesopotamia, and there had been allegations of incompetence against some administrative aspects of surgery in France which reflected badly on Keogh, who, as Director of Army Medical Services had been placed under considerable pressure and was criticised for behaving in an autocratic sort of way, and for never referring to his Army Medical Advisory Board. He felt forced to tender his resignation. Whether or not Keogh's action had been taken in a calculated fashion to rally support, Jones and most of those who had been members of the Provincial Surgeons' Club rallied to support Keogh and ceased to be informal advisors, instead assuming a role of official agents of support and power. Meetings of the Army Medical Advisory Board, as well as Council for Consultants, which had rarely been held until then, finally convened under Moynihan as Chairman of both committees.[77]

Moynihan's chairmanship of these two committees, which had assumed power to help Keogh out of an awkward position, must also have helped to strengthen Jones' position against hostile intervention from the establishment.

After opening the first Orthopaedic Centre in Shepherd's Bush, Jones secured further centres all around the United Kingdom. Apart from the younger orthopaedic surgeons whom he trained as disciples of his methods and philosophy, he called upon his friends of peacetime days to assist him. There was Berkeley Moynihan of Leeds, Harold Stiles of Edinburgh, and John Lynn-Thomas of Cardiff. To those colleagues he owed a debt of gratitude for their support, allegiance and advice.[78] By 1918, twenty special Military Orthopaedic Centres had been established in the United Kingdom under Jones' direction, commanding 20,000 beds. At the hub was Shepherd's Bush.[79]

The fundamental structure of these centres was the same wherever they were located. An orthopaedic centre provided a staff of surgeons with previous experience in operative orthopaedics, who were able to plan a complete course of treatment for a patient. A centre also had surgeons, who though not yet specialising, were interested, and only required experience to enable them in turn to take charge of other new centres. It had young medical officers destined to go overseas, and take best possible practice to forward surgical units, thereby ensuring as much as possible that initial treatment was the best available, and thus preventing development of major problems. Orthopaedic centres also had a curative workshop component. Soldiers undergoing rehabilitation were put to work. Simply exercising a stiff joint repetitively was tedious and demoralising. Movement in association with an occupation was productive, good for morale, and restored movement.[80]

Orthopaedic restorative workshops were also economically viable. They helped to pay for themselves by doing all the maintenance work around the hospital plumbing or joinery workshops or by manufacturing splints and appliances.[81] The outcome from the first 1,300 cases treated at Shepherd's Bush was that 1,000 returned to some form of military service.[82] Overall, some 75% from all centres returned to some form of military service.[83] Table 6.3 summarises the types of treatment available at an orthopaedic centre.

Table 6.3
The functions of an orthopaedic centre

Facilities provided by Orthopaedic Centre	
Orthopaedic surgery-late problems: Delayed union Non-union-bone grafting procedures Tendon transfers Repair of peripheral nerves Fusion of joints destroyed by infection	Curative workshops: Work in a variety of trades; simply moving a joint became tedious; movement in association with an occupation moved the joint, was productive and restored morale

One of the problems Jones had to deal with was the shortage of orthopaedic surgeons to staff his orthopaedic centres. The War Office was faced with the insistent demand that all able bodied men, including medical officers, should go to France. In June 1916 there was an urgent call for five hundred doctors overseas. The medical profession as a whole was against any exceptions. To Robert Jones, however, it was important to retain surgeons under his training who were competent to deal with the clinical problems in orthopaedic centres.[84] As the number of centres progressively increased, so his staffing problem grew. The situation only became easier when Germany introduced unrestricted U-boat activity in February 1917, resulting in the sinking of American merchant ships. As a direct result of this, the United States of America entered the war in April 1917, bringing the prospect of unlimited supplies of men and material to support the allied war effort.

Robert Jones had close associations with orthopaedic surgeons in the United States. American surgeons had been frequent visitors to study Jones' work before the war, and willingly came to his assistance. One of the first things they did after the United States declared war was to send twenty orthopaedic surgeons to Great Britain in May 1917 with Joel Goldthwait, a leading American orthopaedic surgeon. These medical officers were paid by the US Military, but they were assigned to be put at the disposal of Robert Jones, and deployed as he saw fit. After a couple of months, Goldthwait returned to America, and brought another sixty orthopaedic surgeons to Britain.

In May 1917, American Orthopaedic Surgeon Robert Osgood visited those orthopaedic centres with American personnel on their staff, to report on the activities of these personnel, and to describe the work done at the centres. Osgood wrote an account of his visit to one of the centres at Old Mill Hospital in Aberdeen.[85] Old Mill Hospital is still there today, and is now better known as Glenburn Wing, Woodend Hospital.

During his visit to Aberdeen, Osgood noted that the hospital was beautifully situated about four miles outside the city, and was well equipped with a gymnasium, curative workshops, hydrotherapy and electro-therapy units, excellent operating rooms, and a photographic studio. There was an enlisted man, formerly an artist, who made the most beautiful and graphic coloured sketches of important cases. The British officer in charge of the Orthopaedic Centre was Colonel Marnoch, Regius Professor of Surgery in the University of Aberdeen. Osgood saw an interesting collection of knee cases which probably had tuberculosis of the joint; he saw old unrecognised fractures of the tibial spine and injuries to the cruciate ligaments of the knee and injuries of the cartilages within the knee (menisci).

In the curative workshops Osgood observed men making or repairing fishing nets, illustrating once more how orthopaedic centres helped to pay for their costs, while at the same time, men restored movement to stiff finger joints. He observed that there were five hundred auxiliary beds for convalescent cases in the near-by institution, and "most perfect harmony existed between the officer commanding the General Military Hospital and the Orthopaedic Centre".[86]

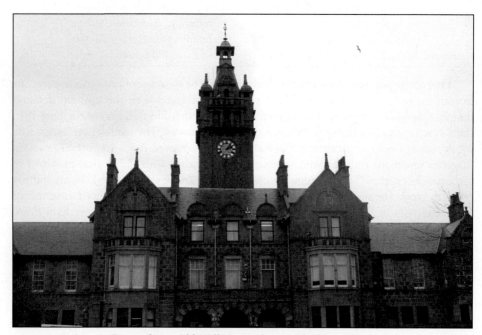

Figure 6.9   Old Mill Hospital, now Glenburn Wing,
Woodend Hospital. (Author's photograph)

The type of work undertaken can be further illustrated by referring to a compilation of works by Robert Jones entitled *Notes on Military Orthopaedics*, published in 1917.[87] Jones tactfully asked Surgeon-General Sir Alfred Keogh, Director-General Army Medical Services, to write the preface to this compilation, first published the previous year in the *British Medical Journal*. Jones clearly hoped that involving Keogh would perhaps help to win over the support of resistant elements within the surgical establishment. Whether it did so or not is debatable.

The chapters deal with many late problems which presented to Jones, and so useful are the techniques described, that the book is still readily available to this day. Jones discussed the problems of mal-union and non union of fractures; tendon transfers and late reconstruction of peripheral nerve injuries; he discussed transplantation of bone and some applications of bone grafting techniques, and provided guidance as to the best positions for fusing joints which had been destroyed by gunshot wounds.

In his introductory note, Keogh stressed just how much the problem of the maimed soldier had leapt into prominence, while in the preface Jones wrote:

> By the time a soldier has passed through various phases of recovery from septic wounds in several different hospitals and is finally transferred to an Orthopaedic Centre for treatment to correct deformity and restore use of injured joints and muscles his spirit is often broken. The shock of injury, frequently itself severe, followed in succession by a long period of suppuration, and then by a wearisome convalescence, during which he receives treatment by massage or electricity, or by monotonous movement with mechanical apparatus of the Zander type*, too often leaves him discontented with hospital life, its monotonous round of routine, and its long periods of idleness. In the orthopaedic centre, he finds his fellow patients busily engaged in employments in which they are doing something, and it is not long before he asks for a job.[88]

One of the specific problems dealt with by Jones in his orthopaedic centres was of course the ongoing management of the compound fracture of the femur.[89] Even by 1918, there remained inconsistencies in management. Those cases treated well primarily in France with a Thomas Splint arrived in the UK with the fracture maintained in good position. Jones believed the management of the compound femoral fracture should be an example of preventive orthopaedics. In other words, if the initial management had been correct, then many complications could and should have been prevented.[90] It remains a fundamental principle of surgery to this day that it is far easier to prevent a problem than it is to treat it once established. Leading on from this, Jones was a strong advocate of specially trained teams looking after compound femoral fractures to provide continuity of care of a uniformly high standard (see Chapter 2). Unfortunately, it still happened that some fractures were badly treated and arrived home in the UK with four or five inches of shortening of the leg as a result of overlap of the fractured bone ends, and every variety of deformity at the fracture site.[91]

By 1918, and the resumption of mobile warfare, patients with fractures of the femur would not infrequently have to be looked after in a tent. In Jones' opinion, it simply

---

* Jonas Gustav Wilhelm Zander (1835–1920) was a Swedish physician who invented a therapeutic method of exercise carried out by means of special apparatus.

was not possible to look after these fractures in an environment unable to support the necessary beams and pulley systems to adequately maintain position of fractures. Even surgeons of good experience were rendered impotent by such conditions.[92]

In patients with significant shortening with overlap, callus (or new healing bone) had to be broken down by manipulation, and traction using weights, with block and tackle used to stretch the muscles, and reduce overriding fragments by two and a half inches.[93] Sometimes open operation would be required, dividing the bone obliquely at the healing fracture site and then applying strong traction to the leg with block and tackle pulley system, gradually pulling the leg out to length. During this time, the leg was kept in a Thomas Splint, which also allowed correction of angulation and rotational mal-position of the fracture. The splint stayed on till the fracture was united. By these measures, more than four inches of shortening could be dealt with.[94]

Writing in 1920, Sir Anthony Bowlby discussed complications of fractures of the femur which had been documented during the last year of the war and he observed the following:[95]

1. With effective splinting, the majority of patients recovered without any significant shortening, only 5% of all cases having more than one inch of shortening.
2. The commonest mal-position was a falling backwards of the lower fragment. 20% of cases had mal-position going on to mal-union.
3. Stiffness of the knee occurred in 20% of patients, although stiffness of the hip joint was never a problem.
4. Nerve injuries were found in 12% of patients.

The statement of fewer than 5% with more than one inch of shortening does not fit with the findings of Jones at the orthopaedic centres, who described so many patients crippled by huge amounts of shortening and mal-union because of inadequate initial management. According to Jones, Orthopaedic Centres were constantly dealing with major deformities following this injury.[96]

Jones opened three orthopaedic centres in Scotland under the direction of Harold Stiles, who was Jones' deputy in Scotland, and was based at Bangour Hospital near Edinburgh. The other two Scottish centres were at the Scottish National Red Cross Hospital, Bellahouston, in Glasgow, and at Old Mill Hospital in Aberdeen. Harold Stiles was an important figure in the development of orthopaedic surgery during the war. He became very involved with the treatment of injuries of the peripheral spinal nerves, and the War Hospital at Bangour was a secondary and tertiary referral centre for the treatment of peripheral nerve injuries. In doing this work, Stiles really became a sub-specialist, in the days before orthopaedics itself had been fully accepted as a specialty.

Harold Stiles (1863-1946) graduated MB CM from the University of Edinburgh in 1885, passing the FRCS (Ed) in 1889.[97] He became assistant surgeon to the Edinburgh Sick Children's Hospital, Royal Infirmary, and Chalmers Hospital. Once established, Stiles moved from the position of surgeon to the Royal Infirmary of Edinburgh to the Children's Hospital, where he made his reputation in bone and joint surgery.[98] When the Mayo brothers from the United States visited the United Kingdom prior to setting up their own orthopaedic unit in the United States, it was Jones and Stiles they regarded as the orthopaedic authorities in the United Kingdom, and visited them both.[99]

After one visit by American surgeons to his unit in Edinburgh, Stiles wrote to his friend Jones:

> I must not close this letter without taking the opportunity of telling you that your name and your work were on the lips of every one of them, and you may take it from me that they were more pleased with your work than any other they had seen. I do not hesitate to tell you this, firstly because I know that it is true, and secondly because I know it will be both an encouragement and a satisfaction to you to know that all your hard and splendid work was greatly appreciated and from what I hear too, the hospitality you showed them was as usual unbounded.[100]

Both Stiles and Jones were original members of the Moynihan Provincial Surgeons' Club, founded in 1909. When Moynihan co-founded the British Journal of Surgery in 1913 with Ernest Hey-Groves, others on the editorial committee were Robert Jones, Harold Stiles, and John Lynn-Thomas.[101]

Stiles followed up his interest in injuries of the peripheral spinal nerves by writing a very informative book entitled *Treatment of Injuries of the Peripheral Nerves*, which was published in 1922. It deals comprehensively with every type of peripheral nerve injury encountered during the Great War, with descriptions of exposure and repair of these injuries. It deals with tendon transfers appropriate for every type of lesion, when repair of the nerve was not an option. No surgeon before or since can have had as much experience in the treatment of peripheral nerve injuries and his book is still available today, having been reprinted for the current generation of orthopaedic surgeons.[102]

Moynihan, too, as consulting surgeon with Northern Command, published work on management of wounds of the peripheral nerves, acknowledging help from his colleagues on the staff of the 2nd Northern General Hospital in Leeds. It was his view that the earliest possible examination be made of a wound with a suspected nerve injury. End to end suture (stitching the two ends of the nerve together) at a casualty clearing station would be the first opportunity to repair a nerve in many cases. If secondary suture of wounds was being performed, then that too would provide an opportunity for repair of nerve injuries. If, because of infection early repair was not possible, then late repair was the only available option. It was important to ensure that joints be kept moving, and muscles kept supple, to allow repair to be performed and yet retain the possibility of a satisfactory functional outcome. Moynihan was of the opinion that nerve grafting was of little value, and tendon transfer was useful when nerve suture impossible.[103]

The various procedures described above all help to illustrate the types of cases likely to be dealt with in an orthopaedic centre. Such patients not only required corrective surgery, but also needed the facilities of the restorative workshop to regain function of their limbs.

Stiles was appointed to be a member of the commission which investigated the administration of military hospitals in France and Britain. Along with Moynihan and Jones, he was a member of the revived Army Medical Advisory Board, which in June 1918 had to withstand an attempt by a committee of the Council of the Royal College of Surgeons to restrict the role of orthopaedics.[104] Presided over by George Makins, President of the Royal College of Surgeons of England, the committee stated that it…

> … regarded with mistrust and disapprobation the movement in progress to remove the treatment of conditions always properly regarded as the main portion of the general surgeon's work from his hands, and place it in those of the "Orthopaedic Specialists"; and thus to educate the layman to the belief that the British surgeon is incapable of dealing with the majority of the most serious injuries the body may sustain.[105]

After the war, Stiles was awarded a knighthood in 1919. He was appointed to be Professor of Surgery, University of Edinburgh, and in the 1920s he played an active role in establishing a Chair of Orthopaedic Surgery in Edinburgh. He was also instrumental in founding a hospital for crippled children, the Princess Margaret Rose Hospital. He was made an honorary fellow of the British Orthopaedic Association.[106] Writing in 1919 about his experience in the war, he emphasised the evolution of the technique of early wound excision as a prophylaxis against sepsis in war surgery, and how it could be used in the treatment of industrial injuries. The Thomas Splint, such an advance in the treatment of fractures of the femur during the war, should become an essential part of the armamentarium of the post-war treatment of fractures of the femur.[107]

Stiles wrote about the experience of the pathologists and microbiologists during the war, and the creation of a new epoch in microbiology, with important research into anaerobic organisms of gas gangrene and tetanus.[108] The chief lesson Stiles learned from the war was the value of team work by young men guided by the wider general experience of their seniors and he stated the following:

> The surgery of the war has been the surgery of young men – men with keen and receptive brains, men who have been trained in the fundamental medical sciences and who have been able to apply their knowledge not merely to the improving of old methods of treatment, but also to the devising of new methods to meet the new conditions they had to deal with and the new environment in which they found themselves. It is largely due to the teamwork by younger men that great advances have been made, not only in wound treatment, but in the early and late treatment of fractures, especially fractures of the femur, in wounds involving joints, in injuries to the nerves, and in military orthopaedics generally.[109]

In the preface to his book *The Early Treatment of War Wounds*, Sir Henry Gray exhibited a very similar sentiment when he expressed the view that this was a young man's war, in surgery as well as military matters. The progress of events demanded that younger men should have every chance in a sphere of action where mental and bodily activity counted for so much.[110]

Gray felt very fortunate and privileged to have been able to make constructive recommendations for management of wounded soldiers. These recommendations were:

... the outcome of concentrated observation and thought by one who has had unusual opportunities, and of discussion with numerous brilliant young surgeons possessed of fresh, active brains and equally dexterous hands.[111]

Reference has already been made to the American contribution to the war, and the important role they had to play in medical manpower in general and in orthopaedic surgery in particular. The Americans made one further major contribution. Before the war ended, the Americans, Osgood in particular, stimulated the necessary confidence and unity among the British orthopaedic surgeons to establish the British Orthopaedic Association. The inaugural meeting was held in the Cafe Royal on 28 November 1917, and the first scientific meeting was on 2 February 1918.

During the war, roughly 6,000,000 British officers, nursing sisters, and other ranks, excluding Indian and Dominion troops, served their country. Of this total, 750,000 or 12.5% had been killed or died of wounds. 600,000 or 10% had been discharged from the service as disabled, with some form of pension or gratuity.[112] By the end of March 1920, demobilisation and discharge had been nearly completed, and a very large number of men had been examined for disabilities claimed as due to war service. Between 11 November 1918 and 31 March 1920, 335,000 men were discharged from army hospitals as disabled by war service, and were awarded a pension or gratuity upon discharge from hospital. A further 485,000 had been granted a pension or gratuity as the result of a successful claim made at the time of demobilisation.[113] Thus by 31 March 1920, 1,420,000 or 23.6% of the total who had served, had been awarded a pension or gratuity.[114]

By 31 March 1930 that figure had risen to 1,664,000, or 27.7%. If one adds the 750,000 deaths casualties, then the total numbers affected by the war by death or disablement was 40.2% of those who served.[115] Of those who were disabled, an assessment was carried out on 31 March 1929. Of 1,595,000 who had been in receipt of a pension, only 1,475,000 were still alive. 120,000 had died. It was estimated that between 60% and 70% of the deaths were either due to, or were related to the pensionable disability.[116] In an analysis of stabilised awards, at 31 March 1929, 46% were the result of ongoing problems with either a wound, mostly, but not exclusively orthopaedic, or by an amputation.[117]

Between the years 1920 and 1929, the Ministry of Pensions issued 95,201 artificial legs, and 20,079 artificial arms. That is not to say there were necessarily fewer upper limb amputees. An artificial leg is a necessity. Without it, walking is impossible. An artificial arm is at best a useful tool, which might contribute a small functional benefit, but is a poor substitute for the extremely complex functions of the human hand. At worse, an artificial arm is a useless encumbrance, fit only to be thrown in the bin![118] [119]

Thus many of the disabilities that persisted after the war were orthopaedic related ones. After the war, Jones had hoped that orthopaedic departments would be attached to hospital departments, but alas, this was not to be. The surgical establishment would not willingly relinquish a sizeable part of its empire. Symbolic of the prevailing mood, in April 1925, Shepherd's Bush was restored to its original function as a workhouse and poor law infirmary.[120] Most other orthopaedic centres met the same fate. The vision of Harold Stiles ensured that Edinburgh established an orthopaedic academic department, but although the British Orthopaedic Association had been born during the war, it would be some years before orthopaedic surgery would be acknowledged as a worthy specialty.

Nevertheless, thanks to the pioneering work done during the war years, the surgical principles of war surgery were firmly established, and are as relevant today in Afghanistan, Iraq, and any other war zone as they were in the years 1914 to 1918. In three and a half years of concentrated experience of war wounds on a scale hitherto unimaginable, and in collaboration with many brilliant young surgeons, Henry Gray defined those principles, and found his destined place.

At a time when civilian practice is lulled into using this or that dressing, and has become used to employing antibiotics to resolve the problems related to infection, it is essential to remember the words of Henry Gray, in his timeless book, *The Early Treatment of War Wounds* when he says:

> The early opening up and mechanical cleansing of severe wounds are necessary preliminaries to any other form of treatment.

Notes

1   Watson, F., *The Life of Sir Robert Jones*. London: Hodder & Stoughton, 1934, p.276.

2   Watson, *op.cit.*, p.26.

3   Lynn-Thomas, J., "A reconsideration of the principles and methods of Hugh Owen Thomas", *British Medical Journal* 1916; 2: pp.71-72.

4   Watson, *op.cit.*, p.63.

5   Cooter, R., *Surgery and Society in Peace and War*. Basingstoke: Macmillan, 1993, p.76.

6   Watson, *op.cit.*, pp.128-129.

7   Dudley, H. & I. Levack, *Aberdeen Royal Infirmary, the Peoples' Hospital in the North East*. London: Baillière Tindall, 1992, p.97.

8   Porter, R.M.M., "Recent Aberdeen Teachers: Sir Henry Gray, KBE, CB, CMG, LLD, FRCS(Ed)", *Aberdeen Postgraduate Medical Bulletin*, October 1971; pp.11-13.

9   Porter, *op.cit.*, pp.11-13.

10   *Ibid*.

11   Smith, F.K., "Sir Henry Gray, KBE, CB, CMG", *The Aberdeen University Review* 1938-39; XXVI: pp.47-48.

12   Gray, Col. H.M.W., *The Early Treatment of War Wounds*. London: Henry Frowde, 1919, p.ix.

13   *Roll of Service in the Great War*. Aberdeen: University of Aberdeen, 1921, p.216.

14   *Roll of Graduates, University of Aberdeen 1926-1955*. Aberdeen: University of Aberdeen, 1960, p.1271.

15   Watson, *op.cit.*, p.158.

16   Gray, *op.cit.*, p.59.

17   Porter, *op.cit.*, pp.11-13.

18   *Royal Army Medical Corps Training Handbook*. London: HMSO, 1911, p.345.

19   Jones, R., "The orthopaedic outlook in military surgery", *British Medical Journal* 1918; 1: pp.41-45.

20   Jones, *op.cit.*, pp.41-45.

21   Bowlby, A., "Gunshot fractures of the femur", *British Medical Journal* 1920; 1: pp.1-4.

22   Whitehead, I.R., *Doctors in the Great War*. Barnsley: Leo Cooper, 1999, p.207.

23   Cooter, *op.cit.*, p.111.

24   Gray, *op.cit.*, p.59.

25   *Ibid*.

26 Marshall, G., "The administration of anaesthesia at the Front", *British Medical Journal* 1917; 2: pp.722-725.

27 Marshall, *op.cit.*, pp.722-725.

28 Gray, *op.cit.*, p.60.

29 *Ibid.*

30 *Ibid.*, p.239.

31 *Ibid.*.

32 MacPherson, W.G. (ed.), *History of the Great War based on Official Documents. Medical Services. General History.* London: HMSO, 1924, Volume 3, p.143.

33 Gray, *op.cit.*, p.246.

34 *Ibid.*, pp.111-115.

35 Dakin, H.D., "On the use of certain antiseptic substances in the treatment of infected wounds", *British Medical Journal* 1915; 2: pp.318-320.

36 Gray, *op.cit.*, p.122.

37 Jones, *op.cit.*, pp.41-45.

38 MacPherson, *op.cit.*, Volume 2, pp.74-75.

39 *Ibid.*

40 Carberry, A.D., *The New Zealand Medical Services in the Great War.* Auckland: Whitcomb & Tombs, 1924, p.399.

41 *Ibid.*

42 *Ibid.*

43 Bowlby, A.., "The mortality of cases of fractured femur", *British Medical Journal* 1919; 1: p.112.

44 Gray, H.M.W., "The mortality of cases of fractured femur", *British Medical Journal* 1919; 1: p.142.

45 *Ibid.*

46 *Ibid.*

47 *Ibid.*

48 Bowlby, A., "Gunshot fractures of the femur", *British Medical Journal* 1920; 1: pp.1-4.

49 Gray, H.M.W., "Hypertonic treatment of wounds", *British Medical Journal* 1915; 2: p.32.

50 Gray, H.M.W., "Early treatment of gunshot wounds of the knee", *British Medical Journal* 1917; 2: pp.278-280.

51 Gray, H.M.W., "General treatment of infected gunshot wounds", *British Medical Journal* 1915; 2: pp.41-43.

52 *Ibid.*

53 Gray, H.M.W., "General treatment of gunshot wounds", *British Medical Journal* 1916; 1: pp.1-7.

54 Gray, H.M.W., "Gunshot wounds of the head", *British Medical Journal* 1916; 1: pp.261-265.

55 Gray, H.M.W., "Early treatment of gunshot injuries of the spinal cord", *British Medical Journal* 1917; 2: pp.44-45.

56 Gray, H.M.W., "Treatment of gunshot wounds by excision and primary closure", *British Medical Journal* 1915; 2: p.317.

57 Gray, H.M.W., "Removal of a bullet from the right ventricle of the heart under local anaesthesia", *British Medical Journal* 1915; 2: pp.561-562.

58 Gray, H.M.W., "An essential principle in the treatment of gas gangrene", *British Medical Journal* 1918; 1: p.369.

59 Lynn-Thomas, J., "A simple modification of the guillotine or flapless method of amputation", *British Medical Journal* 1916; 2: pp.481-482.

60   Lynn-Thomas, J., "A reconsideration of the principles of Hugh Owen Thomas", *British Medical Journal* 1916; 2: pp.71-75, 175-179.

61   Watson, *op.cit.*, p.147.

62   *Ibid*, pp.148-149.

63   Makins, G.H., "Introductory", *British Journal of Surgery* 1918, Vol. 6, Issue 21, pp.1-11.

64   Watson, *op.cit.*, pp.165-166.

65   *Ibid*.

66   *Ibid*.

67   Platt, H., "Moynihan; The Education and Training of the Surgeon. Eleventh Moynihan Lecture delivered University of Leeds 25 May 1961", *Annals of the Royal College of Surgeons of England* 1962; 30 (4): pp.220-228.

68   *Ibid*.

69   *Ibid*.

70   *Ibid*.

71   *Ibid*.

72   MacPherson, *op.cit.*, Volume 1, p.151.

73   *Ibid*.

74   Cooter, *op.cit.*, pp.46-50.

75   *Ibid*.

76   Smith, *op.cit.*, pp.47-48.

77   Cooter, *op.cit.*, p.116.

78   Watson, *op.cit.*, p.170.

79   Cooter, *op.cit.*, pp.105-106.

80   Jones, *op.cit.*, pp.41-45.

81   Watson, *op.cit.*, p.169.

82   Osgood, R.B., "The Orthopaedic Centres of Great Britain and their American medical officers", *Journal of Bone and Joint Surgery (American)* 1918; 2-16: pp.132-140.

83   *Ibid*, p.140.

84   Watson, *op.cit.*, p.171.

85   Osgood, *op.cit.*, pp.134-135.

86   *Ibid*.

87   Jones, R., *Notes on Military Orthopaedics*. London: Cassell, 1917.

88   Jones, R., *Notes on Military Orthopaedics*. London: Cassell, 1917.

89   Jones, R., "The orthopaedic outlook in military surgery", *British Medical Journal* 1918; 1: pp.42-43.

90   *Ibid*.

91   *Ibid*.

92   *Ibid*.

93   Jones, R., *Notes on Military Orthopaedics*. London: Cassell, 1917, p.77.

94   *Ibid*.

95   Bowlby, A., "Gunshot fractures of the femur", *British Medical Journal* 1920; 1: p.4.

96   Jones, R., "The orthopaedic outlook in military surgery", *British Medical Journal* 1918; 1: pp.42-43.

97   Obituary, Sir Harold Stiles, *British Medical Journal* 1946; 1: p.702.

98   Cooter, *op.cit.*, p.43.

99   *Ibid*.

100   Watson, *op.cit.*, p.128.

101   Cooter, *op.cit.*, pp.46-50.

102 Stiles, H.H., *Treatment of Injuries of the Peripheral Spinal Nerves*. London: Henry Frowde, 1922.

103 Moynihan, B., "Injuries of peripheral nerves and their treatment", *British Medical Journal* 1917; pp.571-574.

104 Cooter, *op.cit.*, p.133.

105 *Ibid.*

106 *Ibid.*, pp.42-43.

107 Stiles, H., "Surgical training", *British Medical Journal* 1919; 2: pp.487-489.

108 *Ibid.*

109 *Ibid.*

110 Gray, Col. H.M.W., *The Early Treatment of War Wounds*. London: Henry Frowde, 1919, pp.ix-xi.

111 *Ibid.*

112 Mitchell, T.J. & G.M. Smith, *History of the Great War based on Official Documents. Medical Services. Casualties and Medical Statistics*. London: HMSO, 1931, p.315.

113 *Ibid.*

114 *Ibid.*

115 *Ibid.*

116 *Ibid.*, p.317.

117 *Ibid.*, p.320.

118 *Ibid.*, p.339.

119 Scotland, T.R. & R.J. Galway, "A long term review of children with congenital and acquired upper limb deficiencies", *Journal of Bone and Joint Surgery* 1983; May 65 (3): pp.346-349.

120 Cooter, *op.cit.*, p.131.

7

Abdominal wounds: Evolution of management and establishment of surgical treatments

Steven D Heys

The medical challenges faced by surgeons during the Great War were unparalleled in the history of warfare and were primarily the results of advances in technology and weaponry that had occurred before the war started and also by the pace of scientific development during four years of conflict. The weaponry and munitions, the velocity and characteristics of projectiles and their flight paths, the severe damage inflicted upon tissues (which had been recognised to occur at distances away from where the actual projectile had travelled), the contamination from the soldiers' clothes and the surrounding ground (agricultural land which had been subject to heavy fertilisation with manure etc) were all major factors in the likelihood of severe wounding and death. Furthermore, there was a realisation that the conditions endured by the soldiers, for example, stress and the environment, reduced their resistance to infectious complications of their wounds.[1] Whilst these factors are discussed elsewhere in this book it is important to remember that they are especially relevant with respect to abdominal wounds.

Abdominal wounds have been a major problem in warfare since time immemorial. They comprised approximately 2% of all the wounded who reached a field ambulance in the Great War.[2] Many casualties with abdominal wounds, however, did not survive, and died before reaching surgical help. The most serious nature of abdominal wounds results from damage occurring to the vital organs that lie within the abdomen itself. The abdomen not only presents a large target area on the front of a person but also objects may enter it through the back and buttock areas. Furthermore, penetrating objects entering the body at distances away from the abdomen itself, for example from as far away as the neck down to the knees, have been recorded as being able to track through the body's tissues and locate themselves within the abdomen and cause serious damage. Doctors and surgeons had previously regarded these wounds as fatal and soldiers sustaining abdominal wounds did not undergo surgery and usually died, although there were isolated reported cases where soldiers had survived. This is understandable because of limitations in medical knowledge that existed at the time. But just why is the abdomen so important and why are the consequences of a penetrating injury so severe?

How common are perforating abdominal injuries and what causes them?

The numbers and percentages of casualties who sustained penetrating abdominal wounds has varied over the years in different military conflicts. Based on previous wars it was thought that about 15% of all casualties would have abdominal wounds. It has been stated before that it is often not possible to have accurate and complete data during warfare, and the estimated percentage figure also depends on where the data are recorded. For example, casualties might die on the battlefield and their causes of death may never be documented.

However, carefully recorded data in the field ambulances revealed that only 1.92% of all wounds were in the abdomen, and when documented at the casualty clearing stations this had dropped to 0.72% of all wounds.[3] Although this is a small percentage, in absolute terms it represents a large number of cases given the huge number of wounded who were dealt with during the war. The reasons for these differences in figures may be partly attributable to over diagnosis in the field ambulance. Also some casualties with severe abdominal wounds would not have survived the journey from the field ambulance to the casualty clearing station. This was important information for the Army's medical services because it demonstrated that abdominal wounds were relatively infrequent. Even those surgeons with a particular interest in the management of these casualties understood that when medical services were being delivered in the battlefields it was important that "all arrangements must be made so that the greatest good is done to the greatest number". There was an understanding of the need to provide the best medical care possible but there was as importantly an understanding as to the limitations of what could be provided. The causes of these wounds are shown in Table 7.1; this information is taken from two carefully reported series by Captains Fraser and Drummond.[4] [5]

Table 7.1

Causes of perforating abdominal wounds

Organ wounded	Bullet (%)	Shell/bomb (%)	Bayonet (%)
Stomach	46.2	53.8	0
Small intestine	15.5	16.2	0
Large intestine (colon)	11.9	16.2	0
Rectum	13.2	2.0	0
Bladder	3.6	1.0	0
Kidney	2.6	6.9	0
Spleen	2.3	2.3	0
Liver	49.5	56.1	0.3

Data from Fraser J. & H. Drummond, "A clinical and experimental study of three hundred perforating wounds of the abdomen", *British Medical Journal* 1917; 1: pp.321-330.

A range of bullets was used during the war of varying calibres and velocities. Furthermore, there were differences between the characteristics of British, French and German bullets, but it was the latter, of course, that were most important to the Allied forces. Differences, for example, included their weights and flight characteristics, and that German bullets were more likely to break into their core and mantle components on impact.[6] Experience with large numbers of wounds led to a better understanding of the flight of bullets and how this determined the type and severity of the wound that they inflicted. It was understood that the flight of a bullet leaving the muzzle of the gun has two components, its velocity along the line of the flight and a spin about its longitudinal axis, imparted by the rifling of the barrel. If the bullet impacts on a solid object whether inside or outside the body, it may develop a tumbling motion. It is this which made the effects of rifle wounds particularly unpredictable.

Shell, shrapnel, grenade and bomb fragments were of varying sizes and shapes and caused different types and severity of wounds. Some key features are shown in Table 7.2. Bayonet wounds, as can be seen from Table 7.1, were uncommon. Perhaps this was because bayonets caused so much damage that soldiers wounded in this way died very rapidly on the battlefield and before the medical services had any chance of reaching them to start treatment.

Table 7.2
Features of shell, shrapnel and grenades considered to be important

Type of exploding device	Key characteristics
High-explosive shells	May explode either in the air, on the ground or after burying itself into the ground. Steel case and high explosive variable but included picric acid, TNT, mixtures of TNT and ammonium nitrate. The shape of the fragments of metal varied and moved outwards from the centre of the explosion in all directions.
Shrapnel	Shrapnel shell was usually 75mm in size and contained about 300 lead balls each ½" diameter. It was timed to explode as it was angling towards the ground and balls travelled forwards with the velocity at which it was travelling, determining the extent of the wounds caused.
Bombs and grenades	Varying types but often designed so that on explosion they broke up into quadrilateral fragments of different sizes.
Trench mortars	There were three sizes of German mortars, whose projectiles were designed to come straight down on the enemy. Comprised a high explosive charge around a thin metal shell which exploded just above or on the ground, fragmenting into jagged pieces.

Why are perforating abdominal wounds so important?

The abdomen contains many vital organs that are predominantly concerned with the digestion and absorption of food amongst other important functions. Food enters the stomach through the gullet (oesophagus) and then passes through the stomach, where it is mechanically mixed and the process of digestion begins. It passes to the small intestine where digestion and absorption of the majority of the nutrients from the food is completed. The liver, through the production of bile which is stored in the gall bladder before passing into the small intestine, the pancreas, and the small intestine itself, produce many different chemicals to aid digestion (breakdown) of food and these substances are called enzymes. It is important to note that as long as these enzymes stay within the intestine itself they do exactly what they are intended to do but if they escape

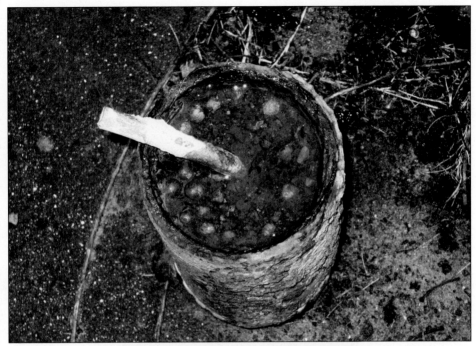

Figure 7.1   A shrapnel bomb, unexploded and found near
Passchendaele, 2009. (Author's photograph)

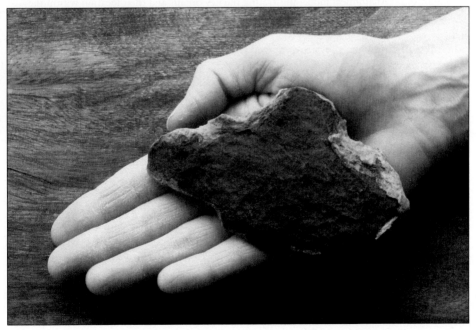

Figure 7.2   Example of a shell fragment found at Serre in 2009; similar
fragments caused penetrating abdominal wounds. (Author's photograph)

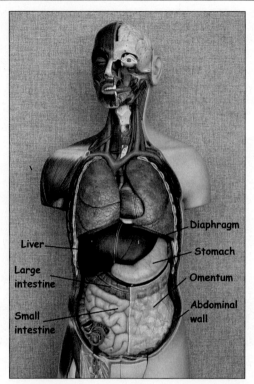

Figure 7.3   Anatomical model illustrating the key organs and their location within the
abdominal cavity. (Ian Brown, Department of Anatomy, University of Aberdeen)

from these organs when they are damaged then they will cause damage to the organs and
body tissues within the abdomen itself.

The material in the small bowel is really like liquid faeces and contains large
numbers of bacteria. These bacteria are helpful to a person as long as they stay within the
lumen of the bowel because they will help in the digestion of food and also themselves
make nutrients to be absorbed and utilised in a variety of body processes. However, if
these bacteria get out of the intestine, for example, because of a hole in the intestine
caused by a penetrating object, they will cause damage by producing inflammation
inside the abdomen which is called peritonitis. These bacteria will multiply and they can
also invade the bloodstream (called septicaemia) and produce chemicals called toxins,
which can damage all the organs in the body and result in many different organs not
working properly and failing. This is called multi-organ failure and usually results in
death, although nowadays with powerful antibiotics, modern intensive therapy units
and the various life support mechanisms, it is possible to make a full recovery if multi-
organ failure happens – but not always, even today.

From the small intestine the liquid material passes into the large intestine (colon)
where absorption of water and some electrolytes such as sodium occurs. This results in
the material now having the consistency of a bowel motion (faeces) and this is evacuated
via the back passage (rectum). Again the large bowel contains many bacteria, more than
the small bowel, and the same consequences will occur if the large intestine is damaged

as happens when the small intestine is damaged. The abdomen also contains other key organs such as the liver, pancreas, kidneys and bladder and their functions are outlined in Table 7.3.

In addition to causing disruption of these organs, the other major effect of a perforating wound to the abdomen is bleeding which is commonly referred to as haemorrhage. These vital organs all have a very rich blood supply which is carried to the organ by blood vessels termed arteries and then away from the organ by the veins. These are large vessels and may carry to the liver, for example, more than a litre of blood per minute. Given that the volume of blood circulating around the body is about 5 to 6 litres in total for the average man, a hole in one of these major blood vessels of only a few millimetres will result in a very rapid loss of blood leading to hypovolaemic shock (lack of volume of blood), where the body's vital organs do not have enough blood containing nutrients and oxygen to maintain their functions.

Death will occur very quickly if loss of blood volume is not restored promptly by giving fluid replacement and if bleeding is not stopped. This requires a surgical operation. In addition to the organs mentioned and their own blood vessels, there are two major vessels termed the aorta and the inferior vena cava which run along the posterior wall of the abdomen. The aorta is the main artery in the body and takes all the blood which the heart pumps out (containing oxygen and nutrients) and distributes it through a series of branches to these different organs. The inferior vena cava is the main vein which returns blood which has come from all the organs in the abdomen and also the legs, to the heart. As the volumes of blood passing through these blood vessels is huge, then damage by a penetrating object results in almost immediate exsanguination and death.

Table 7.3
Key functions of important organs located within the abdomen

Organ	Functions	Consequences of damage
Stomach	Mechanical mixing of food and start of digestion through enzymes produced.	Escape of contents with peritonitis and bleeding.
Small intestine	Breakdown of food into small constituent molecules and absorption into the blood.	Escape of contents with peritonitis and bleeding.
Large intestine	Absorption of water and electrolytes and production of faeces.	Escape of contents with peritonitis and bleeding.
Liver	Manufacture of a range of proteins, carbohydrates and fats for many bodily functions. Production of bile to help digestion of food within the small bowel.	Escape of bile into the abdomen resulting in peritonitis and bleeding.
Gall bladder	On the under-surface of the liver, acting as a reservoir for bile. When food is taken in squirts bile into the small intestine though a tube-like structure called the bile duct.	Damage to the gall bladder or bile duct results in the escape of bile into the abdomen leading to peritonitis.

Pancreas	Produces enzymes for digestion of food in the small intestine and insulin to prevent diabetes from occurring.	Enzymes escape from the pancreas into the inside of the abdomen and may digest the body's own organs. Bleeding may occur with many large blood vessels very close to the pancreas.
Kidney	Production of urine.	Escape of urine into the abdomen and peritonitis, or kidney failure and death if kidney destroyed. Bleeding can also occur.
Bladder	Storage of urine produced by the kidney.	Escape of urine into the abdomen and peritonitis. Bleeding may also occur.

How were abdominal injuries being managed up to the start of the Great War?

A time of great advance in the science and practice of surgery occurred in the 18th Century with major contributions to the understanding of anatomy, and how the body works being made by many surgeons. One outstanding figure was John Hunter, a surgeon and scientist, born in East Kilbride, the youngest of 10 children. He dropped out of school at the age of 13 after the death of his father and spent some time working for a carpenter, where his manual skills were certainly evident from all accounts. At 20 years of age he went to London to work with his brother William, who was an emerging obstetrician and anatomist. John then decided to study medicine, and studied at the Chelsea and St Bartholomew's Hospitals before qualifying. John Hunter pursued his surgical career in London and understood that surgery could only progress and advance with a scientific approach, which he duly adopted in every aspect of his work. He was perhaps considered as one of the first surgeon scientists in the world.

Hunter tackled many of the diseases and problems which were facing surgeons at that time. He developed an understanding of inflammation, blood circulation in the unborn child and its relationship to the mother's circulation. He studied the lymphatic system, diseases of blood vessels and he also developed the understanding of teeth and dentition. He would go to great pains to understand disease and he even inoculated himself with venereal disease to further understand this condition – not that this can have met with the approval of his wife, Ann! He studied anatomy in particular, as this was key to the practice of surgery. He founded his own anatomy school in London as well as being a practicing surgeon at St George's Hospital and being appointed as surgeon to King George III. His interest in military surgery led to his appointment to the British Army as deputy surgeon and then to the post of Surgeon-General in 1790, having been assistant Surgeon-General for a total of four years prior to this.[7]

His great experience led to significant developments in civilian and in war surgery, the latter never more so than in France and Portugal. He wrote about his surgical work there and made original contributions to the literature about gunshot wounds and how they should be treated. His book, *Treatise on Blood, Inflammation and Gunshot Wounds* which was published in 1794, after he died, was regarded as a definitive manual for treatment. However, he advocated that it was not necessary to open and explore wounds

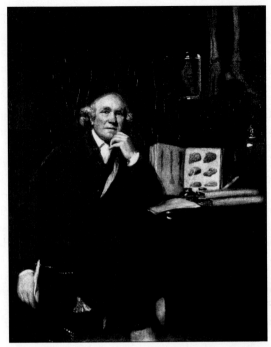

Figure 7.4   Portrait of John Hunter FRCS by Joshua Reynolds. (By kind permission of the Royal College of Surgeons of England)

and like other surgeons before him he was not able to take forwards the understanding and management of casualties with perforating abdominal wounds. He actually wrote that treatment for abdominal wounds should consist of "a tepid bath in order to supply fluid to the general constitution".[8] It is important to remember that anaesthesia was not introduced until the middle of the 19th century and not having anaesthesia played a major role in limiting what surgeons were able to do. Not only that, but at this time there was little understanding of microbiology and infection. Control of infection and knowledge of sanitation was rudimentary. These aspects and the massive impact that all of these had on mortality and morbidity during warfare are discussed in detail elsewhere in this book.

The orthodox surgical view and teaching that continued during the next 100 years and more, through subsequent conflicts such as the American Civil War, Franco-Prussian War, and the American-Spanish War was that casualties with abdominal wounds should be managed without surgery, that is with what was termed "expectant management". The recommended treatment was to put them in the Fowler position (semi-upright with knees straight or bent, so as to relieve tension on the abdominal muscles and assist breathing), to keep the patients warm and not give them anything to eat or drink for three days, to provide morphine, and to administer saline solution given through the rectum (back passage) to combat dehydration.[9] [10] Of course, such wounds were generally fatal.

The general view prevailed that surgery could be harmful in this situation and that if the intestine was damaged then death always occurred. It was therefore better to do nothing. This philosophy was further supported by the observation that some casualties did survive perforating abdominal wounds.[11] Furthermore, there was a school of thought that the intestine could heal itself even if it was damaged and perforated. This does not usually happen and these patients will die except in very rare instances. Those who do survive usually do so because they have not sustained significant damage within the abdomen itself.

The problem facing the surgeon with the casualty on the Western Front, with a perforating abdominal wound, was what to do with such a patient, once significant damage to the contents of the abdomen was suspected.

Unfortunately, by the outbreak of the Great War surgeons were still questioning the value of proceeding to early surgical exploration of the abdomen to identify if wounds had occurred and to repair any damage discovered. Such an exploratory procedure is called a "laparotomy". The British policy at the start of the Great War in 1914 was not to operate on such casualties but simply to treat them as already described above with "expectant management". The basis for this firm position had resulted from an emphasis on the poor results of operative treatment which had been reported by surgeons in the Spanish-American War, the American Civil War, The Balkan conflicts, the French war in Morocco and the Franco-Prussian War, where death was nearly always the outcome for the casualty.[12] [13]

In the USA surgeons had given considerable thought to the matter and had discussed the possibility of early laparotomy but the general consensus, even though some did favour early surgery, was that in the military situation this should not be done.[14] To further fuel the debate, there were reports of small numbers of casualties who had survived significant abdominal wounds without undergoing surgery at all.[15]

This position taken by the medical profession was unfortunate and most certainly resulted in the avoidable deaths of many casualties. Indeed, in retrospect, there were missed opportunities for the earlier development of successful abdominal surgery for perforating abdominal wounds. Firstly, an opportunity was missed during the Boer War (1899-1902). At that time the policy for perforating abdominal wounds was still the expectant management one, although there was some support for earlier surgical intervention. A few surgeons did carry out surgical exploration of perforating abdominal wounds but unfortunately statistical analyses of wounds in this war were limited, incomplete and not considered to be truly representative.[16] However, the results did not seem to be supportive of an operative approach to perforating abdominal wounds. In the whole of the war only 207 abdominal wounds were recorded. Of these, only 26 casualties underwent abdominal surgery and 18 of these (nearly 70%) died.

Unfortunately as far as surgical progress and development was concerned, there appeared to be a significant success rate for those casualties who were managed by the expectant approach in the Boer War. Amongst that number there were two RAMC officers who had both sustained gunshot wounds to the abdomen and who had survived with expectant treatment. This gave even more support to those who viewed expectant treatment as a better option than surgery and who could cite the treatment of doctors themselves as good examples of how expectant treatment worked.[17]

At that time the consulting surgeon to the British Army was Sir William MacCormac. In previous years, MacCormac had been of the opinion that surgery offered the best chance of a successful outcome. That view changed, however, presumably on the basis of poor results reported from other conflicts and from the Boer War itself, and cemented his now negative views as to the value of surgery for perforating abdominal wounds. Perhaps the most often quoted summary of his views became known as MacCormac's aphorism – "In this war a man wounded in the abdomen dies if he is operated upon and remains alive if he is left in peace".[18]

However, there was indeed a missed opportunity, and in retrospect, an indication as to what the problem was. Although the results of surgery were generally poor there was a report of the successful management of two casualties undergoing surgery. In both cases the casualties were operated on within 12 hours of sustaining their wounds. Both these soldiers underwent successful resection and anastomosis (joining together) of the small intestine and survived.[19] [20] So here was a clue that early operation for casualties was going to be crucially important if a successful outcome was to be achieved.

Perhaps the most important piece of work that would have improved the management of casualties with these wounds in the Great War was ignored by British surgeons in particular, and Western surgeons generally. This work was carried out in Russia at the turn of the 20th century during the Russo-Japanese war of 1904-1905 where again the standard care for perforating abdominal wounds was the expectant method. Indeed, Western surgeons and it is thought MacCormac himself, had influenced thinking and practice amongst Russian military surgeons through his membership of the Russian Imperial Military Academy of Medicine. During this conflict, the results of expectant management of perforating abdominal wounds were again poor, with casualties dying in large numbers. One surgeon, however, was not prepared to accept the standard teaching and challenged the orthodox approach by carrying out early abdominal surgery. Her name was Vera Gedroits.

Vera Gedroits was born in Kiev in 1876. She was a Lithuanian princess who was educated in Kiev and St Petersburg and studied medicine in Lausanne, Switzerland. There had been a suggestion that the authorities had been taking an interest in her extra-curricular activities. She had been involved in political activities contrary to the accepted doctrine in pre-revolutionary Russia and she had been sent back to her family's estate and told to remain there![21] She fled the country and moved to Lausanne where she qualified in medicine and practiced initially before returning to Russia. She practiced surgery amongst other areas of medicine.

After the outbreak of the Russo-Japanese War (1904-1905) she led a Russian-supported Red Cross hospital train as chief surgeon. The Russians had more than 75 of these trains, which were equipped with operating facilities and were located close to the front line of the fighting. These trains were fitted out with state of the art medical and surgical facilities and had beds for between 200 and 300 patients. In terms of staffing each train had at least three appropriately trained doctors, up to 10 nursing sisters from the Red Cross Society and up to 40 hospital assistants.[22]

Based on her experience of casualties in this conflict, Gedroits advocated that hospitals should be located as close as possible to the casualty if the best results were to be obtained. This was particularly true for abdominal wounds. Her surgical teams operated on large numbers of casualties. For example, in one month there were 1,255 patients, many of whom had life-threatening wounds. She documented policies for treating particular wounds. In a six-month period she undertook 168 laparotomies for perforating abdominal wounds.[23] She advocated that these casualties should undergo early surgery

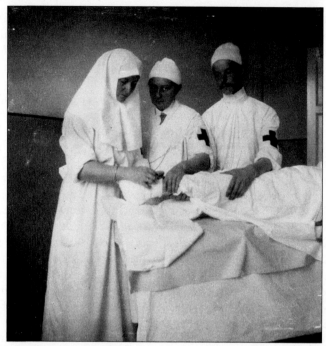

Figure 7.5   Princess Vera Gedroits, Lithuanian princess, surgeon and
poet who became Professor of Surgery at the University of Kiev. (Via
Beinecke Rare Book and Manuscript Library, Yale University)

and the results of her treatment, not reported by her in a formal way but commented on
by her colleagues, indicated that this was correct.[24] After she had presented the results of
her work, the Russian Society of Military Doctors accepted this as the new standard of
care for perforating abdominal wounds. But why did they achieve such results that were
better than those of any other surgeons?

It is likely that this was because of the combination of a strict methodical approach to
surgical care together with her excellent technical skills. For example, one of the criteria
she used was that the casualty had to be operated upon within three hours of sustaining
the wound. When there was a more prolonged delay the results of surgery were very
much poorer.[25] Of course, this policy of operating very early after sustaining the wound
complements the observation from the Boer War. Those who were successfully treated
had surgery within a short time of being wounded. This was to become an important
principle in later years during the Great War.

Following the Russo-Japanese War, she returned to civilian life but then again
returned to military surgery during the Great War, working as a surgeon based with
an army unit in Siberia. Subsequently, she returned to civilian practice once again, but
wanted to pursue an academic career pushing forwards the frontiers of surgery, just
as she had done with her earlier work in abdominal wounds. This she did, and the
culmination of her academic achievements resulted in her appointment as one of the first
female professors of surgery in the world, being appointed Professor of Surgery to the
University of Kiev in 1929.[26]

To the detriment of many soldiers in the Great War, the work of Vera Gedroits and her teams of surgeons was largely ignored in the West, despite the very good results they had achieved. It is difficult to understand why her work was ignored, because the accepted practice in the care for a civilian with a penetrating abdominal injury at the start of the Great War was to undergo exploratory surgery. This principle was not applied to those wounded in battle.[27]

Perhaps of greater concern and for reasons that were not clear, British attention focussed on the management of casualties in Japan. For example, in 1904 there were reports of the high quality of care provided to Japanese soldiers in their wars of the late 19th century from the British military attaché, Sir William Taylor, who later became Director-General of the Army Medical Department.[28]

Further support for Japanese medical care came from the United States medical military observers who commented on the benefits of the non-operative management of casualties of any sort and their transfer back to base hospitals for surgical treatment, including perforating abdominal wounds.[29] Therefore, at the beginning of the Great War, all that had been learned about abdominal wounds by the Russians in an earlier military conflict had gone unnoticed and the lessons as how best to manage casualties with abdominal wounds had to be relearned.

A time of uncertainty and change

The initial experiences of the Allied surgeons who were managing perforating abdominal wounds were analysed. The reported mortality was 70-80% or more using the expectant management policy without surgical intervention, and clearly this was not acceptable.[30]

At this time there was still uncertainty about what treatment should be given and there were other confounding factors which were impacting on the discussions about treatment. Perhaps British surgeons were polarised into two camps – firstly, those who thought that operative treatment should be evaluated further and secondly those who still supported expectant treatment for perforating abdominal wounds. Even though some thought that surgery was the better option, there were concerns as to whether it could actually be carried out close to the front line and whether the time taken to get the casualty to a facility capable of dealing with such wounds would be soon enough.

There was beginning to be a change in attitude towards the management of perforating abdominal wounds and while many surgeons were involved, there were three leading protagonists and key figures in favour of early surgical intervention. These three men were Owen Richards, Cuthbert Wallace and Gordon Gordon-Taylor. Importantly, they had the support of another key figure, Sir Anthony Bowlby, consulting surgeon to the British Expeditionary Force and whose directive that surgery for other types of wounds should be carried out as quickly as possible has been discussed in Chapter 2.

Bowlby had already experienced military surgery, being the senior surgeon at the Portland Hospital in South Africa during the Boer War in 1899, where he had worked with Cuthbert Wallace. Before the Great War he had a distinguished career as a consultant surgeon to St Bartholomew's Hospital, had been surgeon to Edward VII and Surgeon in Ordinary to George V as well as being one of three surgeons appointed to the council of the newly-formed Red Cross organisation by Queen Alexandra. He joined the Army in September 1914 and although initially commissioned as a Major was promoted quickly to Major-General and consulting surgeon to the British Expeditionary Force. In

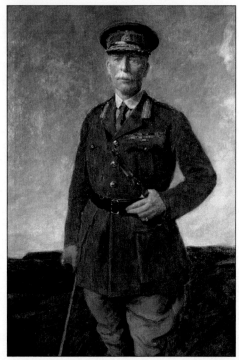

Figure 7.6   Portrait of Sir Anthony Bowlby. (By kind permission
of the Royal College of Surgeons of England)

time it was realised that the work involved as consulting surgeon to all the British forces
in France was too much for one man and Bowlby assumed responsibility for the 2nd
Army with Cuthbert Wallace appointed consultant surgeon to the 1st Army.

As the need for medical care developed with increasing numbers of casualties,
further consultants were appointed but Bowlby retained a position of prominence and
dominance over the other surgeons and was the senior advisor to the Director General
of the Army Medical Services at the front. For Bowlby to support the development of
abdominal surgery being carried out in the casualty clearing stations close to the front
he required evidence to support and facilitate such a change.

Owen Richards was fundamentally important in this respect. A graduate from
Guys Hospital in London, Owen Richards had moved to Egypt earlier in his career
and was appointed Professor of Clinical Surgery at the Egyptian Government School of
Medicine in 1905. Whilst there, he had a particular interest in developing abdominal
surgery and regularly practiced operating on the intestines of cows to understand how
to remove sections of intestine and stitch them back together successfully. This was work
which was fundamentally important not just for civilian practice but also for treating the
abdominal wounds of warfare.[31]

At the outbreak of the war in 1914, he resigned from his post in Cairo and joined
the Royal Army Medical Corps and was attached to Casualty Clearing Station 6, which
was located at various positions including Arras, Merville and Béthune. He persuaded
Bowlby to allow abdominal surgery to be carried out close to the front. After his first

4 months working in casualty clearing stations he had built up some experience of casualties with perforating abdominal wounds and he published (the first surgeon to do so) a paper in the *British Medical Journal* entitled "The pathology and treatment of gunshot wounds of the small intestine" in which he reported on the results of nine patients who underwent immediate surgery.[32] The first patient was dealt with surgically on 28 January 1915; the first successful outcome for such an operation, however, was on 18 March 1915. Richards gave a clear account of the wounds, the surgical intervention and the outcome, although only two casualties survived in his series. Given this poor survival rate, it might have acted as further confirmation that operations were not the most appropriate way of treating these wounds. A summary of the wounds sustained in Owen Richards' series of casualties and how they were treated is shown in Table 7.4 together with the author's own comments about what the most likely reason was for the post-operative death.

Table 7.4
Summary of Owen Richards' initial experience of casualties with perforating abdominal wounds treated by surgery

Wound sustained by casualty	Surgery undertaken	Outcome	What probably happened given today's medical knowledge?
Perforated large intestine with escape of faeces.	A drain was put inside the abdomen to allow the faeces to come out three days after wound occurred.	Died one week later due to "bleeding" but no autopsy.	Infection because part of the damaged large intestine was still inside the abdomen and hadn't been repaired. This would have lead to septicaemia and multi-organ failure.
Perforated large intestine with escape of faeces.	A drain was used to allow faeces out of the abdomen three days after wound sustained.	Died with deteriorating general condition several days later at base hospital.	As above.
Perforated jejunum (upper small intestine).	The hole was stitched closed 2 days after wound sustained.	Died with deteriorating general condition 5 days later.	The cause is likely to have been multi-organ failure because of infection and the major trauma sustained.

Wound sustained by casualty	Surgery undertaken	Outcome	What probably happened given today's medical knowledge?
Perforated small intestine.	Two holes in small intestine stitched closed – time from wounding not given.	Died 2 days later and autopsy showed other damage to small intestine that had been inadvertently not recognised at initial surgery.	The cause is likely to have been multi-organ failure because of infection and the major trauma sustained
Perforated small intestine.	Removal of more than 2-foot length of damaged intestine and anastomosis performed 6 hours after the wound occurred.	Patient recovered and went to base hospital 3 weeks later.	
Perforated small intestine.	Removal of 4 feet of damaged small intestine and anastomosis performed 18 hours after the wound occurred	Patient recovered and went to base hospital 3 weeks later.	
Perforated small intestine.	Removal of 1 foot of small intestine and anastomosis 2.5 days after the wound.	Patient died the following day with no obvious reason at autopsy.	The cause is likely to have been multi-organ failure because of infection and the major trauma sustained.
Perforated small intestine.	Removal of only 1 inch of small intestine and anastomosis but time from sustaining injury not clear.	Patient died a few hours after surgery due to bleeding post-operatively within the abdominal cavity either from injured omentum or the exit wound.	The patient died due to loss of blood from bleeding after surgery, which should have been recognised.
Perforated small intestine.	Removal of 7 inches of small intestine and anastomosis 10 hours after the wound.	Patient died from haemorrhage a week later from the buttock wound – a delayed haemorrhage.	The patient died due to loss of blood from bleeding after surgery, which should have been recognised

Details taken from Richards, O., "The pathology and treatment of gunshot wounds of the small intestine", *British Medical Journal* 1915; 2: pp.213-215.

However, the tremendous interest in his report lay in the fact that the two casualties who survived had sustained injuries to the small intestine, which hitherto had always been considered to invariably result in death. Richards' observations and notes about these casualties were very important because they stimulated discussion and a re-evaluation of how casualties with perforating abdominal wounds should be treated. Although some of his thoughts and statements are now known to be factually inaccurate in the light of subsequent advances in medicine and science, nevertheless his work opened the door to stimulate interest in early abdominal surgery in such wounds.[33] The key points that can be taken from his work, which were vital to improving surgical care of these casualties, are discussed below.

1. *The timing of surgery in relation to when the wound happened* – the time taken for patients to reach his team for surgery could be long and the patients' condition so poor by then that although operation could be undertaken the chances of success were small. The adverse impact of increasing time between when the wound occurred and when surgery took place was a recurring theme in the observations of surgeons treating these wounds. The sooner they were dealt with the better was the outcome.

2. *Selection of casualties for surgery* – not all casualties with abdominal wounds needed surgery. It was suggested that if the casualty did not have any symptoms then there could be a period of observation and monitoring of the casualty's condition. However, it was stated that if any symptoms developed (e.g. increasing abdominal pain and more tenderness spreading across the abdomen), then surgery should be undertaken immediately and appropriate facilities must be on hand to do this. This required an experienced surgeon to be able to make this judgement.

3. *Procedure undertaken* – the surgical incision in the abdominal wall should be in the midline so that all parts of the intestine could be adequately visualised and examined for damage. One of his series of patients had sustained an injury to the intestine but this had not been seen at the time of surgery. The type of procedure carried out then depended on exactly where the damage had occurred. Richards suggested that when the duodenum (first part of the small intestine) and colon were damaged they should be repaired by stitching the hole closed. However, if the small intestine elsewhere was injured then it was considered best to remove the damaged section and join the two ends together (resection and anastomosis).

Whilst Richards knew that this was a limited clinical experience of a small number of casualties, he had contributed to medical understanding with his detailed observations. Other surgeons operating in a similar environment could take his findings into consideration, learn from them, and make further progress.

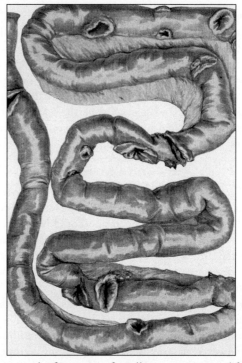

Figure 7.7   Photograph of a section of small intestine removed from a soldier by Captain Owen Richards FRCS. The actual specimen of intestine was kept in the museum in the Royal College of Surgeons of England but was destroyed during a German bombing raid in London during the Second World War. (Private collection)

Table 7.5
Key points considered of vital importance in treating casualties with perforating abdominal wounds identified by Owen Richards

• Time taken to get a casualty back to the appropriate environment where operation can be carried out.
• Surgical teams available.
• Appropriate selection of casualties, observation sometimes before surgery was undertaken.

This work constituted a positive advance in war surgery, but it is important to draw attention to the fact that 10 years had elapsed since the published work of Vera Gedroits, which had been available to all who cared to look. Had her well-documented surgical experience and views been applied on the Western Front at the outset of the war many lives would have been saved. Interestingly, even in a paper in *The Lancet* as late as 1917, Gedroits is only acknowledged as a surgeon in the Russo-Japanese War who "met with some measure of success".[34] It is not clear why her work, accepted as standard in Russia, had been largely ignored and not actively pursued by Western surgeons.

The next stages

Whilst other surgeons had given up carrying out early laparotomy for perforating abdominal wounds, having been discouraged by the results, others were persevering not only in the British sector but also in French hospitals.[35] Cuthbert Wallace was aware of Richards' work in this area and he too believed that early surgery was necessary for casualties with these wounds. He was of the opinion that results of surgery were poor because of the prolonged length of time between the wound occurring and the casualty undergoing surgery in the appropriate facility. Reflecting on what he had seen initially in 1915, Wallace considered that reported cases of successful outcomes for expectant treatment for perforating abdominal wounds were not justified.[36] [37] He thought that casualties who had survived apparently severe abdominal wounds most probably had relatively minor involvement of the abdominal wall. The projectile had not actually penetrated the abdominal cavity. This is a relatively minor wound with a high probability of recovery without necessarily requiring major surgery.

Wallace had a realistic view of casualties who had sustained perforating abdominal wounds. He knew that this was a severe wound and the likelihood of death was high – he quoted figures of some 80% of casualties dying. He had no false expectations of what he might be able to achieve surgically. He declared that there was "no question of revolutionising the mortality" but argued that if he could reduce it by only 10% this would save thousands of lives.

Like Richards, Wallace continued to operate on patients with perforating wounds and was determined to learn all he could by carrying out autopsies when surgery was unsuccessful and the patient had died. By doing so, he made simple but very important observations which did not fit with the views held by those advocating expectant treatment. These were:

- Bleeding was the chief cause of early death.
- Bullets often produced very extensive wounds with multiple holes in the intestine, and concomitant injuries in the abdomen and/or chest – expectant treatment had focused on the mistaken assumption that wounds of the intestine were small and "innocuous" and would heal themselves.
- Expectant treatment had focussed on infection and peritonitis – which occurred at a later stage.

These observations were seminal in re-asserting that haemorrhage was the main cause of early death, which had to be dealt with by surgery, and not by expectant treatment. On the basis of this work Wallace discussed his views with the Surgeon-General, who at this time was W.G. MacPherson, and persuaded him to carry out a small "experiment" where he ensured that some of the field ambulances sent casualties with perforating abdominal wounds immediately to casualty clearing stations. Wallace felt that the results from this experiment were promising and in May 1915 an inquiry was held to determine causes of death after perforating abdominal wounds. Wallace's work was vital in this regard and after a full examination of what was known, three key facts were established by this inquiry are shown in Table 7.6.[38]

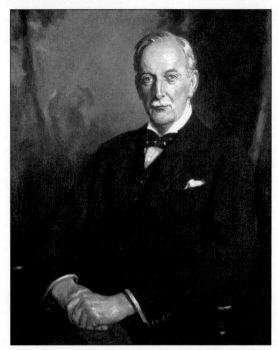

Figure 7.8   Colonel Cuthbert Wallace FRCS. (By kind permission
of the Royal College of Surgeons of England)

Table 7.6
Key facts established by inquiry into the causes of death after perforating abdominal
wounds:

1. That the injuries were as a rule of such a nature that recovery must be a rare event.
2. That haemorrhage (bleeding) was a chief cause of early death.
3. That bullets produce extensive injuries.

Data from Bowlby, A. & C. Wallace, "The development of British surgery at the front", *British Medical Journal* 1917; 1: pp.705-721.

By the beginning of June 1915, there was a movement to be more active in managing abdominal wounds and McPherson ordered that the official policy was to evacuate such cases as quickly as possible and to operate upon them. Haemorrhage had been identified as the primary cause of death. It is difficult to understand why surgeons had not adopted this more vigorous regime earlier, but in all medical correspondence, a key theme was the negative effect of the time taken to get the casualty back to a casualty clearing station and for that facility to have the necessary infrastructure to carry out this type of surgery.[39 40]

However, as entrenchment along the Western Front developed, this resulted in a relative stability in the positioning of medical facilities towards the winter of 1914. This was important because it was possible to establish casualty clearing stations, which were relatively large with quite complex equipment and requirements. It was now possible to develop a rationale for the delivery of treatment, which might involve complex surgery, and demanding care of the patients after surgery until they were fit to travel and be moved to base hospitals.[41] The fixed fighting line of the Western Front was identified as a key factor in allowing a plan of management to become established for casualties with penetrating abdominal wounds. However, whilst distances to the hospital could be only a few miles the time taken to get there under conditions of war could still be long.

Now that official policy had changed, clinical progress could be made. Lieutenant H.H. Sampson RAMC reported his experience treating casualties with abdominal wounds in April 1916, and demonstrated advances that had been made in the understanding of mechanisms of wounding, the type of wounds caused, and how they should be treated.[42]

Sampson had clear priorities when managing such casualties and he made some simple but very important observations. First and foremost, he confirmed Wallace's view that primary bleeding within the abdomen caused by the penetrating missile had to be stopped as quickly as possible to save life. Secondly, and at a later stage, the consequences of infection and peritonitis were likely to result in a fatal outcome. It was crucial that primary haemorrhage be stopped, because there "is little tendency towards spontaneous arrest" and he quoted his experience where bleeding had occurred several hours after wounds had been sustained and showed no evidence of spontaneous arrest.[43] He again emphasised the need for rapid transport to an operating facility after wounding had occurred to stop this bleeding. He also believed that the more quickly the casualty was operated on, the less likely was the risk of subsequent infection.

Other points that he made clear were that multiple injuries occurred commonly and if the intestine was damaged there was often damage to the large veins within the abdominal cavity. Not only could damage to these vessels produce major haemorrhage resulting in immediate death but they could also bleed in a less dramatic way, not apparent initially, but could persist after surgery and also result in death. Therefore, a very careful exploration of the abdomen had to be undertaken to ensure that no coincidental wound in a major vessel was missed. He also noted that wounds of the buttocks and back could be associated with abdominal wounds and so casualties with these wounds should be treated where abdominal surgery was also being carried out in case abdominal wounding had occurred, and the necessary expertise to treat these cases was on hand.

As the war progressed and experience of surgery for perforating abdominal wounds was disseminated amongst surgeons in the casualty clearing stations, other surgeons reported their work with resultant improvements in outcome. Major A. Don, who had previously reported how to gain access to the contents of the abdomen, published a detailed report in 1916 of his surgical experiences in managing perforating abdominal wounds.[44] [45] This reinforced the experience of others that bleeding was the immediate cause of death and peritonitis occurred at a later stage due to the escape of intestinal contents. Don described his surgical technique, and how he explored the abdomen to ensure that no wounds were missed. He also described how specific wounds of each abdominal organ should be treated.[46]

Also in 1916, a larger series of 70 casualties and their wounds was reported by Captain J. Fraser (later to become Professor of Surgery at the University of Edinburgh) and Captain H. Bates. They provided details of their experience and how to manage specific intra-abdominal wounds, the details of which were later updated.[47] [48] The outline of how wounds to specific organs were managed is given later in this chapter.

A time to experiment

Now surgeons were beginning to understand the relationships of the velocity of the projectile and its characteristics in flight, what happens when it strikes the body and the types and severity of wounds likely to be caused. The significance of these determined the severity and type of wound. Therefore, all of this was beginning to affect the way surgeons were thinking about the damage likely to be caused and how to treat it better. Furthermore it was now becoming apparent to the surgeons that damage sustained may not just occur at the exact site of where the projectile struck but could occur at some distance away by mechanisms they were unsure about.

John Fraser, together with another RAMC surgeon, Hamilton Drummond, looked to advance the treatment of abdominal wounds and tried to obtain greater understanding of the clinical problems they were seeing in their daily surgical practice.[49] As well as updating their experience of these wounds by reporting a total of 300 casualties, they questioned themselves as what they were doing and how to do better. They wanted to know the answers to the following questions and conducted a series of experiments using animals.

1. What was the best surgical technique for stitching intestine back together again (for example, end to side anastomosis or side to side anastomosis, which are just different ways of doing the same thing)?

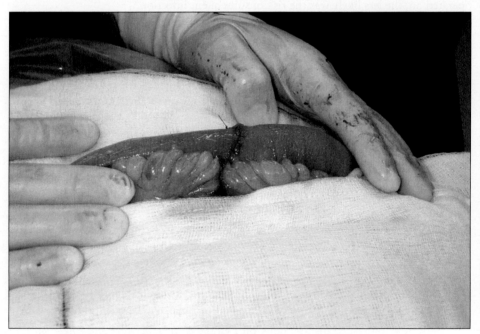

Figure 7.9   A method of stitching the intestine back together is shown here, in which the ends of the intestine are sutured directly together. This is called an "end to end" join or anastomosis. (Author's photograph)

2. Why did the intestine dilate after it had been joined together and didn't work for a period of time after surgery?

3. What were the details of the blood supply to the intestine (important because for intestine to heal it needs a good blood supply bringing oxygen and nutrients to allow healing)?

4. What was the value of omental graft? The omentum is the "apron" of fat found within the abdomen which was used to stitch over a join in the intestine and was thought to help seal it and make it watertight. It was also used to patch and stitch on to other abdominal organs, e.g. the liver, which might help to stop bleeding.

5. How did the position of the wound in the small intestine affect the outcome after surgery?

These were, and still are, key considerations for surgeons undertaking similar types of surgery today. Fraser and Drummond addressed all these questions using a variety of animals including Belgian hares and cats. Whilst these experiments will not be discussed further they were important in providing information for surgeons on which they could base and change their surgical practice when treating casualties with perforating abdominal wounds.[50] Interestingly they recognised the intestinal dilatation occurring after surgery as being important and in some way detrimental to the patient. They considered that it was due to oedema and swelling at the anastomosis where the ends of the intestine had been stitched together and that this caused a mechanical block leading to dilatation of the bowel proximal to this anastomosis.

Unfortunately they had misunderstood and were incorrect, because we now know that after surgery and handling of the intestine (or in the presence of infection and/or damage) the normal spontaneous movement of the intestine, which propels its contents along (called peristalsis) stops and so the intestine dilates and swells up. This condition is called "paralytic ileus" and if there is no underlying damage or infection within three to five days, the intestine will start contracting and normal peristalsis will resume and will move intestinal contents along the length of the intestine.

Recording and audit of casualties treated

Whilst audit and evaluation of every surgeon's work is now regarded as an integral part of everyday surgical practice this was not really the case until a few years ago. During the Great War, the quality of information collected, in general, was poor. However, this was different for patients who had sustained abdominal wounds. Detailed admission and discharge books were kept by the casualty clearing stations dealing with these casualties. This was an important development which provided much information about these wounds leading to better treatment.

However, further more detailed information was wanted in order to constantly evaluate what was being undertaken and learn from previous experiences. Therefore, the casualty clearing stations for abdominal wounds were provided with special books with specific headings as to the data they had to collect and these were provided by the Medical Research Committee.[51] This was different from other casualty clearing stations, which did not specialise in abdominal wounds, where records were kept but to a varying standard and to varying degrees of completeness.

The data obtained was analysed and differences in outcomes and mortality between different casualty clearing stations were evident. However, it was recognised that these figures would be influenced by factors over which the surgeons and their teams had no control. For example, this variability was most likely accounted for by the distance from where the wound occurred and the time it took to get the casualty back to the operating facility and also the severity of the wounds encountered. In terms of time it was shown that the average time taken to get to the casualty clearing station was between 6 and 10 hours after sustaining the wound and after 12 hours mortality increased with a very high mortality if more than 24 hours had passed. It was concluded that if surgery was undertaken within six hours the chances were good and the patient would be more likely to survive. The longest interval from time of wounding to operation where a casualty survived was 36 hours, but this was rare.[52]

Accordingly, the further forward a medical facility was, and the shorter the time it took to get the casualty there, the lower the mortality rate might be expected to be for that reason. However, there would have been men so badly wounded that they would not have survived the journey to a casualty clearing station further back. They would have died before they got there and therefore not be included in the mortality figures. Activity on the front was also important because in quiet times when there was little fighting, the results were better as more time and resource of care was available for each individual casualty. It was also noted that the total mortality of the casualty clearing stations was higher than the operative mortality due to those cases with more severe wounds not making it to the surgeons operating table.

The agent causing the wound was also important in determining outcome. Whilst casualties with bullet wounds and shell wounds had similar mortalities, those who had abdominal wounds caused by grenades and fragment of bombs had a lower mortality, although the reasons for this were not clear. Other factors affecting outcome were identified:

1. Wounds of the small intestine that only required to be sutured closed and with no other associated damage carried the best prognosis,
2. The position of the wound was important, those of the upper abdomen having the best prognosis (least damage), while those below the level of the umbilicus had the worst prognosis (most intestinal damage),
3. Vertical wounds which were associated with penetration of the chest were very serious indeed.[53]

One further factor noted to be of importance in determining the casualties' outcome was the pulse rate. It was noted that most casualties with perforating abdominal wounds had pulse rates of approximately 100 per minute and this was shown to be associated with a good outcome. However, if the pulse rate was 120 per minute, then the chances of survival were reduced. If the pulse rate was greater than 120 per minutes, then there was very little chance of survival. This was a very good observation although the significance was not fully understood at that time. What normally happens when a casualty loses blood is that the blood pressure falls as a result of the reduced circulating blood volume and so what the body does in order to ensure that blood is sent out by the heart to all organs in adequate amounts is to increase its rate of beating to pump more out. So what these surgeons had identified, unknowingly, was that the pulse rate was a surrogate marker for the severity of the wound that had been sustained and which was causing blood loss.[54]

Transport of casualties with perforating abdominal wounds

Therefore, there had developed now amongst the medical services an understanding that the treatment of perforating abdominal wounds required "special arrangements", which were different from those pertaining to the management of other types of wounds. It was now the policy that such casualties should be sent as quickly as possible to the nearest medical facility where abdominal wounds could not only be treated but where the casualty could be managed after undergoing surgery. However, the challenge facing them was how to get the casualty there as quickly as possible.

Although the appropriate casualty clearing station was usually located a relatively short distance from the front line, at around 10,000 yards, getting the casualty there quickly could prove challenging. There were factors which were important in this respect, and which could not be planned for – for example, where exactly the casualty was located (front line or rear), the presence of continued fighting around the casualty or between the casualty and the medical evacuation pathway; mud and poor ground conditions for stretcher-bearers; stretcher-bearers negotiating the trench systems and dangerous open ground and advancing troops in these areas. Furthermore, the time taken to transit the casualty through the more forward medical units (e.g. regimental aid post and field ambulances) back to the casualty clearing station where surgery could be undertaken would all impact adversely on speed of transfer.

The new orders for managing casualties with perforating abdominal wounds meant that they were evacuated preferentially from the regimental aid post to the advanced dressing station, and placed immediately in a motorised ambulance, warmed with hot water bottles, covered in blankets and driven to the appropriate casualty clearing station. Bowlby and Wallace both acknowledged the importance and contribution of the motorised ambulance and development of the petrol engine, as without this it would not have been possible to get the casualties to a safe distance away from shelling quickly enough where they could be treated in relative safety.[55] Care was taken to ensure that the motorised ambulances provided warmth and as much comfort as possible for the wounded. Failure to maintain core body temperature had already been noted to have a detrimental effect, so a system of heated air ducted from around the exhaust pipe was developed to provide warmth and deliver the casualty in the best condition possible.

The time taken to get a casualty to the casualty clearing station could be as little as 30 minutes from the time when the wound was sustained, although it could take up to several hours depending on the factors summarised above and over which there was really no control or way of altering.[56]

Specialised facility for treating abdominal wounds

These were the specially-designated casualty clearing stations which had necessarily become hospitals for abdominal wounds and were equipped to carry out appropriate major surgery. Some of the field ambulances also had developed a specialised advanced operating centre that had the necessary facilities for treating abdominal wounds to enable treatment to be given as soon as possible after the wound had been sustained. For

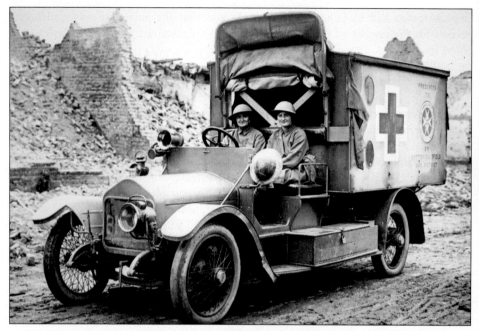

Figure 7.10   Motorised ambulance was the key to the rapid, and most comfortable, method of transport to get the casualty with a penetrating abdominal wound back to the casualty clearing station as quickly as possible and in the best condition to be able to withstand major surgery. (Imperial War Museum Q2660)

example, there were advanced operating centres on the Somme in 1916. Their staffing and administrative control, however, was under that of a casualty clearing station, presumably because their personnel had the requisite experience.[57] It was understood that whilst these special arrangements existed they could, and would, be modified depending on the circumstances that were happening and what was thought to be most appropriate at the time.[58]

Table 7.7
Requirements for a medical facility to treat abdominal injuries:

- Experienced surgical and nursing staff.
- Operating theatre available for immediate use.
- Reachable by motor ambulance within half an hour.
- Treat the casualty after surgery had been carried out.

There were specific requirements if a casualty clearing station was to receive and manage casualties with perforating abdominal wounds. For example, there must be at least one surgeon experienced in the treatment of abdominal wounds, an operating theatre available for immediate use, and experienced nurses available. Furthermore, this medical unit had to be able to be moved quickly should the need exist and without disturbing the patients. For example, after Brandhoek Casualty Clearing Station

Number 44 had been shelled (killing Nellie Spindler) patients with abdominal wounds were evacuated back a distance of three to four miles to Nine Elms, near Poperinge. Details of the casualty clearing stations, how they were staffed and how they functioned are provided in Chapter 2.

Specific wounds of the abdomen and their surgical management

Considerable expertise developed amongst this specialised group of surgeons as to how best to treat wounds of the different organs found within the abdominal cavity. From 1915 many surgeons published their experiences of the wounds they had encountered, what had caused them and how they had learned how best to treat them. One of the surgeons specialising in abdominal surgery was Gordon Gordon-Taylor (a graduate of the University of Aberdeen) who in later years became one of the most respected surgeons both nationally and internationally before his death in 1960 at the age of 82. He produced a book entitled *The Abdominal Injuries of Warfare* and published two papers in the *British Medical Journal* which described very concisely how these wounds should be managed.[59] [60] [61] This was based on the work done by all the surgeons in designated casualty clearing stations and although written in 1939, with the cloud of the Second World War looming and very much in his mind, in many parts is still applicable today to the treatment of perforating abdominal wounds. The following sections will briefly outline the wounds commonly sustained by the intra-abdominal organs and how these were treated by the surgical teams during the Great War.

When should casualties undergo surgery?

The key question that all surgeons, then and now, ask themselves is when is it necessary to operate upon a patient? Does the patient need an operation because of their condition and more importantly when is a patient too ill, or the disease too advanced, to have any prospect of a successful outcome for the patient? The surgeons of the Great War also understood this and were constantly evaluating their own work, and importantly looking for ways of identifying those who should, and who should not, undergo surgery. There was a high standard of surgery practiced in the casualty clearing stations which was well recognised and patient selection for surgery was the key to reducing mortality.[62] Gordon Gordon-Taylor was clear to point out that, unfortunately, "… some men are, from the very first, mortally wounded" and there was nothing that could be done medically to change this.[63] By the later stages of the conflict decision-making was becoming clearer, and Owen Richards, now promoted to the rank of Colonel, published his findings based on a series of 200 casualties with perforating abdominal wounds and others also confirmed these observations.[64] The following are key points which emerged from these and also other surgeons' experiences, and summarise those patients who would not benefit from surgery:

- The casualty's clinical condition was so bad that death would occur if there was any attempt at surgery,
- If the penetrating wound was in the upper right side of the abdomen and the casualty was stable and there was no clinical indication of continued bleeding (from the liver into the abdomen) then this was most likely a liver wound and such wounds had a good prognosis if not operated upon,

- If the wound was located on the left side of the upper abdomen involving the chest and the penetrating object had come out near the armpit then these casualties would do better, in general, if not operated upon because of the high mortality in the early years of the Great War when surgery was undertaken,
- If the wound was more than 24 hours old then an operation would be unlikely to be successful. Those operated on within the first 12 hours did best, but it was still worth operating on the patients up to 24 hours after wounding, although when more than 36 hours had elapsed, the chances of survival were very small. Those who did survive with wounds more than 24 hours old were more likely to have had haemorrhage as the problem rather than perforation of the bowel with severe infection,
- If the pulse rate was more than 120 per minute survival was only 50% of that of those with a pulse rate of less than 120 and so this was also taken into account when deciding if operation should or should not be undertaken.

As in all surgery, preparation of the patient for surgery was vitally important. The role of haemorrhage as the most pressing reversible cause of death had been recognised but there was also a developing understanding that a period of resuscitation prior to surgery was vital. This is important to optimise the patient's general condition, and function of the heart, lungs, kidneys etc before proceeding to surgery – something later generations of surgeons had to relearn.

Although these aspects are discussed in much more detail later, the usual way in which the casualties were prepared for surgery included these specific measures:

- Fluids given directly into veins, into the tissue under the skin (where it was poorly absorbed and of no value but had been given in this way when it was not possible to find a vein because they had collapsed down), or given by a tube placed through the anus into the rectum (fluid is very easily absorbed through the lining of the rectum and into the circulation),
- Use of bicarbonate solutions when a patient becomes "acidotic" – the pH of the blood may become acidic in hypovolaemic shock and this itself can cause an irregular and weak heart beat (see Chapter 3),
- Warming the casualty by hot water bottles or hot air (Chapter 2).

Another interesting observation was that when blood transfusion was given, which most likely increased the blood pressure to a higher level than would occur with the other types of fluids described, further bleeding then occurred which could be detrimental. However, these aspects of medical care were crucial to allow patients to be stabilised and to undergo major surgery and survive (see Chapter 3). Once a decision had been made to undertake surgery it was important to carry this out as quickly as possible in order to have the best chance of survival for the patient. Gordon Gordon-Taylor wrote on the basis of his experiences in his typical language and prose that:

> … speed is the handmaid of success in the operative treatment of gunshot wounds of the belly; there is no place for the surgical sluggard on the floor of the operating theatre in the casualty clearing station … the wasted moments, perhaps half-hours,

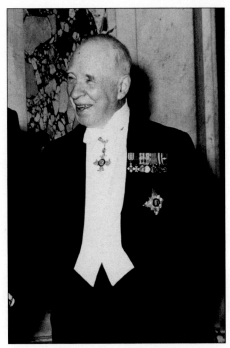

Figure 7.11   Sir Gordon Gordon-Taylor FRCS, who produced an important book, based on surgeons' experiences in the Great War, for those surgeons who would shortly be involved in the Second World War. (By kind permission of the Royal College of Surgeons of England)

of the surgical tortoise are valuable moments dissipated, for surgical aid is therefore deferred, perhaps withdrawn forever, from those who are looking to the operator to save their lives.[65]

Owen Richards had similar views and was quite specific, although stated very clearly and concisely by noting that to get the best results surgeons should be given specific tasks to suit their capabilities and, "... not allowing slow operators to do abdominal work."[66]

In order to gain access to the abdomen, surgeons used a midline (used today) or paramedian incision at least 6-8" in length but were prepared to extend, or use any incision that was deemed necessary, to deal with the damage inside the patients' abdomen. The midline incision gives excellent access to all the contents of the abdominal cavity and this can be seen in Figure 7.12. The first priority was to control any bleeding as this was the chief cause of early death, as noted earlier. Severe bleeding could be encountered from the inferior vena cava or portal vein and techniques are described as to how this could be successfully controlled. After control of haemorrhage had been achieved, a very careful examination of all the organs was made within the abdomen to find all the wounds that might have been sustained.

Although a detailed description of the surgical techniques is beyond the scope of this chapter an outline of the wounds to the different abdominal organs and the outcome from different series that have been reported are show in Table 7.8 and Table 7.9.[67 68 69 70 71 72 73 74] It is important to note however that as the war progressed, developments were taking

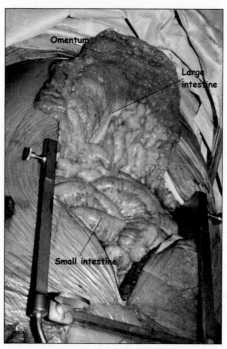

Figure 7.12   This is a mid-line incision showing the excellent access that is achieved, demonstrating that it is possible to access all the intra-abdominal organs. The Omentum is an apron of fat which lies directly underneath the front wall of the abdominal cavity, surgeons used this to position around joins in the intestine or in the repairs of other organs – nature's own filler and glue! (Author's photograph)

place in many fields of medicine, not just surgery. Progress was made in anaesthesia, resuscitation, blood transfusion, antisepsis and radiology which all contributed to the constantly improving survival rates.

Table 7.8

Management of wounds to the gastrointestinal tract

Organ wounded	Types of wounds sustained	Treatment and key points	Outcome
Stomach.	Entrance and exit wounds of anterior and/or posterior surface anywhere. One-third have damage to other organs as well.	Routinely examine posterior wall of the stomach and then suture the holes closed but if stomach is very bruised excise and then suture. Cover the sutured area with omentum.	Mortality 54%

Organ wounded	Types of wounds sustained	Treatment and key points	Outcome
Small intestine.	May present with multiple perforations; damage to blood vessels supplying may occur.	Examine all the small intestine starting at the ileo-caecal junction, identify each perforation and mark and then 3 options: (i) simple suture of perforations; (ii) if extensive damage over a short segment then resect and lateral or end-to-end anastomosis, (iii) resect and anastomosis as before but if concerns about viability of the bowel use a temporary enterostomy (side passage).	Mortality 61%
Large intestine (colon).	Single or multiple perforations and can extend into the retroperitoneal tissues. 40% have other associated injuries in the abdomen.	Usually treated by (i) suture the perforation closed (omentum put around the repair) and initially a proximal colostomy was done to avoid faeces passing through the repaired colon until healed. Later experience suggested that colostomy not required, (ii) if extensive damage and not possible to stitch closed the perforations then a colostomy was carried out and damaged colon removed; (iii) resection of damaged colon and anastomosis with a proximal colostomy/caecostomy; (iii) resection and ileo-colic anastomosis.	Mortality 56%
Rectum.	Uncommon but perforations may be intraperitoneal, extraperitoneal, or both and is a very complex injury.	Explore from within the abdomen, suture perforations closed and temporary colostomy if wound is severe. If extraperitoneal open up the entrance wound and allow drainage and may also need temporary colostomy.	Mortality 70%

Table 7.9

Management of wounds to the solid organs and urinary tract

Organ wounded	Types of wounds sustained	Treatment and key points	Outcome
Liver and gall bladder.	Variable in extent with minor to severe disruption and often associated with damage to lung.	Operated on if casualty showed signs of continual haemorrhage or evidence of damage to other structures in the abdomen or chest. If operation undertaken haemorrhage is controlled by suture and drainage of the liver area established.	Mortality 42%
Spleen.	Variable degree of damage but usually found in association with damage to other organs.	(i) if small wound and not bleeding nothing else required, (ii) if major damage and extensive destruction then remove the spleen, (iii) if repair possible and bleeding stopped then do this and preserve the spleen.	Mortality 35%
Pancreas.	Rare and usually associated with fatal bleeding because of large blood vessels around the pancreas.	If damaged then may try and resect damaged part or if not possible then establish and ensue draining of this area.	Too little experience of this injury to know.
Kidney.	Variable damage from small to complete destruction with haemorrhage often extending extensively retroperitonealy.	Explore the abdomen carefully. May just require draining or a simple suture. If extensively damaged will require removal and often done through a loin incision.	Approximately 40%
Bladder.	Usually with other injuries e.g. fractured pelvis and intestinal wounds and can be intraperitoneal or extraperitoneal.	(i) if intraperitoneal then the perforation is stitched closed and a urethral catheter passed, (ii) if extraperitoneal repair the perforation and place a drain in the suprapubic space. If this hole is not accessible to suture close then drain the area with a suprapubic drain and urethral catheter.	Mortality 41%

Conclusion

Reflecting on what has been discussed in this chapter, it is clear major changes took place in the management of casualties with perforating abdominal wounds during the Great War. In 1914 casualties with these wounds were managed with expectant treatment and the great majority died. However, within two years progress was being made in the understanding of why death occurred and what was necessary to prevent this in terms of the technical aspects of surgery and the development of new operations. Furthermore, the rapid advances in anaesthesia, resuscitation, blood transfusion, microbiology and radiology together with the establishment of an infrastructure of evacuation pathways and medical facilities, in particular the casualty clearing stations with their teams of personal of all types, helped to reduce the mortality from these wounds.

Notes

1 Moynihan B., "An address on the treatment of gunshot wounds", *British Medical Journal* 1916; 1: pp.333-337.
2 Gordon-Taylor, G., "The abdominal injuries of warfare – II", *British Medical Journal* 1939; 2: pp.235-238.
3 Wallace, C., "War surgery of the abdomen", *The Lancet* 1917; 1: pp.561-568.
4 Fraser J. & H. Drummond, "A clinical and experimental study of three hundred perforating wounds of the abdomen", *British Medical Journal* 1917; 1: pp.321-330.
5 Fraser, J. & H.T. Bates, "Penetrating wounds of the abdomen", *British Medical Journal* 1916; 1: pp.509-519.
6 Moynihan, *op.cit.*, pp.333-337.
7 Bowlby, A., "The Hunterian Oration on British military surgery in the time of Hunter and in the Great War: delivered before the Royal College of Surgeons of England on February 14th, the Anniversary of Hunter's Birth", *British Medical Journal* 1919; 1: pp.205-212.
8 Makins, G.H., "Hunterian Oration, 1917, on the influence exerted by the military experience of John Hunter on himself and on the military surgeon of to-day", *British Medical Journal* 1917; 1: pp.213-219.
9 Wallace, *op.cit.*, pp.561-568.
10 Editorial, "The report on the surgery of the Boer War", *British Medical Journal* 1905; 2: pp.1301-1302.
11 Wallace, *op.cit.*, pp.561-568.
12 Bennett, J.D., "Abdominal surgery in war – the early story", *Journal of the Royal Society of Medicine* 1991; 84(9): pp.554-557.
13 Bowlby, A. & C. Wallace, "The development of British surgery at the front", *British Medical Journal* 1917; 1: pp.705-721.
14 Pruitt, B.A., "Combat casualty care and surgical progress", *Annals of Surgery* 2006; 243: pp.715-727.
15 Editorial, "The report on the surgery of the Boer War", *British Medical Journal* 1905; 2: pp.1301-1302.
16 *Ibid.*
17 Wallace, *op.cit.*, pp.561-568.
18 Bennett, *op.cit.*, pp.554-557.
19 Wallace, *op.cit.*, pp.561-568.
20 Bennett, *op.cit.*, pp.554-557.
21 Bennett, J.D., "Princess Vera Gedroits: military surgeon, poet, and author" *British Medical Journal* 1992; 305: pp.1532-1534.
22 "Editorial: Hospital ships and trains", *British Medical Journal* 1904; 2: p.457.
23 Pruitt, *op.cit.*, pp.715-727.

24   Bennett, J.D., "Princess Vera Gedroits: military surgeon, poet, and author" *British Medical Journal* 1992; 305: pp.1532-1534.

25   Wilson, B., "Relearning in military surgery: the contribution of Princess Vera Gedroits", *Clinical and Investigative Medicine* 2007; 30: A32.

26   Bennett, J.D., "Princess Vera Gedroits: military surgeon, poet, and author" *British Medical Journal* 1992; 305: pp.1532-1534.

27   Don, A., "Perforating and penetrating wounds of the chest with severe haemorrhage: a suggestion for treatment", *British Medical Journal* 1916 June 10; 1 (2893): pp.816-817.

28   "Editorial: The Japanese Military Medical Service", *British Medical Journal* 1904; 1: pp.391-392.

29   "Editorial: The treatment of the Japanese wounded", *British Medical Journal* 1904; 2: pp.397-398.

30   Wallace, *op.cit.*, pp.561-568.

31   Anonymous, "Owen W. Richards CMG, DSO, DM, MCh, FRCS", *British Medical Journal* 1949; 1: p.945.

32   Richards, O., "The pathology and treatment of gunshot wounds of the small intestine", *British Medical Journal* 1915; 2: pp.213-215.

33   *Ibid.*

34   Wallace, *op.cit.*, pp.561-568.

35   *Ibid.*

36   *Ibid.*

37   Wallace, C., "The Hunterian Oration", *British Medical Journal* 1934; 1: pp.269-273.

38   Bowlby & Wallace, *op.cit.*, pp.705-721.

39   *Ibid.*

40   Bowlby, A., "The work of the "clearing hospitals" during the past six weeks", *British Medical Journal* 1914; 2: pp.1053-1054.

41   Bowlby & Wallace, *op.cit.*, pp.705-721.

42   Sampson, H.H., "Clinical notes on penetrating wounds of the abdomen", *British Medical Journal* 1916; 1: pp.547-549.

43   *Ibid.*

44   Don, A., "Abdominal injuries in a casualty clearing station", *British Medical Journal* 1917; 1: pp.330-334.

45   Don, A., "Incisions for operations on the upper abdominal organs", *British Medical Journal* 1909; 1: pp.652-653.

46   Don, A., "Abdominal injuries in a casualty clearing station", *British Medical Journal* 1917; 1: pp.330-334.

47   Fraser & Drummond, *op.cit.*, pp.321-330.

48   Fraser & Bates, *op.cit.*, pp.509-519.

49   Fraser & Drummond, *op.cit.*, pp.321-330.

50   *Ibid.*

51   Wallace, C., "War surgery of the abdomen", *The Lancet* 1917; 1: pp.561-568.

52   *Ibid.*

53   Wallace, C.S. & J. Fraser, *Surgery at a casualty clearing station.* London: A & C Black, 1918.

54   *Ibid.*

55   Bowlby, A., "President's Address: On the application of war methods to civil practice", *Proceedings of the Royal Society of Medicine* 1920; 13(Clinical Section): pp.35-48.

56   "Editorial: Abdominal injuries", *British Medical Journal* 1916; 1: p.863.

57   MacPherson, W.G. (ed.), *History of the Great War based on Official Documents. Medical Services. General History.* London: HMSO, 1924, Volume 2, pp.22-25.

58   "Editorial: Abdominal injuries", *British Medical Journal* 1916; 1: p.863.

59   Gordon-Taylor, G., "Abdomino-thoracic Injuries I", *British Medical Journal* 1941; 1: pp.862-864.

60   Gordon-Taylor, G., "Abdomino-thoracic Injuries II", *British Medical Journal* 1941; 1: pp.898-901.

61   Gordon-Taylor, G., *The abdominal injuries of warfare.* Bristol: John Wright and Sons, 1939.

62   Richards, O., "The selection of abdominal cases for operation: with reference to a series of 200 operations", *British Medical Journal* 1918; 1: pp.471-473.

63   Gordon-Taylor, G., "The abdominal injuries of warfare – II", *British Medical Journal* 1939; 2: pp.235-238.

64   *Ibid.*

65   Gordon-Taylor, G., *The abdominal injuries of warfare.* Bristol: John Wright and Sons, 1939.

66   Richards, *op.cit.*, p.471-473.

67   Gordon-Taylor, G., "The abdominal injuries of warfare – II", *British Medical Journal* 1939; 2: pp.235-238.

68   Wallace, C., "War surgery of the abdomen", *The Lancet* 1917; 1: pp.561-568.

69   Fraser & Drummond, *op.cit.*, pp.321-330.

70   Fraser & Bates, *op.cit.*, pp.509-519.

71   Don, A., "Abdominal injuries in a casualty clearing station", *British Medical Journal* 1917; 1: pp.330-334.

72   Gordon-Taylor, G., *The abdominal injuries of warfare.* Bristol: John Wright and Sons, 1939.

73   Gordon-Taylor, G., "The abdominal injuries of warfare – I", *British Medical Journal* 1939; 2: pp.181-183.

74   Wallace, C., "Rectal wounds in the present war", *Proceedings of the Royal Society of Medicine* 1916; 9 (Surgery Section): pp.23-25.

8

Penetrating chest wounds and their management

Steven D Heys

Introduction

Wounds of the chest have been associated with a high mortality throughout the history of war and there had been a general view that there was nothing that could be done to save these casualties. John Hunter, the famous British surgeon with a great experience in war surgery (see Chapter 7), stipulated that the casualty should be laid down on the side of the injury so as to let the blood drain out of the chest through the wound, and this was the only treatment possible. As understanding of the function of the organs in the chest developed and progressed, interest developed in these wounds, allowing the start of a more rational and scientific basis for treatment. Importantly, Patrick Fraser, a surgeon from the Crimean War, realised that fluid within the chest had to be drained and removed because its presence impaired the function of the casualty's lungs.[1] He also noted that it was often better to leave a bullet in the chest if the casualty was reasonably well as there was a possibility that a surgical operation to remove it would potentially cause more damage than leaving it alone.

In the Boer War, penetrating chest wounds were usually caused by a rifle bullet and were managed without surgery and often successfully. In 1914 at the beginning of the Great War, treatment of chest wounds was rudimentary and consisted mainly of trying to drain any fluid within the chest and not to embark on surgical operations within the chest. Perhaps the differing conditions in the Boer War, where wounds were sustained in relatively clean and dry conditions, in stark contrast to wounds sustained in the mud of France and Flanders, contributed to the belief that surgery was not necessary. Indeed surgeons in the Boer War attributed successful result of treatment with only approximately 9% of the wounded and 27% of those with penetrating chest wounds dying to "the climate, the sunshine, and the dry and pure air".[2] Furthermore, a lack of understanding of the physiology and function of the human body led surgeons to believe that it was not possible to operate on the chest without special equipment and that if the lung was touched there would be rapid and unstoppable bleeding.[3] These were, of course, erroneous beliefs.

In the early years of the Great War, casualties with chest wounds had a high mortality in the same way that abdominal wounds had, until surgeons challenged the conventional ways of dealing with them. Several surgeons were instrumental in bringing about change, including Major A. Don, and Captains Roberts, Craig, Hathaway and Gask. These surgeons certainly led the way in the medical literature by reporting their experiences treating chest wounds in casualty clearing stations. Major Don, mentioned in Chapter 7 for his work in patients with abdominal wounds, really led the way and stimulated critical thinking because he was concerned by the "impotency" of the non-operative management of severe haemorrhage in casualties with penetrating chest wounds.[4] In 1916 he began to manage these casualties by considering the way in which the chest wall and the contents of the chest worked under normal circumstances and decided to undertake an early operation to drain blood from the chest and arrest haemorrhage. This was successful and he published his technique straight away for other surgeons to consider and take forward.

All of these surgeons believed strongly that the management of chest wounds should follow the same principles as for wounds sustained elsewhere in the body. This meant surgery at the earliest possible time, to excise the wound by complete removal of all infected tissues and foreign material, and repair of the tissues by primary closure.[5] The results they achieved were an improvement and were an important step towards a more active surgical management policy for casualties with penetrating chest wounds.[6] [7] [8]

Chest wounds were seen less commonly than wounds affecting other areas, due to the high risk of death associated with wounds to the vital structures lying within the chest itself. Around one-third of casualties who died on the battlefield either had an isolated chest wound or a combination of wounds including a chest wound. Chest wounds represented approximately 5% of all wounds requiring initial medical care but because of the deaths that occurred during transfer through the evacuation chain only represented approximately 2% of all wounds arriving at the casualty clearing stations.[9] However, a specific expertise was needed, and developed, to manage these casualties and by 1918 approximately 70-80% of casualties with a chest wound survived if they reached the casualty clearing station.

Penetrating chest wounds were caused by the same projectiles that caused the abdominal wounds described in the last chapter. These were bullets (pistol and rifle), shrapnel balls, or high explosive shells, bombs and grenades. What caused the wound was extremely important because a bullet or shrapnel ball had the potential to go straight through the chest, penetrating the skin and muscle before entering the chest cavity on one side and coming out of the other. However, if it struck a rib or any other bone around the chest such as the scapula (shoulder blade) then due to the changes in its flight characteristics, as discussed in the last chapter, there was the potential to cause much more damage, with greater likelihood of damage and destruction of both the chest wall and the structures inside. In contrast, high explosives and fragments of metal usually caused more extensive wounds at the sites of entry and exit of the projectile and often the projectile dragged with it into the chest large amounts of clothing, soil and debris. Consequently these were much more serious wounds than those caused by a bullet or shrapnel ball, unless of course it had gone through the heart or a major blood vessel and caused a rapid death.

Why are chest wounds so important?

The importance of chest wounds is because of the damage caused to the function of the vital organs and structures which lie within the chest. The organs are enclosed by a semi-rigid protective cage consisting of skin, muscle and bone. The muscles provide a functional as well as protective layer of tissue lying under the skin but outside the chest cavity. They can firstly be categorised into those which are attached at one end to the chest wall and to the upper limb or shoulder blade at the other and have the principal

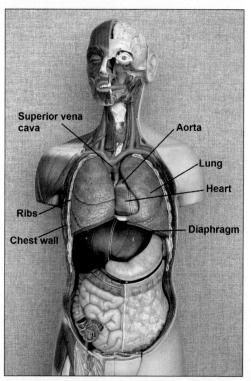

Figure 8.1   Anatomy of the chest, showing the key organs lying within the
chest cavity. (Ian Brown, Department of Anatomy University of Aberdeen)

function of moving the upper limb, for example the large pectoral muscles on the front
of the chest wall. The second group of muscles is attached only to the chest wall, and
act on the chest wall alone. These are the intercostal muscles which are attached to
and between adjacent ribs. There are 12 ribs on each side of the chest in total and their
function is concerned with respiratory movements, i.e. breathing in and breathing out,
because as they rise and fall, contraction of the intercostals muscles swings the ribs out
with a bucket handle type of motion allowing air to move in and out.

Lying directly underneath and on the inside of the chest wall and between the
chest wall and the lungs, is a small potential space called the pleural cavity which is
lined by a membrane (very thin lining on the surface of the lung and on the chest
wall). These two layers normally stick together and this keeps the lung fully expanded.
If, however, air gets into this potential space then the lung will collapse and this is called
a pneumothorax and if blood gets into this space it is called a haemothorax. The lung(s)
cannot then function and expand normally until the air or blood is removed from the
pleural space.

The two lungs lie on either side of the chest cavity and are spongy in texture
comprising thousands of air sacs. Air which is breathed in through the mouth and/or
nose passes through the back of the throat into the airway called the trachea (windpipe)
which runs inside the chest between the two lungs and then splits into two main branches
one to take air to the left and the other to the right lung. The lung is where the air that

is breathed in containing oxygen (which is necessary for all the body's cells), comes into contact with the blood and oxygen diffuses into the blood stream. The blood flowing to the lungs contains a large amount of carbon dioxide, which has been produced by the body's cells and needs to be removed. This gas diffuses from the blood into the air within the lungs' air sacs and is breathed out.

Another major organ is the heart, which is simply a mechanical pump for the blood and divided into two halves, each with a different role but still nevertheless each is a pump. Blood returns to the heart having been returned from all the body's tissue through two main blood vessels which are veins, called the superior and inferior vena cava. This blood needs to be oxygenated so this right side of the heart pumps it to the lungs through the pulmonary arteries where oxygen is taken into the blood and carbon dioxide is removed. The blood then comes straight back from the lungs through the pulmonary veins to the left side of the heart and the left side of the heart pumps this blood out through the aorta, which is the main artery running through the chest and the abdomen (see Chapter 7). Branches from the aorta are numerous and through these blood reaches all the body's tissues before being returned to the heart through the vena cava as described above.

The oesophagus (gullet) also runs with the trachea from the back of the throat running along the length of the chest cavity at the back and lying behind the heart where it then passes through the diaphragm to enter the abdominal cavity and join with the stomach. The diaphragm separates the abdominal and chest cavities and is actually a thin sheet of muscle which contracts, moving upwards and downwards and helps to draw air into and out of the lungs. The structures in the centre of the chest, i.e. the heart and large blood vessels, the trachea and its branches which enter the lungs (trachea and bronchi) and the oesophagus (gullet) together with a variety of nerves are termed the mediastinum, and this is a commonly used anatomical term.

Very simply, therefore, as a result of trauma to the chest the three most immediate problems that the casualties faced were, lack of oxygen in the blood necessary to supply all the tissues and organs in the body, haemorrhage (bleeding) and failure of the heart to pump adequate amounts of blood around the body. However, a review of the deaths occurring in casualties with chest wounds categorised them as generally falling into one of three groups as shown in Table 8.1[10][11] and this information was particularly important for developing a rational plan of management for life-threatening and potentially life-threatening wounds (see Table 8.2).

Table 8.1
Causes of death after penetrating wounds of the chest

Time of death	Cause of death
Death on the battlefield or within a few hours of admission to medical facility.	Injury to the large blood vessels in the chest or a massive wound that was too extensive to be treated surgically.
Death after 48 hours from sustaining the wound.	Usually infection within the pleural cavity.
Deaths at the base hospital seven days or more after the wound occurred.	These were due to infection.

Taken from Stevenson, W.F., "Notes on surgical experiences of the Boer War", Journal of the Royal Army Medical Corps 1903; 1: pp.93-8.

Table 8.2
Commonest life-threatening and potentially life-threatening situations

Life-threatening	Potentially life-threatening
Obstruction of the airway Tension pneumothorax "Sucking" pneumothorax Large haemothorax Flail chest segment Cardiac tamponade	Simple pneumothorax Haemothorax Perforation of the trachea and or bronchi Tears of the oesophagus (gullet) Rupture of the diaphragm

How were these wounds classified and how did the surgeons of the Great War approach these wounds?

The approach taken by the surgeons to perforating wounds of the chest was a very simple and understandable one. Wallace and Fraser[12] recognised that simplicity was the key in being able to understand and treat the damage that had occurred, and they considered that the wound may be to:

- the chest wall at the site of the penetration,
- the lung underlying the chest wall, and
- the lung on the opposite side of the chest together with the structures in the mediastinum.

Working classifications of the different types of chest wounds evolved during the Great War and were found useful by all the teams in the evacuation pathway chain for management. Commonly, casualties were categorised on being admitted to the casualty clearing station as follows:[13]

- Type A – closed entrance and exit wounds and no foreign body retained
- Type B – open wounds with entrance and exit wounds or with entrance wounds and a retained foreign body
- Type C – open tangential wounds at the periphery of the chest circumference.

A further refinement was that those with Type A wounds were then categorised into those where the blood within the chest was infected and a second group where it was considered that the blood within the chest was not infected. This formed a basis for clinical management because those casualties in groups B and C proceeded to urgent surgery which had become recognised as the best treatment, whereas the patients in group A in whom it was felt did not have any infection within their chest did well without having to have any surgery performed on them.[14] Other surgeons and teams had different ways of classifying chest wounds. An example is shown in Table 8.3 and perhaps this describes not just the structural damage but gives us more information about the effect the wound had on the patient.[15] A "sucking" wound was one where air entered the chest through the hole in the chest wall each time the casualty breathed in and air within the chest cavity (air should be within the lungs themselves) then couldn't get out again due to a tissue flap valve, so that pressure within the chest cavity increased greatly, compressing both lungs and stopping them from functioning. This was a potentially life-threatening wound.

Table 8.3
Alternative classification of penetrating chest injuries

Class	Description	Occurrence
1	"Open" or sucking wounds with free air entry.	19%
2	"Closed" wounds with large septic laceration of the chest wall.	16%
3	"Closed" wounds with early signs of infection of haemothorax.	10%
4	"Closed" wounds with no evidence of intrapleural infection.	50%

Data from Don, A., "Perforating and penetrating wounds of the chest with severe haemorrhage: a suggestion for treatment", British Medical Journal 1916; 1: pp.816-817.

Damage to the chest wall at the site of, and around, the penetration
Perhaps the simplest of all wounds was the bullet (or shrapnel ball) which passed straight through the chest and did not have its flight characteristics altered in any way! However, as already explained, a fragment of metal from a shell or grenade was of variable size and often caused more damage to the chest wall. In addition, often the underlying ribs were broken and fragments of the ribs and the skin and muscle of the chest wall, or large segments, would be lodged inside the chest cavity. Clearly some of these wounds would be instantly fatal or not survivable from the time they were sustained.

Damage to the underlying lung
The lung is a relatively large structure and with two occupying the majority of the chest these were nearly always damaged to a greater or lesser extent. The physical nature of the lung is very spongy as it comprises sacs containing air as explained above and it is relatively easy for projectiles to pass through causing damage. Damage was not limited to the track that the projectile had followed but there was also often bruising and bleeding of the lung further away and with wounds that had been sustained at a closer range then whole areas of lung could be affected in this way. If the larger blood vessels in the lungs were damaged then bleeding could be substantial and this might accumulate in the pleural cavity. This would compress the lung and impair its function to a varying degree. This is called a haemothorax.

Damage to other structures in the chest and the opposite lung
It became apparent that it was not only the lung underlying the damage to the chest wall that was at risk but also the lung on the opposite side of the chest could suffer damage. This varied from a mild bruising to extensive changes throughout the lung which resembled a pneumonia (infection of the lung) when autopsies were performed on those who died. Nowadays, we recognise a condition known as adult respiratory distress

syndrome (ARDS), which occurs at 24-48 hours after an injury or major trauma. When this happens there is an inflammation throughout the lung with fluid accumulating in the lung, impaired lung function and impaired exchange of gases within the lung substance which can result in death. Nowadays these patients are managed in an intensive care unit, and frequently need to have a period when they are put on a ventilator, a machine which breathes for a patient when breathing becomes too difficult. This allows the lungs to maintain oxygen levels in the blood stream until the inflammation resolves in the lung, but often these patients also have failure of other organs such as the kidneys and heart. Even today there is a significant mortality rate for such patients and this is probably what was happening to these casualties. The features of ARDS are summarised in Table 8.4 It is likely that many of those soldiers who survived the carnage of the Great War but died of the complications of Spanish flu in 1919 would also have died of ARDS occurring.

Table 8.4
Adult respiratory distress syndrome (ARDS)

Causes (examples)	What happens in the lung?	Effects on the casualty
Major trauma Infections Pneumonia After surgery Drug reactions	The body releases a variety of chemicals that cause inflammation in the lungs. Cells called macrophages and polymorphs (normally to fight infection) accumulate in the lungs and then release a further series of chemicals. This causes even more inflammation, fluid accumulation and damage to the lung.	The lungs become swollen and fluid accumulates in the air sac where inspired air would normally be. The patient cannot then take into the body oxygen and so the levels of oxygen in the blood stream fall. The patient will become breathless and struggle to breath and even becomes so exhausted trying to breathe more deeply and more quickly that they stop breathing. The lack of oxygen in the bloodstream may lead to dysfunction in many other organs, leading to death.

Initial treatment on passing through the evacuation chain to the casualty clearing station

The casualties with penetrating chest wounds were usually in quite a distressed condition by the time they had gone through the chain of evacuation and arrived at the casualty clearing station. Not only were they generally very anxious, but they had varying degrees of respiratory distress and breathlessness due to impaired pulmonary function arising from damage to the chest wall, pleura or lung, or of any combination of these. This leads to a lack of oxygen in the blood stream (hypoxia) and failure to expel carbon dioxide resulting in dysfunction of all the body's tissues and organs. In addition, they had often sustained blood loss with resultant hypovolaemic shock, which itself could lead to dysfunction of other organs and death (discussed in earlier chapters).

Prior to the casualties arriving at the casualty clearing station where the definitive and life-saving surgery would be undertaken, initial treatment would have been given at the regimental aid posts and advanced dressing station. It was standard practice to begin treatment by warming and resting the patient, and if there was an open wound involving the pleural cavity this was closed either by stitching the skin closed over the hole or by filling the hole with gauze and then applying a strong strapping over the top.

A detailed physical examination of the casualty would have been undertaken to ascertain how severe the chest wound was and to identify any other areas of the body that had been wounded, especially the abdomen and spine. There was awareness that the chest wound might have been caused by a projectile entering the body elsewhere and so this was carefully sought. The physical signs looked for, and detected when present, depended on the type of wound, and were exactly the same signs we would look for today. The casualty then had a chest X-ray taken in the casualty clearing station. This was particularly important to locate the position of any, or multiple, foreign bodies and fragments of bone within the chest. The surgeons could also see if a haemothorax and/or a pneumothorax was present and how severe these were, and also looked at the opposite lung and at the heart to determine if there was any suggestion of damage or displacement of these organs. They also observed how the diaphragm was moving as this could also indicate important features of the wound.[16]

A well defined plan for treatment after the casualty's arrival at the casualty clearing station was as follows:[17] [18]

- Casualties were put into a special ward, warmth was provided and they were allowed to rest for about an hour.
- If there was a sucking wound which had not been closed previously, this was covered by a dressing (or temporary stitches) and checked to make sure that air was not being sucked in when the casualty took a breath in.
- If casualties were distressed, which was usual, they were given a small amount of a morphine-like drug (omnopon) by injection under the skin.
- Fluids were given to the casualty by administering one pint of hot coffee with 1 ounce of glucose – given by the rectum (back passage).
- A mixture of camphor, olive oil and ether might also be given by an intramuscular injection – to relieve distress.
- The casualty was positioned in bed sitting up in Fowler's position (see Chapter 7).

The next step in the management was to decide whether or not the casualty required surgery. There emerged a consensus that the wounds shown in Table 8.5 could be managed without chest surgery.

The casualties who had a relatively small amount of blood lying within the pleural cavity, between the inside of the chest wall and the surface of the lung (fitting into the categories shown in Table 8.5) could have this removed without undergoing an operation. The usual treatment was to aspirate this by inserting a needle between the ribs through the chest wall to suck out the blood, after first rubbing a small amount of bismuth, iodoform and paraffin into the wound and surrounding skin to disinfect the area.[19] These casualties were then carefully observed for signs of ongoing bleeding or difficulty in breathing, with regular monitoring of their pulse, blood pressure and respiratory rate. If the casualty's clinical condition deteriorated, it was clear this conservative management was not working and that surgery was necessary.

Table 8.5
Casualties with wounds not requiring surgery

Casualties with chest wounds who did not require surgery
• If there was a small wound which looked clean and there was no other evidence of there being serious damage in the chest. This included wounds where the projectile had gone straight through the chest.
• If the missile was still in the chest but of a very small size and the casualty also did not show evidence of serious damage in the chest.
• If there was a large foreign body in the cavity and it was thought that it would be too difficult and dangerous for the casualty to attempt to remove it.
• If there was a haemothorax (blood in the pleural cavity as explained above) without there being infection in it.

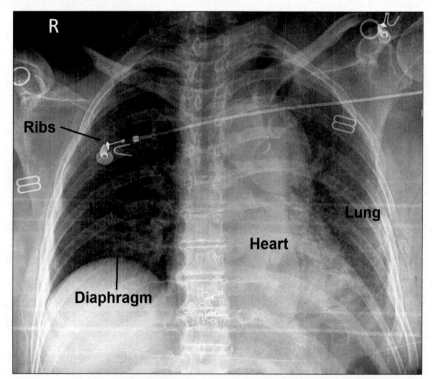

Figure 8.2   Chest X-ray indicating a serious injury to the underlying lungs as a result of chest trauma. The lungs should appear as a uniform black colour (due to air inside the lung) but here there is a "fluffy" white appearance indicating the accumulation of fluid within the lung stopping it from taking in oxygen for the body and possibly resulting in the death of the patient. (Courtesy of Dr Alan Denison)

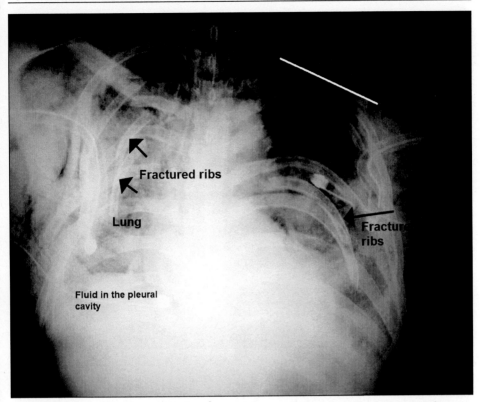

Figure 8.3   This chest X-ray shows several abnormalities as a result of trauma to the chest. There are fractures ribs on both sides (arrows) and on the right a segment of the ribs has become displaced inwards causing extensive damage. The underlying lung appears a white colour (instead of a uniform black appearance) indicating extensive damage to the lung itself. In addition there is some fluid inside the chest on the right side and on the left side at the uppermost area of the lung (indicated) there is a very black appearance (blacker then normal lung) that indicates that there is some air outside the lung but in the pleural cavity. (Courtesy of Dr Alan Denison)

Although surgery could be avoided in some cases by simply draining the chest, not only did some patients need operating on as outlined above but others, who seemed to settle initially, went on to develop an infection in their chest cavity, because blood was an excellent medium in which bacteria could grow. If the casualty developed a rising pulse rate with a high temperature and the amount of fluid in the chest increased, this was highly suggestive of infection and the fluid from the chest was examined microscopically to detect any bacteria. If it was decided that infection was present, an operation was then necessary to open up the chest and drain the remaining blood and any pus which may have accumulated. This dangerous complication led to the suggestion that all casualties should undergo surgery in order to prevent it happening, but this was not adopted as the standard policy. A strong advocate of immediate surgery was Major George Gask, who believed that it was important to remove any blood from within the chest cavity and thus hopefully prevent infection.

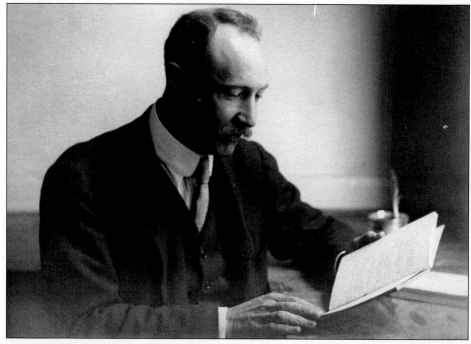

Figure 8.4   Professor George Gask. (Courtesy of the National Portrait gallery)

George Gask was one of the most important contributors to the development of chest surgery in casualty clearing stations. He was consulting surgeon to the 4th Army and developed great expertise in the management of casualties with chest trauma. He published his results for treating 500 patients with penetrating gunshot wounds of the chest and these are discussed later.[20] After the Great War, he returned to London and became Professor of Surgery at St Bartholomew's hospital, establishing an academic unit of surgery there.

Management of casualties requiring surgery

Whilst the patients described above did not need to undergo surgery initially, the following categories of patients were identified as needing to proceed to immediate surgery in the casualty clearing station:

Table 8.6
Casualties requiring urgent surgery

Casualties with chest wounds who required urgent surgery
• If there was marked "ragged" damage of the chest wall.
• Compound fractures of the ribs (the broken rib was exposed to the environment).
• Bleeding from the chest wall.
• "Open" wounds of the chest wall where air was being sucked in when the casualty breathed and could not escape because of a valve-like effect.

Casualties with chest wounds who required urgent surgery
• The presence of a foreign body that was in a position where it was accessible to remove safely.
• Large amounts of bleeding inside the chest.
• Damage to the diaphragm.
• Pain due to splinters of fractured ribs which were rubbing against the surface of the lung when the chest moved during breathing.

Taken from Roberts, J.E. & J.G. Craig, "The surgical treatment of severe war wounds of the chest", British Medical Journal 1917; 2: pp.576-579.

Pre-operative preparation for surgery

As expertise developed in the management of casualties with chest wounds, there was a growing recognition that a short period of time to begin treatment of "shock" was required (see Chapter 3 where this is explained in detail). Casualties were warmed up and kept quiet. This usually took about an hour but could take up to six hours. There was also recognition that casualties with chest wounds could not be operated on, if as well as having one directly damaged lung, the opposite lung was also collapsed. Operating on such casualties resulted in death.

Surgeons today will spend long periods of time with patients before surgery explaining what the operation will entail and then obtain informed consent before surgery can proceed. Whilst the situation was obviously different almost 100 years ago in the setting of war, the following is an interesting insight into what surgeons might want to tell the casualty before surgery:

> … the patient should be warned in a tactful way that he may feel extraordinarily distressed and apprehensive during the operation … but that he should try to lie and breathe quietly, that struggling and excitement will only increase his distress, and that the symptoms will pass off very quickly once the operation is finished.[21]

How did the surgeons treat the wounds in the operating theatre?

The surgeons had priorities of treatment. They had to try to ensure that the lungs were allowed to function as well as possible to provide oxygen to the body. They had to stop bleeding thus preventing hypovolaemic shock and death, and they had to do everything possible to reduce the subsequent risk of infection developing in the pleural cavity and chest. This third factor was the main cause of later death if the casualty survived the initial wound and/or surgery. The reason for the development of infection was the same for any type of wound a casualty might have sustained. It is worth remembering from Chapter 2 that wound excision was the single most important surgical intervention at a casualty clearing station. There was always a high risk of bacteria being carried straight into the wound on the projectile, fragments of bone, or on clothing contaminated with mud and debris. Only by removing all this material completely could the risk of infection be reduced.

While the principles for treatment of chest wounds were the same as any wound, there had to be some specific modifications given the vital nature of the lungs and heart within the chest. Surgeons knew that speed was essential if the patient was to survive because the casualty's general condition meant that he could not withstand long periods of anaesthesia (Chapter 3). Everything should be planned and an important piece of advice from experienced surgeons was that "the operator must not lose his head when things become alarming".[22] It had been believed that the techniques required for working in the chest were possessed by all experienced surgeons working in the casualty clearing stations and the surgical instruments required were no different from normal instruments for every day purposes.[23] Whilst this is true, as in all branches of surgery, specialism in chest surgery and developments in techniques and better instruments enabled surgery to be performed more efficiently and with better results as time progressed.

Interestingly the surgeons may have begun the operation under local anaesthetic after giving the patient a "premed" (similar to today's "premeds" as it comprised omnopon and scopolamine designed to reduce the lung and airway secretions). The technique used was designed to anaesthetise the chest wall initially by injecting a local anaesthetic called novocaine (similar to today's ones which are used in hospitals and by dentists) into the wound and surrounding area and also around the intercostal nerves which run along the under surface of each rib. This provided very good anaesthesia for the chest wall and a similar technique may be used today to relieve pain in patients who have fractured ribs.

When the surgeons got inside the chest cavity, they then needed a general anaesthetic which was nitrous oxide and oxygen. It may have been supplemented with chloroform in some patients. An interesting description in one of the reports of these wounds and written by a surgeon states that the patients may also be given "a few whiffs of chloroform and ether".[24] Other surgeons thought the patients should be "well doped" and "be made very drowsy" although still capable of cooperating with the surgeon's instructions.[25] Perhaps surgeons didn't fully appreciate the importance of appropriate anaesthesia in the management of their casualties! Nitrous oxide is still used today although in combination with other anaesthetic agents, to provide better and safer general anaesthesia. The specifics regarding the use of anaesthetic agents and developments in anaesthesia has been discussed in more detail in Chapter 3.

First, damaged tissues around the entry wound to the chest wall were excised, being sure to remove all damaged and dead tissue, debris and foreign material, down to the level of the underlying ribs. Surgeons knew that unless this was done there was a high risk of infection developing subsequently in the post-operative period. If there was damage to the underlying ribs this was carefully assessed and any ragged pieces of bone were smoothed off, and loose bits of devitalised bone splinters were removed. If the wound extended into the chest the surgeon would explore this manually, putting his hand into the chest feeling for and removing any bits of bone that had been driven inside the chest, evacuating any blood and inspecting the surface of the lung. Pre-operative chest X-rays were not always available, so the surgeon had to be vigilant in feeling for foreign bodies. If there was bleeding from the lung this was stopped using fine sutures. The surgeon then had to decide whether to open the chest more extensively so as to formally inspect all the structures or whether the exposure undertaken to accomplish wound excision was enough. Some surgeons stopped and closed the wound at this stage if they thought there was no damage to the structures within, although others always thought it necessary to go further and have a really good look inside the chest for unsuspected damage. This, of course, prolonged the surgery and was a bigger operation for the casualty to withstand.[26][27]

The more severe chest wounds, however, did require more extensive surgery, for example, if there was major bleeding or if there was a large foreign body within the chest and it had been decided that it should be removed (as explained previously). Large fragments of metal nearly always carried fragments of contaminated clothing into the chest, which always gave rise to infection if not removed. Depending on where the pre-operative X-ray indicated the fragments of metal to be, it was sometimes possible for the surgeon to gain access inside the chest by working though the hole in the chest that the projectile had caused. Sometimes, however, this did not provide adequate exposure for the surgeon or the projectile was located some distance away within the chest from where it had entered. This meant that the chest had to be cut open in a different place and in a specific way. This operation is termed a "thoracotomy" and is strategically placed to give optimum access to the area of the chest requiring attention.

The way this was done was to make an incision some 6 inches long along the line of the 5th or 6th ribs and running from the side of the chest towards the front wall of the chest. After cutting through the muscles overlying the chest wall the underlying rib was reached. A 4 to 6-inch segment of rib was removed by cutting it off at the front where it is attached to the cartilages which lie between the rib at its front end and the breast bone (these act like a buffer under normal circumstances) and cutting straight through the rib at the back end of the incision. The lining on the inside of the chest (called the pleura) was then cut open and the surgeon had entered the chest. Alternative techniques were developed by some surgeons to avoid removing a section of rib. These included splitting a rib down the centre and then opening it up like the leaves of a book with an upper and lower half of the rib still being attached to the intercostal muscles on either side.[28]

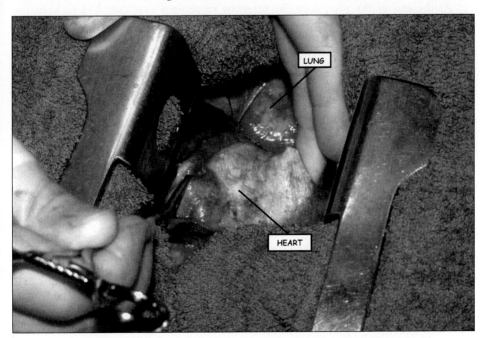

Figure 8.5   The incision used in a thoracotomy operation to gain access to the structures within the chest. (Courtesy of Mr George Gibson FRCS)

To see what he was doing, an instrument called a "rib spreader" was then inserted between the ribs (or between the two halves of the rib if it was retained) spreading them well apart giving the surgeon a good view of the lungs and the heart.[29]

Any foreign body identified using this technique could easily be removed. If however, it lay within the lung tissue itself it would require to be located by touch during a careful examination of the lung. It was removed from the lung either through the hole it had caused on the way in, or by making a new cut in the lung to get it out – a relatively easy procedure. The lung was carefully repaired by stitching it and any bleeding was stopped. If any lung tissue was considered to be too damaged to survive then it was removed and the remaining lung stitched back together. The chest cavity was carefully examined to make sure that there was no further bleeding. Then it could be washed out with saline solution or perhaps even an antiseptic solution, for example Eusol, Dakin's solution or flavine depending on the surgeon's preference, to try to reduce the risk of infection developing later.

The layers of the chest would be closed separately just as they had been cut open, pleura being stitched to pleura, muscle to muscle and skin to skin. The surgeons considered that the most important layer to stitch together very precisely was the pleura lying on the inner layer of the chest wall and to do this they used catgut, which is a material still used in present surgical practice. Sometimes, depending on the extent of the damage done to the chest wall or where there was an inadequate amount of muscle to repair, then just the skin was stitched closed. Techniques were also developed to deal with cases where there was insufficient skin left after the chest wall (muscle layers) had been closed.

At the end of the procedure the surgeons recognised that they had to keep the pleural cavity free of blood and/or air as the lung would collapse down if this was not the case. To expel any air lying between the surface of the lung and the inner wall of the chest, if necessary they often aroused the casualty, although there must still have been a degree of anaesthesia present, with the casualty drowsy and hopefully not fully aware of what was happening. The casualty was then told to purse his lips, hold his nose, and make a strong expiratory effort so as to expel the air and so the lung would fully expand just as the last stitch was being tightened![30] This is no longer necessary, the reader will be pleased to know, as the anaesthetist has a tube passed into each lung and can inflate the lung fully when the surgeons are closing the layers of the chest wall and whilst the patient is still anaesthetised.

There was great discussion about whether or not drains should be put into the chest at the end of surgery to allow the drainage of any fluid that might accumulate within the chest after such procedures. Indeed, there was controversy as to whether they should be used anywhere because it was recognised that infections could get into the body through the drainage tube.[31] The generally accepted policy for chest wounds was that drains were not used unless the chest wall could not be closed or if there was a well-established infection inside the chest. The drain used was a rubber tube of about a half-inch diameter which was positioned just inside the pleura and attached to a glass bottle containing boric acid which was on the floor. The tube was actually in the boric acid so this allowed a negative pressure to be maintained within the pleural cavity (because as air left the chest cavity it could not be replaced) and so encourage the lung to remain expanded. Such a drainage system is called an "underwater seal" and is used today but usually with water and not boric acid. It has already been pointed out in Chapter 2 that delayed closure was not an option with chest wounds. Not to close the wound would almost certainly mean the death of the patient.

Post-operative care and complications that occurred after chest surgery

After surgery patients were nursed initially semi-recumbent and then partially sitting up. One of the most important things was to keep their lungs clear of secretions by coughing up sputum. If they could not do this it would accumulate in the lungs and predispose to pneumonia and death. After an operation either on the chest or abdomen, trying to breathe deeply or to cough could be extremely painful unless adequate pain relief was administered. Morphine was used for this and it is still used as the basis of pain relief after surgery today. The substances used to aid coughing and help the patients to get rid of their lung and bronchial secretions included tincture of camphor, syrup of Tolu, ammonium carbonate, creosote and potassium iodide – none of these, however, would be used now.

It was recognised that there might be an accumulation of fluid (or air) in the pleural cavity as detected on clinical examination and/or with a chest X-ray. If this occurred then it was drained by inserting a needle into the chest (called an aspiration) using local anaesthetic for the skin and muscles and using a tube which was large enough to allow the fluid out without blocking. If the fluid re-accumulated, then repeated aspirations were performed. However, if there was blood in the fluid and this had clotted then it was not possible to aspirate and an operation had to be done to open the chest and scoop all the blood clot out manually. This had to be done because it was recognised that clotted blood was an excellent medium for harbouring and growing bacteria leading to serious infections.

Infection developing in the chest after surgery was the most serious complication. Although surgeons believed in "the natural power of the pleura to deal with infection"[32], unfortunately this power frequently failed the patient and infection occurred. If the fluid within the chest did become infected (and there was no clotted blood) then a tube was placed into the chest by removing some of the stitches. If it was not possible to drain the infected fluid through the tube then an operation was required to open up the chest and remove all clotted blood and infected material. This is similar to what would be done now although the needle would be positioned very accurately through the chest wall into the fluid lying in the chest using an ultrasound (sound wave) scanner to guide the needle into the correct position and we would also use antibiotics for the infection. Antibiotics were not available during the Great War, and consequently patients with chest wounds complicated by sepsis often died.

The mortality for chest wounds admitted to the casualty clearing station fell to approximately 20%. The surviving casualties would remain at the casualty clearing station for varying periods of time before being transferred back to base hospitals. For example, if the wound was a small haemothorax but they were well, then they would be kept for 72 hours whereas those undergoing major surgery would stay for at least 10 days or until any post-operative complications that occurred had been treated. The reasons for this are that it was just not safe to transfer the casualties unless their clinical situation was stable. The complications of these wounds may result in collapse of the lung with accumulations of air or fluid (pus and/or blood) and these can very quickly become life-threatening without immediate treatment,

The outcomes following surgery depended on the severity of the wound inflicted. Roberts and Craig analysed 199 casualties who were admitted to their casualty clearing station to try to learn more and to improve management. They categorised the deaths according to the severity of the injury as shown in Table 8.7.

Table 8.7
Outcomes of surgery for penetrating chest wounds

Class	Description	Number of operations	Survival rate
1	"Open" or sucking wounds with free air entry	29	34%
2	"Closed" wounds with large septic laceration of the chest wall	23	43%
3	"Closed" wounds with early signs of infection of haemothorax	15	93%
4	"Closed" wounds with no evidence of intrapleural infection	0	-

Data from Don, A., "Perforating and penetrating wounds of the chest with severe haemorrhage: a suggestion for treatment", *British Medical Journal* 1916; 1: pp.816-817.

They carefully analysed their data and their results, and published it in the medical literature to share and learn from their experiences. Of the 199 casualties who were admitted during the time of their analysis, 108 were evacuated to base hospitals without undergoing an operation, 24 died without having surgery and 67 casualties underwent chest surgery at the casualty clearing station. They described these 67 soldiers as "forlorn hopes" but 34 recovered to be evacuated to base hospitals with the other 33 dying. However, about half of those who died had major "gross" injuries elsewhere, most commonly in the abdomen, and they considered that no deaths were attributable to the chest injury itself.

Another series of 365 casualties with chest wounds who were admitted to the same casualty clearing station between June 7 1916 and August 31 1917 was detailed by Gask and Wilkinson.[33] Not only is this a very large experience to learn from but the data they collected gives a fascinating insight into their management of these wounds. Of these casualties 76 died but 45 of these had significant associated wounds of the head, abdomen, spine, heart blood vessels or combinations of these. However, when they specifically focussed on those soldiers with chest wounds only there were 31 deaths out of 320 cases, which gave a mortality rate of only 9.6%. The causes of death were shock and blood loss or infection as had been found previously. The details of the operations undertaken in the 104 casualties who proceeded to surgery are shown in Table 8.8.

Table 8.8
Operative details and mortality for casualties undergoing chest surgery

Type of operation	Number of operations	Survival rate
Excision of wounds of chest wall	36	94%
Thoracotomy for repairing the chest wall/lung with draining haemothorax	24	63%
Thoracotomy with removal of foreign body, repair of lung and draining haemothorax	16	81%
Thoracotomy for infected haemothorax	15	67%
Combined abdominothoracic operations	12	83%

Date from Roberts, J.E. & J.G. Craig, "The surgical treatment of severe war wounds of the chest", *British Medical Journal* 1917; 2: pp.576-579.

But perhaps what also gave great insight into the risk of death with chest wounds and how they should be managed were the figures which they provided where wounds were broken down according to their cause. It was clear that the rifle bullet passing through the chest was associated with the very best chance of survival. It must be remembered however, that all these figures refer to a selected group of casualties because these are the ones who made the journey back to the casualty clearing station satisfactorily. Those with more severe injuries died either on the battlefield or during the evacuation pathway.

Table 8.9
Mortality from chest wounds according to cause of the wound

Cause	Mortality
Bullet with entrance wound only (bullet remains in chest)	17%
Bullet with entrance and exit wound (passed through the chest)	10%
Shell fragment with entrance wound only	21%
Shell fragment with entrance and exit wounds	47%
Shrapnel ball	9%

Date from Roberts, J.E. & J.G. Craig, "The surgical treatment of severe war wounds of the chest", *British Medical Journal* 1917; 2: pp.576-579.

Wounds of the heart

Wounds of the heart were almost universally fatal with casualties dying very quickly on the battlefield due to bleeding – even today they are unlikely to survive. However, there were reports in the medical literature of a small number of casualties from the Great War who survived after undergoing surgery for wounds to the heart! One was alive and well nine months later, the other survived the surgery but died a few days later. These are discussed below in view of their rarity and the surgical skill needed to do this:

Case I

A soldier had sustained a wound with a fragment from a bomb penetrating his chest close to the nipple on the side of his breast bone. The casualty was clearly seriously wounded from his general appearance and his pulse and when a small probe was put into the wound it pulsated with a "cardiac rhythm".[34] The surgeon, Captain Fraser, removed a portion of the casualty's rib and after identifying the lining around the heart called the pericardium (this forms a sac within which the heart is contained), he cut it open and blood came out. He saw that there was a small hole in the muscle of the heart wall of the right atrium and he succeeded in stitching this closed. What was actually happening was that blood was escaping through this hole in the wall of the heart but blood was being contained within the sac surrounding the heart thus putting pressure on the heart and not allowing it to pump blood properly. This casualty recovered well.

Case II

The second case was more complex. The casualty had been wounded eight days previously, with a small wound to the right side of the lower part of his breast bone. However, chest X-rays suggested that a bullet was actually in the muscle wall of the heart, as it moved as the heart was beating. The surgeon here was Colonel Henry Gray (later Sir Henry Gray) who had made a hugely significant contribution to the treatment of casualties with wounds of bones, joints, soft tissues and head as discussed in other chapters, contributions which, most importantly, were acknowledged by his surgical colleagues who were operating in the casualty clearing stations.[35]

Colonel Gray decided to operate under local anaesthetic and made an incision on the front of the chest wall over the breast bone trying to follow the track he thought the bullet would have followed. He operated skilfully, identified the heart and with his finger felt the bullet which was thought to be either in the wall of the right ventricle of the heart or possibly lying in the cavity of the pumping chamber of the heart. With the patient feeling no pain and not in any distress he took hold of the heart and cut into the heart muscle to remove the bullet and then stitched the heart muscle back together whilst holding it between his finger and thumb![36]

The casualty was well for four hours after the surgery but then his respiratory rate was observed to be 48 breaths per minute (normally 12-16) and he died almost five days later. At post-mortem examination the heart was well healed, there was no blood in the pericardial sac. However, there were some clots of blood in the cavity of the right heart (probably because of the damage to the heart) and these had become dislodged and travelled to the lungs blocking the lungs' circulation and causing death. This is called a pulmonary embolism and also occurs when clots of blood from within the veins of the leg (for example, after long aeroplane journeys) become dislodged, travelling to the right ventricle and then to the lungs, as happened in this casualty's case.

Combined wounds of the abdomen and chest (thoraco-abdominal wounds)

An even more serious wound than either that of the chest or abdomen was the penetrating wound involving both the chest and the abdomen. This occurred in approximately 12% of all abdominal wounds[37] and about 9% of all chest wounds[38]. These wounds were often fatal but when casualties did survive they presented a complex management problem for the surgeons of the Great War, and indeed, this wound is still a very complex one for the surgeons of today, almost 100 years later. Whilst the concern was the damage to the organs in both the abdominal and chest cavities these wounds also involved the diaphragm, which was nearly always damaged on one side, as bilateral injury to the diaphragm was usually fatal.

The diaphragm is not only important in breathing, as explained earlier, but it also acts as a partition between the chest and abdomen. The abdominal organs (most commonly the stomach, small intestine and large intestine) can pass into the chest through any holes in the diaphragm, usually on its left side because on the right side the liver sits under the diaphragm and is immobile and attached in its position. This extrusion of the abdominal viscera into the chest is called a diaphragmatic hernia and can cause major problems for the patient, interfering with breathing or the intra-abdominal organs can become damaged at a later stage. It was crucial, therefore, for the surgeons to try to work out where the projectile had entered the body, where it had gone after entering, and where it had come out, to be able to operate with a chance of success.

Careful planning for surgery was essential and X-rays of the chest and abdomen taken pre-operatively were extremely important to help determine where the damage was most likely to have occurred, and also provide information regarding location of any foreign bodies. Judgement was required in deciding which of the wounds required addressing the most urgently. Wallace and Fraser[39] made the following clear and simple recommendations (re-iterated some 20 years later and recommended to surgeons preparing for the Second World War):[40] [41]

- Disregard the thoracic wound if it is small and concentrate on the abdominal wound.
- If there is an "open" sucking wound of the chest then this should be the first priority before attending to the abdomen.
- If the abdominal wound is extensive and there is little damage to the chest the abdomen should be explored through an abdominal incision first.
- In those wounds of the chest which are close to the lower margin of the rib cage then access to the abdomen can be obtained by cutting through the lower part of the rib cage.
- If the foreign body lies higher up and closer to the diaphragm and it is thought that the rest of the abdomen is alright, then the surgeon can gain access to the upper abdomen when working in the chest by working through the hole in the diaphragm.

Generally, if at all possible the diaphragm was repaired by stitching it together, because it improved the casualty's breathing post-operatively and helped to prevent an immediate, or subsequent, diaphragmatic hernia from developing.

This type of surgery was a major undertaking in the Great War. Even today, with intensive care units providing specialised ways of supporting the functions of the heart, lung and kidneys, these wounds have a substantial risk of death. However, during the Great War, the mortality of thoraco-abdominal wounds fell quite dramatically; this is shown in Table 8.10. Whilst these casualties could be regarded as a very select group, given that they were fit young men who had already survived the journey to the casualty clearing station, nevertheless there had been important developments in surgical techniques, anaesthesia, and pre- and post-operative care which had contributed to the improved survival of these patients. Perhaps the most important development in reducing the mortality was the introduction of blood transfusion in 1917.

Table 8.10
Survival for casualties undergoing combined surgery on the chest and abdomen during the Great War

Year	Recovery rate
1916 (Battle of the Somme)	18%
1917	49%
1918	67%

Data from Wallace, C., "War surgery of the abdomen" *The Lancet* 1917; 1: pp.561-568.

Summary

In parallel with the changes that were taking place in the management of casualties with all types of wounds during the Great War, there were major developments in the treatment of chest wounds. At the start of the Great War, treatment was based largely on experiences in the Boer War, where a rifle bullet was the main wounding agent. If this had passed straight through the chest and the soldier had not died, there was a reasonably good chance of surviving without further surgery. However, this did not happen in France and Flanders. It was recognised that this was inappropriate treatment given the nature of the wounds and the environment in which the fighting was taking place. Surgical experience resulted in the development of clearly defined categories of casualties depending on whether they did or did not require surgery, and a rational management plan for those with chest wounds was developed. As with abdominal wounds, the increasing success rates were also due very much to the developments in anaesthesia and blood transfusion, which played a critical role in supporting the types of major chest surgery being undertaken in casualty clearing stations.

Notes

1   Fraser, P., *A Treatise Upon Penetrating Wounds of the Chest*. London: John Churchill, 1859.

2   Stevenson, W.F., "Notes on surgical experiences of the Boer War", *Journal of the Royal Army Medical Corps* 1903; 1: pp.93-8.

3   Gask, G.E., "Gunshot wounds of the chest", *British Medical Journal* 1939; 1(4089): pp.1043-1045.

4   Don, A., "Perforating and penetrating wounds of the chest with severe haemorrhage: a suggestion for treatment", *British Medical Journal* 1916; 1: pp.816-817.

5   Roberts, J.E. & J.G. Craig, "The surgical treatment of severe war wounds of the chest", *British Medical Journal* 1917; 2: pp.576-579.

6   *Ibid.*

7   Gask, G.E. & K.D. Wilkinson, "Remarks on penetrating gunshot wounds of the chest, and their treatment", *British Medical Journal* 1917; 2: pp.781-784.

8   Hathaway, F.J., "The early operative treatment of penetrating gunshot wounds of the chest", *British Medical Journal* 1917; 2: pp.582-583.

9   Herringham, W., "Penetrating wounds of the chest at the casualty clearing stations", *British Medical Journal* 1917; 1: pp.721-722.

10 Gask, *op.cit.*, pp.1043-1045.

11 Gask & Wilkinson, *op.cit.*, pp.781-784.

12 Wallace, C.S. & J. Fraser, *Surgery at a casualty clearing station*. London: A & C Black, 1918.

13 *Ibid.*

14 *Ibid.*

15 Roberts & Craig, *op.cit.*, pp.576-579.

16 Gask & Wilkinson, *op.cit.*, pp.781-784.

17 Roberts & Craig, *op.cit,* pp.576-579.

18 Anderson, J., "The surgical treatment of severe penetrating wounds of the chest in a casualty clearing station", *British Medical Journal* 1917; 2: pp.575-576.

19 Roberts & Craig, *op.cit,* pp.576-579.

20 Gask & Wilkinson, *op.cit.*, pp.781-784.

21 Roberts & Craig, *op.cit,* pp.576-579.

22 *Ibid.*

23 Anderson, *op.cit.*, pp.575-576.

24 Hathaway, *op.cit.*, pp.582-583.

25 Roberts & Craig, *op.cit,* pp.576-579.

26 Gask, *op.cit.*, pp.1043-45.

27 Hathaway, *op.cit.*, pp.582-583.

28 Cowell, E.M., "Plastic transcostal thoracotomy", *British Medical Journal* 1917 Nov 3; 2 (2966): pp.581-582.

29 Hathaway, *op.cit.*, pp.582-583.

30 Roberts & Craig, *op.cit,* pp.576-579.

31 Hathaway, F., "The abuse of drainage tubes", *British Medical Journal* 1918; pp.1718-1720.

32 Hathaway, F.J., "The early operative treatment of penetrating gunshot wounds of the chest", *British Medical Journal* 1917; 2: pp.582-583.

33 Gask & Wilkinson, *op.cit.*, pp.781-784.

34 Bowlby, A. & C. Wallace, "The development of British surgery at the front", *British Medical Journal* 1917; 1: pp.705-721.

35 Hathaway, F., "The abuse of drainage tubes", *British Medical Journal* 1918; pp.1718-1720.

36 Birkbeck, L.H., G.N. Lorimer & H.M. Gray, "Removal of a bullet from the right ventricle of the heart under local anaesthesia", *British Medical Journal* 1915; 2: pp.561-562.

37 Wallace, C., "War surgery of the abdomen", *The Lancet* 1917; 1: pp.561-568.

38 Gordon-Taylor, G., *The abdominal injuries of warfare*. Bristol: John Wright and Sons, 1939.

39 Wallace & Fraser, *op.cit.*

40 Gordon-Taylor, G., "Abdomino-thoracic Injuries I", *British Medical Journal* 1941; 1: pp.862-864.

41 Gordon-Taylor, G., "Abdomino-thoracic Injuries II", *British Medical Journal* 1941; 1: pp.898-901.

9

Wounds of the Skull and Brain

David Currie

Early development of neurosurgery and understanding brain function

Before the 20th century, most surgery which was carried out on the head was limited to simple treatments of those who had suffered some sort of trauma and injury to the head. In 1815, in Guthrie's textbook *Gun-shot Wounds*, the focus was on the management of wounds to the limbs and the surgery of methods of amputation.[1] However, shortly after, in 1829, John Hennan included a chapter on head wounds in his textbook *Principles of Military Surgery*.[2] He was pessimistic about the prognosis of these wounds, but described surgical procedures to realign skull bones that had been fractured, to remove bone driven into the brain, and more complex procedures to remove bullets lodged within the brain.

Hennan also described an operation to remove a blood clot lying between the skull and the fine membranes which cover the surface of the brain (called an extra-dural haematoma). He made multiple holes in the skull bone to allow the blood to be evacuated, therefore removing pressure on the brain, and stopping the source of the bleeding. The soldier went on to make a full recovery after a long post-operative course which was complicated by infection.[3]

In the Crimean War (1853-56) and the American Civil War (1861-1865) deaths from infectious diseases far exceeded the numbers of deaths from wounds sustained in battle. Head wounds in the Crimea were associated with a mortality rate of almost 100%. In the American Civil War some attempts were made to treat soldiers with penetrating wounds of the head surgically, but usually they were considered to be "inoperable" and surgery was withheld. For those undergoing surgery, mortality rates were still in excess of 80%. However, it has been accepted that the quality of surgical services during the American Civil War was poor, with badly trained surgeons operating in unhygienic conditions. They were working before the time of Lister's introduction of antisepsis into surgical procedures. Almost inevitably, post-operative infection complicated treatment of penetrating head wounds. George Otis, a skilled surgeon, later to become Surgeon General, noted that there had been limited progress made in the treatment of head injuries.

Knowing the structure and function of the brain was an important pre-requisite for understanding and treating head injuries, and at the end of the 19th century, topographical neuroanatomy, or the mapping of the brain to understand which parts of the brain were responsible for particular functions, was poorly understood. In 1861 the French anatomist and physician, Paul Broca, gave a description of his observations on a ten-year old boy with a tumour in the left frontal lobe of the brain. The patient presented with dysphasia (loss of ability to speak) and a right-sided limb weakness leading Broca to conclude that speech and the function of the right limbs were localised in the left frontal area of the brain. Other publications followed, establishing which areas of the brain

234

controlled particular functions (cerebral localisation). However, the subject remained controversial and Arthur Lynch wrote:

> Students in medical schools and universities all over the world have been taught the story of centres of localisation – even as a student I ventured to doubt this theory.[4]

Continuing on this theme, Hughlings Jackson, a London neurologist, contributed to the understanding of neurophysiology, laying the foundations of clinical diagnosis based on the topographical mapping of the brain, and its application to localising and surgically treating cerebral lesions. In 1876 William MacEwen, in Glasgow, was able to localise a brain abscess by means of clinical examination and his knowledge of topographical anatomy. This was very important for the development of neurosurgery. Victor Horsley, a surgeon working at Queen Square in London, collaborated with Hughlings Jackson, and could use this new knowledge to develop the science of clinical localisation and surgery for brain tumours.

Whilst advances were taking place in the clinical practice of neurology and the beginnings of neurosurgery, researchers were carrying out further experiments to unravel the complexities of the structure and function of the brain. In 1898, Scagliosi had investigated what happened to the brain when it was injured. To do this, he subjected rabbits to a head injury and then examined their brains after the rabbits had been killed, taking sections of the brain for microscopic examination to study what had occurred within the brain tissue.[5]

Further experiments along these lines were carried out by researchers who studied monkeys. One of their key findings was that brain swelling due to the accumulation of fluid within the brain tissue occurred and this is called "cerebral oedema". Victor Horsley was particularly interested to understand what happened when the brain was subjected to a bullet wound, and he carried out ballistic experiments by firing bullets into wet clay (to simulate body tissues) and focused on the behaviour of the bullet and its likely effects on the surrounding tissues. Further work in this area revealed that when the brain was injured damage could be more extensive and may occur some distance from the site of injury.

Horsley was recognised as a key figure in the early development of neurosurgery – his name is synonymous with early neurosurgery in England. However, other surgeons took a particular interest in this area, including Percy Sargent and his team at the National Hospital for the Paralysed and Epileptic at Queen Square in London. They were also doing pioneering research and clinical procedures. They demonstrated that it was possible to remove brain tumours using neurosurgical techniques that were available at the time, although with a high mortality. Not all was plain sailing in the early development of neurosurgery, as was illustrated by some public reactions. An example of this occurred in London, when Rickman Godlee carried out one of the early resections of a brain tumour from a patient in 1884.[6] The patient died of post-operative complications, resulting in public disquiet about interfering with the brain. Fortunately there had been support for the development of this type of surgery, with an editorial in the medical journal *The Lancet* commending the venture into a new area of surgery.

Whilst these advances were taking place in England similar advances were being made elsewhere in Europe. Surgeons such as Kohler, Wagner and Borchardt, working in

Germany, had also reported the successful removal of brain tumours. Surgeons attempted ever more challenging procedures, with Horsley, Goodlee and Benett at the National Hospital for the Paralysed and Epileptic, and Wagner in Berlin, all trying to develop neurosurgical treatments for epilepsy – advancing to another grade of complexity for surgery on the brain.

Head injuries were far more common than brain tumours and most surgery for head injuries was still carried out by general surgeons who had no specialist interest in neurosurgery. Sargent, however, was an exception, and operated mainly on such patients. He was involved in the Great War as a neurosurgeon all over the Western Front and especially at a general hospital at Boulogne, where his skills were frequently required.

An important development in operative neurosurgery was made by Wagner in Berlin, who introduced a new technique called the osteoplastic craniotomy flap, to allow the surgeon to gain better access to the brain.[7] Before then, a hole was bored through the skull with a trefine, and then the margins of the hole nibbled away until it was big enough to see and work through. The problem was that once made, there was no putting it back! Wagner's procedure was much less destructive, but was more complicated to carry out and also resulted in a greater blood loss for the patient. He used a mallet and chisel to fashion a bone flap which could be lifted up away from the skull itself (raised), but was still attached by a hinge at one end, and could be replaced in the correct position after the operation had been completed with no resultant defect in the bone of the skull.

It was recognised by surgeons, however, that this was a major procedure associated with heavy blood loss. Therefore many recommended carrying out cranial surgery in two stages – firstly, performing the craniotomy and delaying the resection of the tumour until the patient had recovered from the blood loss created by the first procedure. A refinement of this surgical technique occurred when Leonardo Gigli developed and used a wire saw to cut through the skull more easily and his technique has been used until the present day. It is only recently that its use been surpassed by the introduction of the powered craniotome, which does the job more quickly.

Developments in neurosurgery and the Boer War

During the Boer War (1899-1902), some progress in the management of casualties with head wounds was made. Of those soldiers with head wounds who reached hospital, the mortality was 33%. The essential improvement resulted from gaining wide access to the track of the wound, identifying and removing in-driven fragments of bone and blood clots, suturing the dura, and closing the wound primarily.

Interestingly, the young surgeons performing this surgery were Cuthbert Wallace (Chapter 7), Anthony Bowlby (chapters 2, 3, 6, 7) and George Makins (Chapter 6).[8] Surgeon-General WF Stevenson expressed the opinion that:

> Even the most severe cases of gunshot fracture of the skull should be given the chance of recovery afforded by operative intervention.[9]

Stevenson's book *Wounds in War* was one of the most important textbooks of military surgery prior to the Great War. His book included a chapter on experimental work on bullet wounds as well as a chapter on wounds to the head. He observed that:

Owing to the improved methods of wound treatment the pendulum of opinion is swinging perhaps to the other extreme and we find Mr Victor Horsley (surgeon) recommending operation in all cases of depressed skull fracture (fractures in which the bone fragments have been driven inwards).[10]

The situation with respect to the medical literature then changed and there were frequent references in the medical journals of the day to the management and complications of wounds of the head and spine. There was a growing interest and enthusiasm about neurosurgery as a speciality and in 1902 the French surgeon Chipault published the first part of a three volume text, the other two parts being published in 1903, bringing together international experience in the field of neurosurgery. *L'état Actuel de la Chirurgie Nerveuse* was an account of the experience and opinions of 50 contributors from around the world.[11] There was a bibliography of 1230 references, representing a significant and growing literature on the subject.

The Great War

One of the enduring images of the Great War is the soldier with a head bandage or soldier bandage – an image synonymous with bravery. Another is the "Tommy", the British soldier wearing the characteristic Great War steel helmet. Behind these images is the story of suffering caused by an unprecedented epidemic of severe head and spinal wounds, and the surgeons whose task it was to deal with wounds that were as much of a challenge then, as now in the 21st Century. The wounds of those involved in the Great War were often devastating and frequently fatal, none more so than wounds of the brain.

At the start of the Great War, there were senior surgeons with experience in the management of head injuries, although there was no specific organisation of neurosurgical services or even a specialty called neurosurgery. Lessons learned during the Boer War had to be re-learned, a familiar theme in the history of surgery.

Of course, military surgeons were mainly confronted by head wounds, and by penetrating head wounds in particular, caused by bullets, shrapnel balls and fragments of shell casing. It was the surgeon's usual practice simply to raise (or "elevate") bone fragments that had been driven inwards inside the skull. The surgeon then explored the brain itself and removed bone fragments or bullets and debris. If the skull had to be cut open more formally, to allow greater access and a better view of what damage had occurred, a disc of skull bone was removed using an instrument called a trephine. Then, if it was necessary for the surgeon to get even more access to the brain, he used bone nibblers to enlarge the opening in the skull. The result, of course, was an even greater defect in the skull bone than the one caused by the initial wound!

An important figure in the development of neurosurgery before and during the Great War was Harvey Cushing. He was from Cleveland, Ohio, and had initially obtained an arts degree at Yale University before going on to study medicine at Harvard University. Cushing graduated in 1895 and his first post was in medicine at the John Hopkins Hospital in Baltimore. After completing his surgical training he was appointed later to the post of Professor of Surgery in Boston in 1912. He was especially interested in the nervous system and set about studying both the pathology of brain tumours, and the various factors that were responsible for the high operative mortality in neurosurgical

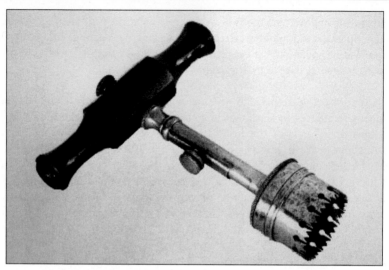

Figure 9.1   Trephine used in early neurosurgery. (Reproduced
with permission from Alan Peck Medical Antiques)

patients. One major contributory factor to this high mortality was excessive bleeding, and this was one that Cushing addressed.

He collaborated with Dr W.T. Bovey, a physicist, to develop a novel method for controlling bleeding. This resulted in the introduction of the "Bovey Electrocautery Tool", which was actually a diathermy machine. This used a high frequency electric current to coagulate blood vessels and is still used today by surgeons in all specialties to stop bleeding. When this machine was applied to neurosurgical operations together with excellent surgical technique, he was able to improve significantly the survival of patients undergoing surgery for brain tumours. Cushing presented his results to a meeting of the American College of Surgeons in 1919. This was a key paper and was greeted by William Mayo with the words "Gentlemen, we have this day witnessed the birth of a new specialty, neurosurgery" and with that neurological surgery was declared to exist as a specialty. Cushing's work had been of international significance and he had already been awarded an honorary fellowship of the Royal College of Surgeons of England in 1913, which is the highest honour that can be bestowed by the College.

Cushing's developments in neurosurgery were also applicable to the surgical management of patients with head injury and in particular those occurring during the Great War. He served as a surgeon with the American Base Hospital Unit Number 5 from Harvard, which took over the running of Number 11 General Hospital from the British in 1917. At the end of 1917, the Harvard Unit moved to British General Hospital Number 13, when Number 11 was transferred to Italy. In 1918 Cushing became senior consulting neurosurgeon to the American Expeditionary Force. While serving as a Colonel with the Harvard Unit working with the British Expeditionary Force, it is reported that in a letter to his wife he had firmly criticised a British surgeon. Unfortunately this was read by a French censor, who handed it over to the British authorities! There were some anxious moments for Cushing, as he was threatened with a court martial, but the matter was resolved and he was transferred to American command.

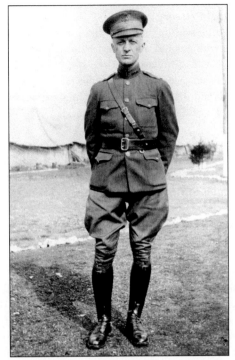

Figure 9.2   Harvey Cushing in France. (Courtesy of the
Cushing/Whitney Medical Historical Library)

The understanding of head wounds at the beginning of the Great War

The surgeon of the Great War was particularly concerned with open wounds of the skull and brain.

The patho-physiology of gunshot wounds had been studied by Horsley in the 1890s when the .303 rifle was introduced to the British Army, and as previously indicated, he had studied the patterns caused by rifle bullets as they were fired into wet clay. He extended his findings to describe the forces involved when a bullet penetrates the head. His work was published in 1915[12], and was of great importance to surgeons working in advanced medical units and in base hospitals.

Horsley detailed this very clearly in a key paper published at the beginning of 1915, which served as the basis of his presentation on this subject to the London Medical Society on 8 February 1915. His observations are summarised as follows:[13]

1. Concussion

Patients had died where there had not been any penetration of the skull and he attributed this to a paralysis of the respiratory and cardiac centres located in the brain stem. He likened this to the death caused by a cricket ball striking the skull. Others had also demonstrated that following trauma there is the development of oedema and tissue fluid lying within the brain substance which also contributes to a rise in intra-cranial pressure.

2. Rise in Intracranial Pressure

There might be bleeding within the brain and a rise in the intracranial pressure which, if not dealt with, would cause death by pressure upon and failure of the respiratory centre and stimulation of the vagal centre. This would result in deteriorating consciousness, slowing of the pulse rate and death of the casualty. It was becoming understood that reducing intracranial pressure was a necessary part of the management of a casualty with a head wound.

3. Sepsis

This was stated to be due to the "incomplete disinfection of the original wound" and "leaving head cases alone". Many surgeons were leaving patients to die after sustaining these wounds as they did not believe surgical intervention to offer any hope of success. Horsley described this as "a wicked practice". He pointed to the operative interventions pioneered during the Boer War as the way forward for the management of these wounds.

4. Hernia cerebri

This was the extrusion of a part of the brain to lie outside the skull due to a rise in the pressure within the skull. He considered this to be due to either the direct effects of the brain injury or to infection subsequently arising within the brain. To deal with this problem before death of the casualty occurred, he recommended trimming away these parts of the brain or the use of absolute alcohol or formaldehyde.

Protections against head wounds

During the Boer War, soldiers wore a pith helmet, which was coloured khaki, and only gave protection from the sun!

During the Great War, head wounds were seen in large numbers by all combatant nations. Wallace and Fraser attributed the frequency of head wounds to the fact that trench warfare exposed, in particular, the upper parts of the body to enemy fire.[14] In the first year of the war all combatant nations wore soft headgear. The French Army introduced steel helmets for their soldiers, called M15 Adrian helmets, named after the person thought responsible for their development (General August-Louis Adrian). They were very light (0.76kg) and were designed to protect against shrapnel from exploding shells. However, they were not effective at stopping bullets. Nevertheless they formed the basis for most military helmets well into the 1930s.

Following the French lead, the British Army and later the United States Army introduced the steel Brodie helmet which began production in 1915 but was not issued to troops in large numbers until as late as 1916. The Brodie helmet, designed by John L. Brodie of London (also known by various names including Tommy helmet, shrapnel helmet, tin hat, battle bowler) was a different design thought to confer advantages over the French Adrian helmet. For example, it was made from one sheet of thick steel giving greater strength to the shallow bowl structure, had a wide brim, a leather chinstrap and was more resistant to metal fragments and bullets. Modifications were made during the Great War to increase its effectiveness in preventing wounds. including making a wider brim and the addition of manganese to the steel which increased its strength. Despite the availability of helmets, head wounds still remained a major surgical problem

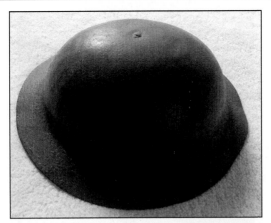

Figure 9.3 British Steel Helmet – the Brodie Helmet.
(Reproduced with permission from Robert Reid)

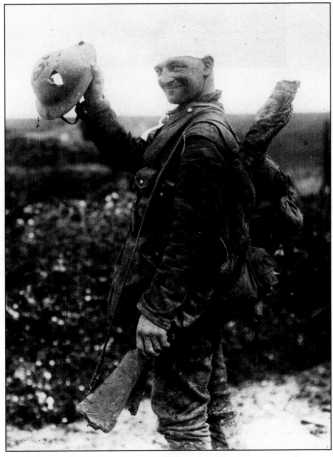

Figure 9.4 "Saved by the Helmet". (With thanks to the
Trustees of the National Library of Scotland)

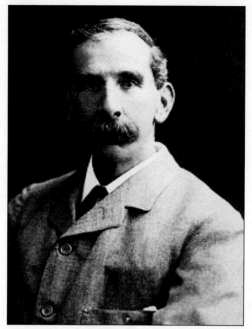

Figure 9.5   Sir Victor Horsley FRCS. (Wikimedia Commons)

throughout the war as the helmets did not withstand all insults. Also, soldiers who sustained head wounds had not always been wearing them at the moment of wounding. The development of the German helmet is discussed in Chapter 3.

Training in the treatment of head wounds

The British surgeons with the task of treating this epidemic of head injuries were, for the main part, general surgeons who had not had any prior experience of the management of such patients. The American medical services, entering the war later, were better prepared.

In the United States, Harvey Cushing had been lobbying for specialist surgical teams to treat casualties with head injuries. American Army Surgeon-General, William Gorgess, learned that about 15% of casualties at the Western Front had sustained head wounds. Volunteer surgeons with experience in neurosurgery were sought and it was estimated that 300 such specialists were required to go to the Western Front. It became clear that there were insufficient numbers of surgeons with the desired level of experience, so educational courses were established to bring specialist knowledge to the volunteers. Training took approximately 70 days and these surgeons were known as the "70 day neurosurgeons". As a result of these efforts the Americans formed specialist neurosurgical units in France. Little organisation took place in Britain, principally because of the limited numbers of surgeons who could be described as "specialist neurosurgeons". Horsley (regarded as the doyen of British neurological surgeons) had been able to make little contribution to the care of head injured troops and even before his deployment overseas he was to write, of some real concern, that:

I have not been permitted to see any cases in the present war, except for a few exceptional instances which happened to be referred to me unofficially.[15]

Horsley, a Territorial Force officer, had volunteered his services on the Western Front where his experience would have found its best outlet. Instead, in 1915 he was sent to Egypt, where surgical demands were quite different. His radical political views and his confrontational manner with colleagues did not perhaps aid his cause and he died of heat stroke in Mesopotamia in 1916.

Problems facing surgeons treating casualties with head wounds

The problems facing surgeons dealing with head wounds were soon apparent. Wound contamination and wound infection presented on an unprecedented scale, as described in Chapter 2, and affected patients with head wounds just as it did other wounds elsewhere in the body. It had to be decided when and where surgery should be carried out (there were differing views on this), and on the management of intra-cerebral foreign bodies including how to locate them and how best to remove them. There was much to learn about the prognosis of casualties with severe head wounds and their complications.

By its nature, trench warfare and a landscape of barbed wire determined the feasibility of retrieval of the wounded and their transportation to medical facilities. In the case of head injured patients the difficulties of retrieval were increased when patients were unconscious or confused. The filthy conditions endured by the troops and the heavy contamination of wounds that was inevitable in these surroundings has been referred to in previous chapters. Henry Gray of Aberdeen, in his important textbook *The Early Treatment of War Wounds* observed that:

The greatest obstacle to successful treatment of wounds in France is the virulent inflammation which is prone to intervene from infection with organisms of the most noxious type which have their habitat in the highly manured soil on which fighting takes place.[16]

With specific reference to head wounds, Gray went on to say:

Infected gunshot wounds of the skull and brain require more careful consideration and prompt attention than similar wounds of any other part.

Percy Sargent, a colleague of Horsley's in London (before the Great War started), was the most experienced British surgeon to serve in France and had an extensive experience of neurosurgery. He wrote both an analysis of his experience of head wounds and reviewed the outcome for soldiers with head wounds returning to England. He reported 5 months' experience in a base hospital in 1915 and observed that:

Owing to modern methods of warfare, and especially to trench fighting, the proportion of head injuries to the total number of wounded is surprisingly large.[17]

The injuries referred to included penetrating head wounds caused by bullets or shrapnel and the concussive effect caused by exploding shells, grenades and bombs,

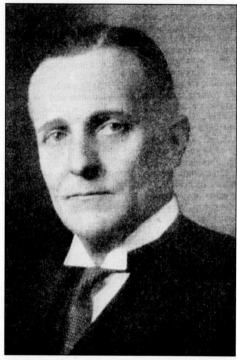

Figure 9.6   Percy Sargent FRCS. (Reproduced from the *British Medical Journal* January
28 1933 with permission from the *British Medical Journal* Publishing Group)

which caused damage without any signs of wounding. The challenge to the surgeons
came largely from missile wounds.

Sargent classified head wounds into three categories, which had implications for
treatment:[18]

- Those due to a glancing blow or where the entry and exit wounds lay close
  enough together to be considered as one,
- A missile had entered the cranial cavity and was still there,
- The missile had traversed the cranium.

Initial management of casualties with head wounds

The soldier with a head wound arriving at a regimental aid post could only expect a field
dressing before he was passed on to an advanced dressing station. There are accounts of
surgical procedures for head injuries being carried out at advanced dressing stations but
this was exceptional. The complexity of the surgery meant being transferred to a casualty
clearing station and then, if necessary, to a base hospital. We know now that the time
interval to treatment is one of the most important factors determining the outcome
of head injuries and development of complications. The merits of early treatment of
penetrating head wounds at designated casualty clearing stations instead of delayed
treatment until transfer to a base hospital were clear and became standard practice.
Thus, during the Third Battle of Ypres, all head injuries were dealt with at Mendinghem

Casualty Clearing Stations west of Poperinge (see map of casualty clearing stations in Chapter 2).[19]

Henry Gray concurred with this view. He recommended that only non-urgent cases should be referred on and be taken back immediately to the base hospital. His textbook of surgery (*Early Treatment of War Wounds*) contained a chapter on wounds of the brain and its coverings and gave clear instructions on pre-operative assessment, anaesthesia and surgical procedures.[20]

The value of early definitive surgery was illustrated by Horsley in 1915. A patient was transferred to his care in London after surgery in France for a severe penetrating head wound. The patient presented in an unconscious state at a dressing station. Major Sherran RAMC operated on him immediately, cleaning the wound and evacuating a haematoma (blood clot). The wound healed without sepsis and the patient survived to be returned to England and a gradual return to independence. Horsley, who held strong views about the importance of early surgery for head wounds, expressed his admiration for the prompt action of his RAMC colleague:

> We may hope, therefore, that the brilliant surgery of officers like Major Sherran will prevent cases arriving in England under conditions hopeless for restoration both of life and function.[21]

Treatment of minor head wounds

One of the achievements of the wartime experience of head wounds was the lesson that apparently minor head wounds carried potentially lethal complications. Captain J.E. Roberts published a series of 140 casualties with "minor" head wounds who were treated at base hospitals in France and he stated:

> As their injuries are apparently superficial and their symptoms are few or none, they frequently come down as "sitting" cases and on arrival there is a tendency to overlook the fact that among them is a fairly high percentage of cases with definite injury to the skull or to the skull and brain.[22]

Roberts emphasised the need to explore such apparently minor penetrating head wound in every case. That dogma is still emphasised to present day students of medicine and surgery throughout the world. Another RAMC officer, Captain George Tabuteau, with experience of 95 casualties with head wounds, wrote in 1915:

> Preconceived ideas that severe injuries inflicted on the skull or brain are bound to be accompanied by definite symptoms have been shown to be wrong. Frequently one sees men with severe damage to the skull and brain walking into hospital ... It appears almost impossible to be able to diagnose the degree of severity of the injury without carefully watching the patient for some time.[23]

This thinking was the basis for the treatment of head injuries in civilian life for many years and it became routine in the modern era of neurosurgery to detain patients with apparently minor head injuries for a period of a least 24 hours observation so that deterioration, if it occurred, was recognised at an early stage.

Management of casualties with skull fractures and penetrating head wounds

General aspects

Patients with penetrating head wounds included those with depressed skull fractures with an overlying wound, wounding of the brain with or without retained fragments of bone, bullet or shrapnel and "through and through" wounds where a missile had passed right through the head, as Sargent had usefully classified.[24] It was accepted that all penetrating wounds should be explored. The main reason for surgery was to prevent infection by removing contaminated tissues and foreign bodies. Once a brain abscess or meningitis (inflammation due to infection of the thin membranes surrounding the brain) was established, the mortality was very high, probably greater than 90%. Surgery was indicated to remove blood clot, and it was also thought that disability and epilepsy would be reduced by removing damaged brain and other debris.

While cranial surgery was indicated mainly to treat a large number of penetrating head wounds, patients could present with simple skull fractures and possible intracranial bleeding. Shocked patients tolerated poorly both a general anaesthetic and the blood loss entailed in surgery (see Chapter 3 for more details). Consequently much of the surgery was carried out under local anaesthetic, even although such patients might be restless, coughing and straining as well as being distressed. General anaesthesia with ether or chloroform caused the brain to swell with a resultant rise in intracranial pressure. This has hazardous effects for the patient and can result in death, as has been explained earlier in this chapter. Harvey Cushing certainly favoured local anaesthetic for this reason, and used local anaesthetic in conjunction with sedation with opiates (morphine-like drugs) as he believed this to be the safest approach. This policy was followed by most surgeons, who were in agreement with Cushing's views.

Severe blood loss was a contributory cause to continuing high mortality in both civilian neurosurgery (as explained earlier) as well as in wartime surgery. Scalp wounds bleed heavily due to the rich blood supply of the scalp. Furthermore, bleeding from the brain can be difficult to control. Therefore, surgeons infiltrated adrenaline around the skin wound margins to diminish bleeding, because adrenaline causes constriction of the blood vessels thus reducing blood loss. Other surgeons tried their own novel ideas to reduce blood loss including the use of scalp tourniquets.

Clinical Examination

Percy Sargent had the benefit of working in base hospitals in France with Gordon Holmes, who was a neurology colleague at Queen Square in London. To Holmes is attributed the routine method of carrying out a neurological examination that remains in use today. Sargent emphasised the importance of carrying out a detailed neurological examination in head injured patients in order to be able to recognise the need for surgery. Since, in his experience, most wounds were already infected, there was a serious risk in opening the membranes surrounding the brain – the dura is the outermost and thickest of the three membranes covering the brain – to evacuate a suspected intracranial haematoma, because infection might be introduced. He described the clinical features of raised intracranial pressure (increasing headache, vomiting, declining consciousness, slowing of pulse, a rising blood pressure and a changing breathing pattern) and he thought it important to balance the risk of meningitis against the risk of death or greater neurological impairment if surgery was not carried out. He concluded that surgery to evacuate a haematoma and so decompress the swollen brain was justifiable as being the lesser of two evils, despite the risk imposed by an already contaminated or infected wound.

Pre-operative X-rays

Of particular importance for these casualties was the development and introduction of X-rays for locating intracranial bone fragments and foreign bodies (see Chapter 5). X-rays also enabled surgeons to recognise closed skull fractures, i.e. where the skull is fractured but the skin overlying the bone has not been lacerated or opened up by the wounding agent. This was of particular value when patients presented with head wounds complicated by intracranial bleeding where there was no visible surface wound on the scalp or head to indicate where to operate. Of course, subsequent generations of surgeons have had the benefits of developments in radiology allowing the use of contrast radiology (ventriculography and cerebral angiography, in which some form of contrast material is injected into the ventricles of the brain or the arteries of the brain); most importantly and used nowadays are CT and MRI scanning. Interestingly, indirect imaging of the brain in the form of ventriculography was first suggested in 1918 by Walter Dandy, who was a close contemporary and fierce rival of Harvey Cushing.

Views about skull fractures and impact on management

The casualty's neurological signs such as dysphasia (speech impairment) or limb weakness on one side gave an indication of which side of the head the surgeon should operate on. X-rays showing a fracture gave additional valuable information, allowing the surgeon to have a better idea as to where the damage was most likely to be. Most surgeons recommended the routine elevation of depressed fractures of the skull, even if there was

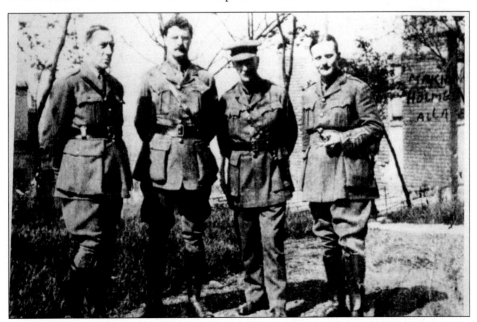

Figure 9.7   Gordon Holmes (second left) and Percy Sargent (right). (Private collection)

no overlying wound to the skin. There were notions that impingement of bone fragments on the brain or laceration of dura and brain might cause neurological damage that could be reduced or prevented by surgery. Some surgeons even advocated this approach when fractures lay over the great venous sinuses (large veins which lie at several locations within and around the brain) because of the hypothetical risk of "disturbance of venous drainage" of the brain. The very serious risk here is of difficult venous bleeding if these sinuses are damaged by the surgeon's knife during surgery. Henry Gray reported the results from 14 such patients who were operated on after one battle of whom "only one died".

This drew a critical response from Sir Edward Farquhar Buzzard, Regius Professor of Medicine at the University of Oxford, who criticised what he clearly saw as the "gung-ho" attitude of surgeons, commenting:

> I am tempted to inquire whether the removal of the depressed bone is attended by the return of the venous circulation or whether the surgeon is not forced in the course of this operation to promote further thrombosis in order to check the alarming haemorrhage which may occur when the sinus is exposed. The only harm caused by the depressed bone may be the interference with the circulation in the lacunae and the cortical veins and the remedy proposed is likely to make this condition irremediable ... I should like to show him (Gray) the remarkable recoveries which are made by some of these cases which have never been operated on. Nothing has impressed me more in connection with the cranial surgery of the war than the success of the conservative methods adopted and advocated by many British and French surgeons, not only in these cases but in dealing with depressed bone and foreign bodies as a whole.[25]

Management of Foreign Bodies in the Brain

Penetrating head wounds were commonly accompanied by foreign material and, in particular, fragments of metal and bone deep within the wound. In the earlier stages of the war there was some doubt and confusion about the merits of attempting to remove foreign bodies. Captain W.E. Tyndall reported that:

> The necessity for the examination of the brain for foreign bodies, and their removal, is a subject of some controversy among the surgeons who are working in the clearing stations.[26]

Furthermore, Sargent and Holmes, who were developing a great experience in the management of these casualties, stated that:

> It seems extremely doubtful if surgical intervention other than that necessary for the drainage and the healing of the wounds diminishes appreciably the risk of later complications ... our records show that many patients with foreign bodies lodged deeply in the brain recover and are scarcely more liable to serious complications than men in whom the brain has been merely exposed and lacerated.[27]

However, this view was not held by all. It was generally accepted that removal of bullets, shrapnel and contaminated bone fragments was necessary in order to prevent infection from subsequently developing. In addition, Henry Gray believed that foreign material should be removed because it was harmful. He explained this as follows:

> A direct effect on the delicate pulsating of brain tissue ... by interfering in a rather obscure way in the circulation of the brain ... by causing, when they become encapsulated a localised connective tissue mass which may act as deleteriously as a tumour.[28]

Gray's view was that removal of a foreign body resulted in more complete and more rapid recovery. Similarly, Cushing supported the view that foreign bodies should be removed wherever possible, although he acknowledged the difficulties in safely locating deeply-placed objects and noted that sometimes symptoms did not result if the foreign body was not removed.[29]

It is important to remember that it can be difficult to locate an object within the brain even in practice today. As early as the 1890s attempts had been made to do this by taking X-rays rays in two planes (see Chapter 5 for details). By the time of the Great War, a variety of other devices to allow detection of metallic foreign bodies in the brain had been developed. One idea was to use a battery with one pole connected by a wire to a metal probe and the other to a plate in the patient's mouth. If a bell was included in the circuit it would ring if the circuit was completed by contact with the metal fragment or bullet. Another device employed a similar circuit but was attached to an electro-magnet. On contact with the metallic foreign body, there would be a buzzing sensation in the probe. An entire textbook was published in 1918 on the subject of 'The Localisation and Extraction of Projectiles' by Ombredanne and Ledoux-Lebard, with an account of the various devices available.[30]

Henry Gray recommended that the operation to remove a foreign body from the brain should, wherever possible, be carried out under local anaesthetic. After X-ray localisation the track of the bullet within the brain should be explored with the index finger until the foreign body was located. A scoop could then be passed along the finger to deliver the object and remove it. The patient was encouraged to cough in order to help to expel blood clot, bone fragments and necrotic tissue. This would not, of course, be done today!

Cushing was concerned that surgeons might be too preoccupied with removal of the foreign body, omitting to remove necrotic and contaminated brain tissue from the track of the bullet. He did not favour digital exploration because of the increased neurological damage it might cause and described, instead, the gentle use of a soft catheter to irrigate the track and suck out debris. He had an interesting turn of phrase to express these concerns in one of his papers:

> But we must recognise that the surgical profession contains its "Little Jack Horners" and it is better, on the whole, for all of us to keep our fingers out of the brain so far as possible![31]

Operative Techniques

The general surgical principle of early wound excision, involving removal of all devitalised tissue to minimise the risk of infection applies equally to wounds of the brain. There is, of course, a major problem, in that the brain is a vital organ. One can remove all dead muscle from a thigh, with the prospect of a good recovery, apart from a slight limp. Removal of all necrotic brain from a head wound, however gently, may necessitate irrigating away practically the entire brain and clearly this is not the situation any surgeon (or patient) would want to be placed in.

It is also very important to obtain primary skin closure over the site of the craniectomy (the hole in the skull).

Because there is little "give" in the scalp it was often difficult to obtain closure where there had been loss of skin. A simple surgical technique to achieve skin closure was to make "releasing" incisions on either side to allow the main wound to be closed without tension.[32]

Instructions were given to the American neurosurgical teams in 1918; an example is given below:

> If a case is operated on and a penetration found, the operation must be completed, with a primary closure following the special debridement applicable to these injuries. In this respect wounds of the nervous system differ from other wounds which in times of rush should not be subjected to primary closure. 'All or nothing' is a good rule to apply to the cranio-cerebral injury – in short, evacuate these cases untreated to the nearest base (except for shaving and the application of a wet antiseptic dressing) rather than do incomplete operations … The chief source of the high mortality in cranial wounds is infection – infection of the meninges; direct infection of the brain leading to encephalitis; infection of the ventricles.[33]

Control and Management of Raised Intracranial Pressure

Before the war it had been recognised that one of the consequences of brain injury was swelling resulting in raised intracranial pressure and that this both contributed to the harmful effects of head injury and made surgical operations more difficult. Directly or indirectly, the treatment of serious head wounds is about controlling intracranial pressure. The means to do this were very limited in 1914. Foremost, it was important to recognise that the patient might have increasing intracranial pressure and that this might be due to intracranial bleeding which might be amenable to surgery. Where this was due to an intracranial blood clot, urgent surgery was required. Continuing high pressure within the skull due to brain swelling or infection could be reduced by decompressive craniectomy or subtemporal decompression. This involved removing an area of skull to allow the brain to swell unimpeded. The practice was used widely during and after the war but was abandoned in the later 20th century only to have found favour again in recent years.

Intracranial pressure could also be lowered by carrying out a lumbar puncture and draining a quantity of cerebrospinal fluid. There are dangers that in doing this the brain will be displaced downwards resulting in compression of the brain stem containing the centres that control breathing and the circulation and, ultimately, breathing stops and death of the patient ensues. The hazards of over-draining cerebrospinal fluid, causing deepening coma and respiratory arrest, were recognised by the doctors of that time. As well as mechanical means of lowering pressure hypertonic saline was used, usually introduced rectally, to bring about a state of dehydration and thereby reducing brain volume.

Complications of head wounds
Brain Hernia

Surgeons had long been aware that defects in the skull due either to skull injuries or to trephining tended to result in brain herniation or "fungus cerebri" where brain tissue bulged out of the skull defect. Sir George Ballingall described this complication in *Outline of Military Surgery* as early as 1852.[34] Because of a persisting sense of fatalism towards severe head injury, surgical inexperience and the lack of accepted protocols for managing head wounds in the field, this remained a major problem in the Great War. When the wound was left open the injured brain herniated through the defect. When this became infected the hernia increased. The process increased the local neurological damage and the whole process was likely to lead to brain abscess, meningitis and death. Sargent reported that of 600 patients with penetrating head wounds identified in France and returned to hospitals in London, 120 had cerebral hernia.[35] The mortality amongst these patients was almost 25%. Once the problem was established the only solution was to treat the wound with antiseptic dressings and then to amputate the herniating brain before closing the wound. Brain herniation could be reduced by carrying out a craniectomy on the other side of the head in order to reduce the intracranial pressure or by lumbar puncture and cerebrospinal fluid drainage. Horsley, Cushing and others stressed the importance of primary wound closure in layers as a means of avoiding brain herniation.

Infection

There was general agreement that early treatment of head wounds offered some chance of reducing the risk of subsequent infection developing but the debate around the value or otherwise of antiseptics applied to wound surfaces was extensive. It even reached the level of personal abuse, with Victor Horsley, as one of the prominent participants, doing battle with other surgeons including Sir R.J. Godlee and Sir W. Watson Cheyne. Horsley wrote:

> I proved in your last issue, by quoting Lister's own words, that Sir R.J. Godlee's statement was a complete misrepresentation of the facts and of true Listerian antiseptic surgery. Though, fortunately, the younger generation of surgeons cannot be deceived by this perversion of Lister's science there remains a public duty to be done, and that is, the immediate withdrawal by the authorities of Sir R.J. Godlee's misleading and erroneous leaflet.[36]

Godlee had worked as Lord Lister's assistant, had made the first observation of streptococci from a wound swab and was, perhaps, worthy of greater respect. Watson-Cheyne was senior surgeon at Kings College Hospital and another student of Lister's who held strong views and expressed them without much obvious concern about whose feelings he hurt.

A high proportion of cases, however, arrived in base hospitals with already infected wounds, in contrast to head wounds in civilian practice, and the standards of surgery were questioned. However, the *British Medical Journal's* war correspondent stated that:

> Teeming, therefore, as was the soil with anaerobes and contaminated with the former as are the men's clothes, it is inevitable that every wound caused by a relatively slow travelling missile should be instantly, and for the time being, irremediably infected.[37]

Of those who survived to be transferred, there was a 3.7% death rate – the majority died of infection. All deaths from sepsis had wounds that penetrated the dura, the membrane covering the brain. Large numbers were still being transferred with open wounds and 10% had retained foreign bodies in the head. Approximately 10% of returning casualties in this group required further surgery in England.[38] Secondary surgery was indicated, amongst other things, for the treatment of cerebral abscesses and subdural empyaema (abscess). Septic granulating wounds were dressed variously with magnesium sulphate, potassium permanganate or "salt sacks" – gauze sacks containing salt – which were packed into the wound until a delayed closure was possible or the wound healed spontaneously. Remarkably, these patients could recover despite the absence of antibiotics.

Skull Defects
One of the effects of a large number of penetrating head wounds and the surgical practices of the time was the number of returning soldiers with skull defects. Some of these were sufficiently large to constitute a risk to the patient or a "cosmetic" problem due to the destructive nature of these wounds. Various suggestions had been made about suitable materials for repairing and filling in the defect in the skull bone (an operation called cranioplasty). Both gold and silver plates were used and put into the skull to cover the bone defect but the favoured technique was to use bone taken from the patient themselves from another site of the body. Bone from the iliac crest (the rim of the pelvis) and ribs were the most commonly used. The results were successful but this was a major procedure with a substantial morbidity and complication rate. In the last years of the war both aluminium and celluloid plates began to be employed and used to repair these skull defects.

Longer-term symptoms after head wounds
It is now recognised that apparently relatively minor closed head injuries with loss of consciousness can be followed by disabling symptoms which include headache, depression, dizziness and fatigue. Some recognition of the nature of acute and chronic anxiety states was beginning, but still required to be distinguished from notions of "hysteria" and "shell shock".

The latter term was applied both to the effects of close proximity to an explosion – what we would now recognise as a diffuse closed head injury followed by post-concussional symptoms – and to anxiety states that may now be recognised as "combat stress reaction".

Transporting casualties with head wounds

Patients with head wounds did not tolerate transport in the post-operative period. The reasons were not analysed but might include the risks in transit of dehydration and hypotension (low blood pressure), hypoxia (shortage of oxygen) and supine posture which results in raised intracranial pressure.

If surgery was to be carried out at a casualty clearing station, then it should be complete and the patient only be transferred to the rear after about 10 days. Tabuteau advised a delay of 3 weeks before transporting a patient[39] and Gray, with his considerable experience, advised a similar policy, which was to operate at the casualty clearing station and keep the patient there for three weeks prior to transfer to a base hospital.[40]

Prognosis of casualties with head injuries

Given the devastating effect of a bullet on brain tissue, it is little wonder that severe morbidity might follow "successful" treatment of severe head wounds. Henry Gray, with his experience of managing head wounds in South Africa, commented that:

> There was a considerable number of men injured in the head during the South African War who afterwards became a burden to the state owing to derangements of the brain and it must be remembered that the maiming effects of sepsis in that campaign were not apparent to anything like the same degree as in this one.[41]

After the Boer War Stevenson had observed that the possibility of recovery from head injuries, if properly managed, should encourage surgeons to take an optimistic view. This message was repeated by surgeons in the Great War. Gray wrote that:

> The power of the brain to accommodate itself to extraordinary conditions … has also been very striking. But who can foretell that, later on, such cases are to be free, as never before, of sequelae which experience has shown to be so frequently inevitable. Because of that experience and because no one can foresee how soon trouble will arise it is surely right that we should do all in our power to prevent trouble.[42]

Gray continued:

> We can prevent permanent disability in most cases by systematically removing foreign material or displaced bone from the surface or substance of the brain whenever these are accessible to legitimate surgery.[43]

The optimistic views of surgeons about the indications for surgery and the possibility of good outcomes were met with some scepticism by others. Professor Buzzard expressed considerable doubt about this, and there was some scepticism again as on his part towards the value of surgical intervention when he stated:

> This is a remarkable statement as it stands, and still more remarkable when we realize that "permanent disability" must include various forms of paralysis, disorders of speech, disorders of the special senses, and traumatic epilepsy, as well as mental

derangement, and that no evidence is offered as to the permanent condition of his cases after the "complete" operation he so strongly advocates. It is the permanent condition of these unfortunate victims of the war which chiefly interests us, and upon which claims for the superiority of any particular method of treatment must surely be based. Those of us who are watching and treating these patients after their removal from the base hospitals may form in the course of time some opinion as to the accuracy of Colonel Gray's claim. Meanwhile, I cannot help feeling that some of his principles are founded on the old fallacy that the presence of foreign material rather than the injury to brain substance is the origin of such disorders of function as paralysis and epilepsy.[44]

Poor prognostic factors were recognised by surgeons, including severe compound wounds due to shell fragments, low blood pressure and a rapid pulse, "through and through" injuries and established infection of the brain. Meningitis then, as now, carried a very poor prognosis but there were case reports of recovery even from this feared complication.[45]

Summary

Neurosurgery was developing as a specialty before the Great War and continued to do so, with the war influencing development. The wartime experience of brain wounds also provided the opportunity to make studies of basic neuroscience. Drawing on this experience, the French surgeon Chatelin published a book on functional neuroanatomy based on a study of 5,000 cases of brain wounds. Gordon Holmes, working as a neurologist in France and collaborating with Percy Sargent at General Hospital Number 13, had the opportunity to study soldiers who had suffered gunshot wounds of the occipital lobes. The occipital lobe of the brain is responsible for vision and Holmes carried out detailed charting of the fields of vision of his patients. The data obtained provided valuable knowledge of the anatomy of the occipital lobes. Cushing visited Holmes and Sargent and expressed his admiration for the quality of their work with head injured patients. He also observed that "these two men have an unparalleled opportunity not only to be of service to the individual wounded but, when all this is over, to make a contribution to physiology, neurology and surgery which will be epochal.[46]

Notes

1   Guthrie, G.J., *On Gun-shot wounds of the extremities*. London: Longman, Hurst, Rees, Orme and Brown, 1815.

2   Hennan, J., *Principles of Military Surgery*. London: John Wilson, 1829, 3rd edition, pp.281-343.

3   *Ibid.*

4   Lynch, A., "Cerebral localization", *British Medical Journal* 1915; 1: p.141.

5   Scagliosi, G., "Ueber die Gehirnerschütterung und die daraus im Gehirn und Rückenmark hervorgerufenen histologischen Veränderungen. Experimentelle Untersuchungen", *Virchows Archiv* 1898; 152: pp.487-525.

6   Kirkpatrick, D.B., "The first primary brain-tumor operation", *Journal of Neurosurgery* 1984; 61: pp.809-813.

7   Buchfelder, M. & B. Ljunggren, "Wilhelm Wagner (1848-1900). Part 2: The osteoplastic flap", *Surgical Neurology* 1988 Dec; 30 (6): pp.428-433.

8   Gordon, D.S., "Penetrating head injuries", *Ulster Medical Journal* 1988; 57: pp.1-10.

9   Stevenson, W.F., "Notes on surgical experiences of the Boer War", *Journal of the Royal Army Medical Corps* 1903; 1: pp.93-8.

10 *Ibid.*

11 Chipault, A., *L'état Actuel de la Chirurgie Nerveuse*. Paris: J. Rueff, 1902.

12 Horsley, V., "Remarks on gunshot wounds to the head: made in opening a discussion at the Medical Society of London on February 8th, 1915", *British Medical Journal* 1915; 1: pp.321-323.

13 *Ibid.*

14 Wallace, C.S. & J. Fraser, *Surgery at a casualty clearing station*. London: A & C Black, 1918, pp. 211-228.

15 Horsley, *op.cit.*, pp.321-323.

16 Gray, H.M.W., *The Early Treatment of War Wounds*. London: Henry Frowde, 1919.

17 Sargent, P. & G. Holmes, "The treatment of cranial injures of warfare", *British Medical Journal* 1915; 1: p.537.

18 *Ibid.*

19 MacPherson, W.G. (ed.), *History of the Great War based on Official Documents. Medical Services. General History*. London: HMSO, 1924, Volume 3, pp.143.

20 Gray, *op.cit.*, pp.68, 174-212.

21 Horsley, *op.cit.*, pp.321-323.

22 Roberts, J.E., "The treatment of gunshot wounds of the head, with special reference to apparently minor injuries", *British Medical Journal* 1915; 2: pp.498-500.

23 Tabuteau, G.G., "The treatment of gunshot wounds of the head, based on a series of ninety-five cases", *British Medical Journal* 1915; 2: pp.501-502.

24 Sargent & Holmes, *op.cit.*, p.537.

25 Buzzard, E.F., "Gunshot wounds of the head", *British Medical Journal* 1914; 1: pp.432-433.

26 Tyndall, W.E., "Early complications resulting from retained bone fragments in a case of gunshot wound to the head", *British Medical Journal* 1917; 1: p.423.

27 Sargent & Holmes, *op.cit.*, p.537.

28 Gray, *op.cit.*, p.191.

29 Cushing, H., "Notes on penetrating wounds of the brain", *British Medical Journal* 1918; 1: pp.221-226

30 Ombredanne, L. & L. Ledoux-Lebard, *Localisation et Extraction des Projectiles*. Paris: Masson & Cie, 1917.

31 Cushing, *op.cit.*, pp.221-226.

32 Gray, H.M., "Observations on gunshot wounds of the head", *British Medical Journal* 1916; 1: pp.261-265.

33 Ireland, M.W., *The Medical Department of the United States Army in the World War* Volume XI. Washington DC: Government Printing Office, 1927.

34 Ballingall, Sir G., *Outlines of military surgery*. Edinburgh: Black, 1852, 4th ed.

35 Sargent, P. & G. Holmes, "A report on the later results of gunshot wounds of the head", *Journal of the Royal Army Medical Corps* 1916; 27: p.300.

36 Horsely, V., "The treatment of wounds in the present war", *British Medical Journal* 1914; 2: p.901.

37 Anonymous, "Medical arrangements of the British Expeditionary Force", *British Medical Journal* 1914; 2: p.848.

38 Sargent, P. & G. Holmes, "A report on the later results of gunshot wounds of the head", *Journal of the Royal Army Medical Corps* 1916; 27: p.300.

39 Tabuteau, *op.cit.*, pp.501-502.

40 Gray, H.M.W., *The Early Treatment of War Wounds*. London: Henry Frowde, 1919, pp.174-212.

41 Gray, *op.cit.*, p.175.

42 Gray, H.M., "Observations on gunshot wounds of the head", *British Medical Journal* 1916; 1: pp.261-265.

43 *Ibid.*

44 Buzzard, *op.cit.*, pp.432-433.

45 Gray, H.M., "Observations on gunshot wounds of the head", *British Medical Journal* 1916; 1: pp.261-265.

46 Cushing, H., *From a Surgeon's Journal 1915-1918*. Boston: Little, Brown & Co, 1936.

10

Development of Plastic Surgery

John D Holmes

War is the best school for surgeons.

Hippocrates

Everything has been thought of before, but the problem is to think of it again.
Johann Wolfgang von Goethe (1749-1832)

The definition and history of plastic surgery

Since ancient times man has devised surgical procedures to alter appearance, mostly for reconstruction after injury. Rhinoplasty (reshaping or reconstructing the nose) and treatment of burns were described in Egypt in 3000BC and nasal reconstruction (the "Indian rhinoplasty") was described by Shushruta in 800 BC for restoration of the nose following its amputation as a punishment for crime.

The original technique used tissue taken from the cheek but this was modified later to use skin from the forehead. "Cosmetic" operations were recorded in Roman times to remove scars and to reshape nasal profiles. Celsus (Aulus Cornelius Celsus, ca 25BC to ca 50AD) even described circumcision reversal and correction of gynaecomastia (abnormal enlargement of male breast). Galen (Aelius Galenus, AD129-199/217), an accomplished philosopher and surgeon, also described various procedures but, during the Dark Ages, these writings were lost to the West, although some survived in the Arabic world. Superstitious beliefs during this time held back further surgical advances but, during the Renaissance, surgery was rediscovered, therefore allowing surgeons such as Tagliacozzi (1546-1599) to develop techniques to reconstruct the nose using a pedicled flap (see later) from the upper arm.[1]

This reconstruction however was not particularly robust and even Tagliacozzi himself regarded it as "virtual", being in danger of falling off if blown too hard! The attitude of

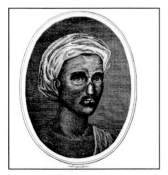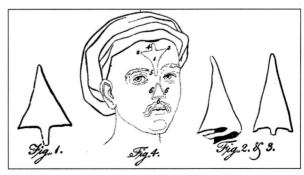

Figure 10.1   Two images showing the "Indian Rhinoplasty". (Private collection)

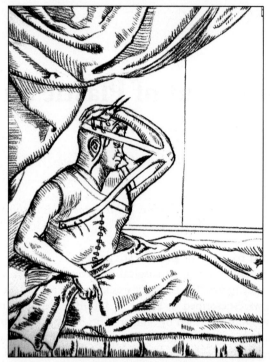

Figure 10.2   Taggliacozzi Flap. (Private collection)

Tagliacozzi, however, was one of scientific and medical interest in the condition of the patient rather than the judgemental opinions of society at the time, which held that patients who had lost their nose as a result of syphilis or trauma were "punished by God".

Again, largely because of these types of beliefs, no further progress took place, until in 1794 a group of British surgeons observed an Indian rhinoplasty using a forehead flap. This was described in a letter to the *Gentleman's Magazine*[2] and provoked interest in Europe. The word "plastic" in surgery was perhaps first used around this time by the German surgeon Carl Ferdinand von Graefe (1787-1840) in his paper on this subject, "Rhinoplastik" in 1818.[3]

The term "plastic" (the Greek word πλαστικός is the past participle of the verb πλασσειν, to mould or to form) is frequently misunderstood. In modern usage it tends to mean something artificial, but in surgical terms it means the moving of tissue into a defect, permanently, to correct it. A definition of plastic surgery is "a remedying of a deficiency of structure (and function): reparative of tissue."[4]

Defects in the surface of the skin can be repaired by various methods. The simplest is by direct (primary) closure – bringing the edges of the defect together and closing by sutures. If necessary, surrounding skin can be undermined and loosened to allow it to slide enough to close the defect. This method can be applicable for some large defects on the trunk and thigh. For other, perhaps even larger defects, for defects where there is insufficient local skin, or for smaller defects on the face which cannot be closed by this method, other ways of correction are needed. A simple and traditional technique employed was to allow the wound to heal by secondary intention (Chapters 2 and 6).

It was left unclosed and nature's own healing mechanisms caused the wound to shrink and allow the surface cells to grow over. This was, to a large extent, uncontrollable and wounds, especially those of the face, healed with a poor aesthetic and functional outcome (scars heal with shrinkage and distort the surrounding tissue).

In the early to mid 19th century, experiments were performed to "transplant" skin from one part of the body to another. These were largely successful, and by 1869, Reverdin[5] was able to report useful application of tiny areas of epidermis (pinch grafts) onto a granulating bed of an ulcer, so allowing it to heal. Granulation tissue is a velvety tissue with a rich blood supply which grows over the surface of a wound or ulcer, and represents efforts of the body to heal itself. Its rich blood supply means it will readily allow a graft to "take". This technique was developed further by Thiersch in Germany and Ollier in France[6], who took larger areas of thin graft using a modified shaving blade and applied these to wounds. These grafts form the basis of modern split skin grafting. Free grafts depend for their survival on having a blood supply in the bed onto which they are put. In contact with an appropriate bed, after a few days, the vessels connect up with the residual vessels of the free graft, so allowing "take".

There can, however, be considerable scar tissue around the bed, and this can lead to shrinking of the healed wound and graft causing contracture, giving unsatisfactory results, especially around the face. To a certain extent, this can be avoided by using a "full thickness" graft, one that contains the whole of the depth of the skin. By taking this extra tissue, scarring and contracture is less. "Split skin" grafts are thinner and only take the top layers of the skin. The donor sites heal by the epithelial (skin) cells remaining in the hair follicles and sweat glands in the donor site spreading over its surface. Full thickness grafts include these skin elements and the donor site cannot heal spontaneously in this manner. The donor defect needs to be closed directly or grafted with a further split skin graft to achieve healing. This, and the fact that getting it to "take" is more difficult, limits the useful size of full thickness grafts. Free grafts, also, are not suitable to cover defects without a viable blood supply in the base.

Exposed bone, cartilage or tendon, an open joint after a major wound or exposed foreign material, for example metal-work to hold a fracture in place, will not accept a free graft because there are no blood vessels to grow into the graft, which will consequently not regain a blood supply, and will turn black and fall off. In these cases it is necessary to move tissue with its own blood supply from elsewhere to close the defect. This tissue is known as a flap. The first flaps described (India and Italy) were not based on known anatomical blood supplies and can be said to be "random pattern". The length/breadth ratio could not normally be extended beyond 1:1. The distal end (the free unattached end) of any flap made with dimensions beyond this ratio would be at high risk of dying. These flaps could be moved "locally" either by simple advancement directly into the defect or by transposition from an adjacent area of healthy non-injured tissue and are widely used in reconstruction to this day.

Tissue could also be brought in from a "distant" location. A skin flap was raised, leaving it attached at one end. The other end was then taken to a defect. After three weeks or so the moved component of the tissue would have acquired a blood supply from the bed into which it had been put, and the tissue joining it to its original site could be safely divided and returned to fill the donor defect or excised. This technique forms the basis of the "Indian" forehead flap for nasal reconstruction and can even be used,

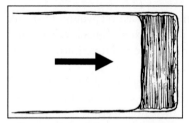

Figure 10.3   Advancement flap principle. (Author's collection)

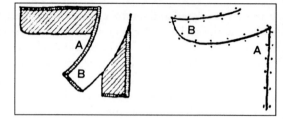

Figure 10.4   Transposition flap. (Author's collection)

for example, to transfer tissue from one leg to the other as a "cross-leg" flap. A further development of this was the tube pedicle. Flaps were constructed in an area remote from the defect and two 1:1 ratio flaps raised in continuity end to end so making a rectangular flap with a 2:1 ratio. The edges of this flap were sewn together to form a tube and this was allowed to settle for three or so weeks.

The blood supply by this method was redirected within the flap into a longitudinal orientation. In other words, the blood vessels gradually realigned and adjusted to supply the flap in a longitudinal orientation from each end of the flap, which was not the orientation of vessels in the skin before the flap was raised. One end could then safely be detached and sewn into the defect in one or more stages. After two to three weeks, new vessels entered this part of the flap from the recipient bed. At this stage the donor end of the flap could be divided and the flap tissue moved to cover the defect. Several operations were often required to provide refinement to the end result. Importing uninjured tissue in this manner allowed an improved functional and aesthetic outcome than that provided by direct closure alone or by the use of skin grafts, especially around the face.

In 1889 Manchot[7] had described the anatomy of blood vessels to the skin, and, if flaps had been based on these known blood vessels perfusing that area of skin, this 1:1 ratio could have been greatly extended. This would have given much greater flexibility to the use of these flaps as they could have been used further from the donor site. Although some mention of the vascularity (blood supply) at the base of some of these flaps was made by Gillies (superficial temporal artery at the base of the forehead flap allowing it to be made beyond the 1:1 ratio[8] and Manchot's diagrams being included in Davis's textbook of 1919)[9], the great leap forward into basing flaps on known blood vessels did not occur until much later (later 20th century) with the work of surgeons such as Ian McGregor in Glasgow[10] and Ian Taylor[11] [12] in Melbourne, Australia and many others.

Technical advances in surgical microscopy and suture materials have allowed tissue based on single increasingly small vessels to be transferred as free flaps using micro-vascular anastomosis (joining up the two ends of tiny blood vessels), so avoiding the need to "waltz" pedicle flaps to their eventual site. For example, a muscle from the back called latissimus dorsi can be taken, and transplanted to the leg, most commonly to cover an exposed knee joint. The vessels which supply the muscle are carefully preserved, and then stitched (anastomosed) to equally small vessels in the leg, thereby providing healthy, richly vascularised tissue to cover the defect. These flaps were not used in treating casualties during the Great War. Patients with exposed knee joints, as a result of bullet or shrapnel wounds would have required an amputation (Chapter 6).

Religious and social taboos continued to influence developments in surgical techniques to correct or alter appearance. The wounds sustained in various conflicts, however, profoundly changed the attitudes of society at large and allowed a foundation for progress in methods of reconstruction. The Great War brought a new range of weapons to inflict damage on the soldier, sailor, and later airman, such as had not been seen in previous conflicts. These have been extensively discussed in previous chapters (chapters 2 and 7), so no further mention need be made of them here. Suffice it to say, that the type of trench warfare seen produced much greater numbers of wounds to the head and neck than had occurred in warfare before.

Early radical wound excision was a fundamental surgical principle established during the Great War, and has been discussed at length in chapters 2 and 6. For wounds of the head and neck, however, wound excision produced large defects that could not be closed by traditional techniques. It became necessary to devise methods of restoring casualties with these wounds back to as near normal an appearance as was possible.

Establishment of plastic surgery in the United Kingdom

At the beginning of the Great War, there was not an established plastic surgery specialty either in Britain or America. Any "plastic surgery" was performed by general surgeons as part of their overall repertoire of operations which they could perform. Although there was a good deal of medical literature, it was confusing and often contradictory, offering little help to the surgeon faced with what seemed to be an overwhelming number of casualties. Large defects of the face were closed primarily to achieve healing as soon as possible, with no real attention given to the functional or aesthetic result. Wounded servicemen (especially in Germany) were returned to the front as soon as possible, and this was sometimes with wounds that had not completely healed. The resulting disfigured appearance of these returning soldiers (mostly) had the effect of lowering morale not only in the patients, but also in his comrades with whom they had to live and fight.

The management and evacuation of wounded military personnel was streamlined during the Great War. Medical officers worked as appropriate in various locations in relation to the front (Chapter 2). In January 1915 an ENT Surgeon, Harold Delf Gillies, a New Zealander of Scottish descent, then aged 33, was sent to France.* At the 83rd (Dublin) General Hospital, Wimereux, just north of Boulogne, he met Charles Auguste Valadier, a flamboyant French "dental practitioner".

Valadier was born in Paris on 26 November 1873 to a French pharmacist. As a child he went to live in America and became an American citizen. He went to Dental School in Philadelphia, qualifying in 1901, and gained his New York and Pennsylvania state examinations which enabled him to practice dentistry later. He practiced in New York and took on a French assistant (Robert Vielleville). Returning to France in 1910 he set up practice in Paris but, because he was without French qualifications, he had to use those

---

* Harold Delf Gillies was born in Dunedin, New Zealand on 7th June 1882. He was sent to school in England at the age of eight and went to study Medicine at Caius College, Cambridge and St. Bartholomew's Hospital, London, qualifying in 1908.

   He was appointed OBE in 1919, CBE in 1920 and Knighted in 1930. He continued to work as a Plastic Surgeon and in the Second World War was again involved in treating injured servicemen. In 1946 he became the first president of the newly formed British Association of Plastic Surgeons. He died in 1960.

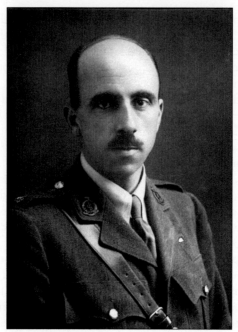

Figure 10.5   Harold Delph Gillies in 1916. (Courtesy of British
Association of Plastic, Reconstructive and Aesthetic Surgeons)

of Vielleville in order to continue practicing. In the meantime Valadier enrolled with the Ecole Odonto-Technique de Paris to qualify as *Chirurgien-dentiste* from the Faculty of Medicine of Paris University in 1912. Thus he became a dentist fully qualified to practice in France.

At the outbreak of the War he volunteered for service. For various reasons, perhaps because he was not by then a French National, he was taken on by the British Red Cross, rather than by the French. He reported for duty on 29 October 1914. He probably, thus, became the first dentist appointed for British troops. His, however, was only an honorary appointment, although he was given the rank of lieutenant.

By early 1915, Valadier had established a 50-bedded dental and jaw unit at the 83rd General Hospital at Wimereux, just north of Boulogne. He was by all accounts a wealthy man and much of the equipment that he used was provided by him. He gained a reputation for being rather flamboyant, especially as he had his own personal Rolls-Royce fitted up as a mobile dental surgery, from which he treated a large number of senior British and other Allied officers. He did, however, treat a large number of casualties using innovative techniques, and was experimenting with moving tissue around the face to repair defects as well as using bone grafts to replace damaged jaws.

His treatments remained controversial but he recognised that early closure of wounds wherever possible prevented undue scarring and contracture. He also advocated the retention of teeth around mandibular (lower jaw) fractures to allow the easier fitting of splints[13], although this was disputed by others at the time[14]. Infection was prevented by draining the area through a sub-mandibular stab incision (incision below the lower jaw) and irrigation using a pump apparatus. Another technique was to close the remaining fragments of the mandible deliberately using temporary wires and cap splints after closure of the skin. The splints were connected by a jack screw which was turned to close the ends of the mandible. When callus (new bone, produced in response to a fracture, as part of the healing process) formation was seen on X-ray, the screw was reversed and the fragments distracted (pulled apart through the callus).

It was noted that new bone continued to form between the ends. When an adequate arch was established, a permanent plate was used to hold the position[15], since the new bone was fragile and soft and would not have been able to withstand the stresses imposed upon it without the additional support of a metal plate. This, perhaps, was an early description of what today is known as distraction osteogenesis, a technique later described by a Russian, Ilizarov[†][16], and now being developed widely in several areas of reconstructive surgery. Valadier's standing locally necessitated the presence of a qualified medical practitioner for him to continue working. Harold Gillies was assigned to this task in early 1915.

This experience caused Gillies to develop an interest in facial reconstruction. He was lent a book written by a German surgeon (Lindemann) and was further inspired by some of the few illustrations in it. He wrote:

It was rather an informal war. The enemy did not seem to mind our learning of the good work they were doing in jaw fractures and wounds about the mouth.[17]

In June 1915 he went to see Hippolyte Morestin, an eminent and innovative plastic surgeon working in Paris. Morestin had a profound influence on Gillies.[18] Morestin would have been better known had he survived into the peace at the end of the Great War. Unfortunately, he died at the age of 49 in the influenza pandemic of 1919 without having had the opportunity to report his wartime activity and experiences. What Gillies saw in Paris made him realise that there was a need for specialist treatment of casualties with wounds of the face. Through various political connections, Gillies enlisted the help of senior Army medical authorities Sir Anthony Bowlby, Consulting Surgeon to the BEF, and Sir George Makins, President of the Royal College of Surgeons 1917, to establish a dedicated unit for the treatment of servicemen with these injuries.

In late 1915, Sir Alfred Keogh, was Director General at the War Office, having gained military medical experience in the Boer War (1899–1902). He had radically reorganised medical services to improve sanitation and effectively prevent communicable disease. He also tried to break down the barriers that existed between civilian and military medical practice, integrating the training of military personnel into civilian medical schools, as has been discussed in Chapter 1. As far as plastic surgery was concerned[19], Keogh had already promoted the idea of establishing units to treat patients with specific individual wounds, for example, head injuries and orthopaedics. With large numbers of casualties, their needs would be best served by having all the experts in one place. Thus, the seeds for a specialist unit had already been sown, and it did not take much persuasion to set up a dedicated unit for the treatment of facial injury.

---

†   Gavril Ilizarov (1921–92) was a Soviet surgeon who, in 1944, was sent to the city of Kurgan in Western Siberia to treat soldiers with broken legs. He developed an apparatus to hold fractured bones in place from horseshoes and bicycle spokes and noticed the device could also be used to lengthen the bones if there had been loss.

In January 1916 Gillies was ordered to report to the Cambridge Military Hospital, Aldershot "for special duty in connection with plastic surgery". Thus the first Plastic Surgery unit in the UK was founded. There was a delay in equipping the new hospital so Gillies took the opportunity to visit France again to continue his observations on facial wounds. During this visit he observed a number of men who would have need of the new service but who were not being recognised as such. He himself purchased luggage labels onto which he put his own name and "c/o Cambridge Military Hospital". These were sent out to advanced medical units and within a few weeks casualties were arriving in Aldershot with the labels attached. 200 patients were expected, 2,000 arrived! The opening of the unit had coincided with the beginning of the Somme Offensive in July 1916.

It soon became obvious that there was a need for rehabilitation facilities for treated servicemen and a house was acquired in Aldershot. This quickly became inadequate, and, after intervention by the Red Cross and the Order of Saint John, Frognal House, Sidcup was made available as the Queen's Hospital. It was realised that a multidisciplinary

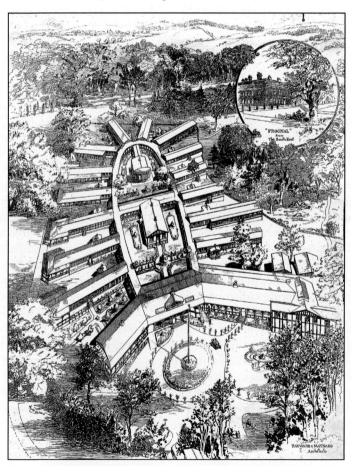

Figure 10.6   Architect's drawing of Queen's Hospital,
Sidcup. (Courtesy of the Gillies Archives)

team[20] (perhaps not a term that would have been used then) would be required to treat these difficult and challenging cases. Gillies himself was closely involved in the design of the new hospital. A central admissions block had wards (each with 26 beds) radiating from it.

Accommodation for operating theatres, and dental, X-ray, radiography, photography and psychotherapy departments was arranged around the circumference of the site. There were also studios for the artist Henry Tonks, who painstakingly documented each case by drawing, and the sculptor J.W. Edwards, who made the plaster casts used for planning reconstruction. The hospital opened in August 1917 and initially had 320 beds, expanding to 600 by the end of the war. Queen Mary's Hospital Sidcup, as it became, still exists, although not with a Plastic Surgery Unit. By July 1918, at least five satellite hospitals had been established in the Home Counties bringing the total number of beds available to Gillies and his team up to 1,000. With the increased number of beds came an expansion of medical, dental and nursing staff who came from all parts of what was then the British Empire – namely Canada, Australia, New Zealand and South Africa, as well as the United States of America, all of which supplied troops to the war. Men from each country therefore, had care from their own homelands, which added greatly to the efficiency of working and morale as well as adding a certain amount of competition between the teams. Gillies later wrote:

Our wounded had call upon surgical skill from the whole Anglo-Saxon race.[21]

Many of the records of the activity at this time were lost as result of bombing in the Second World War and the exact number of patients admitted is not known. The official statistics record that approximately 16% of the wounded admitted to casualty clearing stations had injuries of the face, head and neck[22] and it is thought that around 5,000 were admitted to Queen's Hospital, Sidcup. It is known, however, that up to the Armistice in November 1918, 11,752, operations took place at Queen's Hospital (a rate of nearly 100 operations a week) and that after the Great War the work continued, with nearly 3,000 further operations being performed between March 1920 and April 1925 (until the Queen's Hospital was closed in 1929, 18,135 military personnel were treated there; 8,000 of these had facial injuries).

Table 10.1
Numbers of wounds of the face, head and neck amongst 48,290 admissions to casualty clearing stations

	Number of wounds admitted			Percentage of total admitted		
	Severe	Slight	Total	Severe	Slight	Total
Head, neck and face	2,804	4,905	7,709	5.81	10.16	15.96

Data from Mitchell, T.J. & G.M. Smith, *History of the Great War based on Official Documents. Medical Services. Casualties and Medical Statistics.* London: HMSO, 1931, pp.40-42.

Although Gillies was conversant with French developments in facial reconstruction, by his own admission[23], he was unaware of historical descriptions of techniques and previous developments in plastic surgery describing plastic surgery as a "strange new art"[24]. As far as he was concerned he had to devise new operations to deal with the problems with which he was confronted. The vast numbers of casualties requiring treatment forced him and his team to improvise on a massive scale. Unfortunately, presumably because of the pressure of work, none of this "new" surgery was recorded at the time, and, whilst other specialties regularly published the results of their work in the *British Medical Journal* and other journals, there seems to have been almost nothing written about plastic surgery. A collection of case reports was put together and published as a now classic text book *Plastic Surgery of The Face based on selected cases of War Injuries of the Face including Burns* after the end of the war.[25] In this he expounded his techniques, many of which were innovative, but perhaps more important were the innovations he brought to the total management of the patients. He by then had the chance to look at other work and wrote:

> There is hardly an operation – hardly a single flap – in use to-day that has not been suggested a hundred years ago.[26]

All was brought together and analysed more in his two-volume work (*The Principles and Art of Plastic Surgery*) co-authored with one of his pupils, D. Ralph Millard, in 1957.[27]

The Problem of Tissue Loss

Gillies noted that many casualties arrived at the hospital in a very poor condition with wounds far worse than anything he had seen before. Men arrived from the front through different clearing stations and base hospitals. They were wrapped in bandages, sometimes blind, poorly nourished and often unable to eat or speak because of the loss of function of the mouth, lips and tongue. Many were depressed and in a poor psychological state, and having seen their facial injuries did not wish to be seen by, or to communicate with others.

Infection was common and potentially fatal secondary haemorrhage from wound breakdown was a constant problem. Some casualties survived the difficult journey only to perish when in reach of definitive treatment. Evacuation from the Front was often in crowded transport requiring casualties to be moved sitting up. Once away from the frontline, where there was more space, well meaning but misguided attempts to alleviate apparent suffering and provide comfort by lying them down resulted in death due to asphyxia. Voluntary control of the tongue was lost as a result of the damage to the face and mouth and fell backwards into the pharynx so obstructing the airway with fatal consequences. This sequence of events was easily avoidable and perhaps these lessons had been learned by the end of the War.

Thus, many hurdles needed to be overcome before any corrective surgery was undertaken. Poor nutrition had to be corrected, infected wounds cleaned, fractured mandibles stabilised and basic dental work performed. In the early days at Aldershot, management was hastily thought out without recourse to description of previous techniques other than those seen by Gillies on his trips to France. Simple wounds were closed directly using existing anatomical landmarks, but gunshot and missile wounds usually involved complex loss of both soft tissue and skeletal elements (bone). Many wounds at that stage were closed by pulling tissue together with local advancement flaps, when new tissue should have been introduced. As time went on, however, more was learned and more complex methods of replacing lost tissue were used.

The most fundamental, and now perhaps the most obvious (but often forgotten) principle for planning treatment was one of diagnosis. Observation and accurate assessment was mandatory. A full history was taken, and a thorough physical examination was performed. Then, with the assistance of X-rays, photographs and sketches, the extent of each individual patient's defect could be assessed and a treatment plan decided upon. Many members of the team were involved in this full assessment. The surgeon himself, nursing staff (who could observe difficulties in day-to-day living), dentists and technicians, radiologists, artist and photographer, all made a contribution to the overall case discussion. Early on, Gillies realised that it was difficult to relay in words an exact description of complex facial wounds. He, therefore, enlisted the help of Henry Tonks, a Fellow of the Royal College of Surgeons who had given up surgery to become an artist and had latterly been the Professor of the Slade Art School. With his help, sketches of the injuries were made and patterns made for any reconstructive procedures. Gillies himself also enrolled for an art course. Tonks had once told Gillies that:

Never is there a really fine architectural structure that is not functionally correct.[28]

Thus it came to be realised that, by correcting the lost functions of speech and eating, the appearance of the face would also improve.

Part of the diagnostic process was to understand the original defect. Patients could take up to a year from time of injury to be admitted to the unit, and by then the facial wound could have healed but with considerable scarring and resultant distortion of the surrounding tissue. There was often tissue loss, and before reconstruction could begin, the extent of this loss had to be ascertained. The healed wound would be taken apart and tissue returned to its normal position. At this stage, patients often looked worse than they had on admission (mirrors were banned on the wards so that patients avoided seeing themselves). If skeletal elements were missing, temporary prosthetics were made and the soft tissues mobilised over these to keep them in the correct position relative to surrounding structures.

The story of George Florence and his wounds

George Napier Florence was born in Peterhead, in the north-east of Scotland on 12 May 1898, the fourth son of Robert and Bridget Florence. His father was a cooper/fish curer and it is thought that George had followed him into the trade. He was 16 (enlistment age was 18) when he followed three of his older brothers into the 1/5th (Buchan and Formartin) Gordon Highlanders in January 1915.[29] In May 1917, the 5th Gordons, as part of the 51st Highland Division, were involved in the action around Arras in taking (and retaking) the chemical works at Roeux. The fighting was fierce and both German and British forces suffered heavy casualties (the 5th Gordon's lost 11 officers and 234 other ranks).[30] George Florence was listed as wounded in the Regimental Diary on 16 and 17 May 1917.[31]

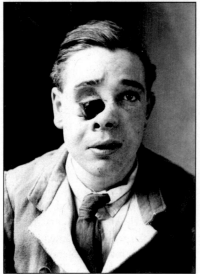

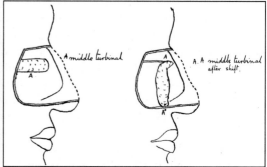

Figure 10.7   G.N. Florence on admission to Queen's Hospital, Sidcup, on 12 November 1917. (Courtesy of the Gillies Archives)

Figure 10.8   Operative diagram of first operation, septal and turbinate swing. (Adapted from original, courtesy of the Gillies Archives)

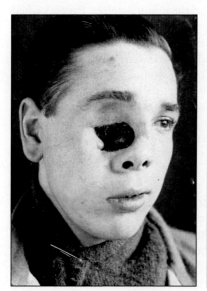

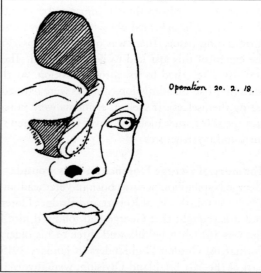

Figure 10.9   G.N. Florence 14 January 1918, after the first operation. (Courtesy of the Gillies Archives)

Figure 10.10   Operative diagram 2 February 1918 – forehead flap brought into orbit. (Adapted from original, courtesy of the Gillies Archives)

The details of George's repatriation are not known, but, as he had sustained buttock

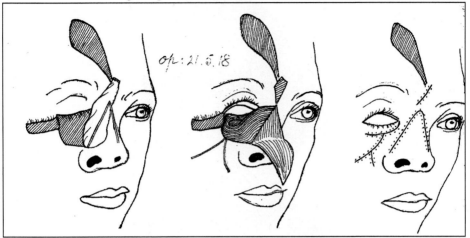

Figure 10.11   Operative diagram 21 May 1918 – forehead flap pedicle detached. (Adapted from original, courtesy of the Gillies Archives)

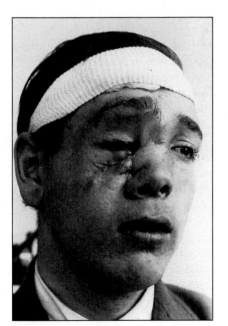

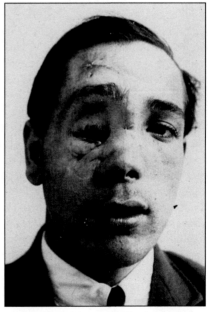

Figure 10.12   G.N. Florence 23 May 1918, two days after the second operation. The forehead flap donor site is unhealed. (Courtesy of the Gillies Archives).

Figure 10.13   G.N. Florence 8 June 1918, eighteen days after the second operation. The forehead flap donor site is dressed, presumably after grafting. (Courtesy of the Gillies Archives).

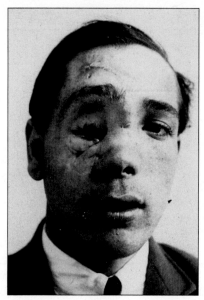

Figure 10.14   G.N. Florence 1 August 1918 – almost at the stage of
discharge from Queen's Hospital. (Courtesy of the Gillies Archives).

wounds as well as the facial injuries, he may have spent some time at the Royal Herbert
Hospital in Woolwich, which was a centre for orthopaedic injuries. The story goes that
when he was in hospital the King visited and spoke of him to the doctors, saying, "you
must help this young man". It is believed it was as a result of this intervention by King
George V that he was moved to the Queen's Hospital.[32]

The following is taken from the admission and operation notes written when George
was a patient in Queen's Hospital, Sidcup (courtesy of the Gillies' Archives).

He was admitted 6 November 1917 (six months after injury) with a gunshot wound
to the nose and right eye. A full assessment would have been undertaken, not only of
the wound, but also of his general and nutritional condition as well as his psychological
state. Photographs were also taken to record the pre-treatment state.

George's wounds had healed but left him with an open nose and eye socket. On
19 November 1917 he underwent what was to be the first of seven or more operations.
Lieutenant G. Seccombe Hett (an ENT surgeon, later to become Physician to Queen
Mary and highly thought of by Gillies for his techniques of nasal reconstruction) moved
the nasal septum (the central strut of the nose) and right middle turbinate (part of the
lining of the nose) as flaps and closed the lateral side of the nose.

There was a period for this to heal and it is next noted, on 8 February 1918, that this
septal swing and turbinate shift had been successful.

A flap was now prepared by introducing a skin graft under the skin of the forehead to
form a lining for the inside of the nose. Twelve days later Seccombe Hett (now promoted
to Captain) brought the flap down. The graft had taken well on the underside of this
flap but had not taken on the donor forehead wound, the edges of which were closed as
much as possible with tension sutures. A flap was mobilised moving the lower eyelid up

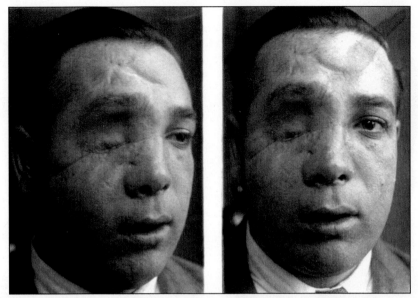

Figure 10.15   G.N. Florence 6 June 1924, in the middle of revision
operations after the war. (Courtesy of the Gillies Archives)

to produce the slit of the eyelids. Cheek flaps were also moved to help fill the cavity on
the side of the nose

By 21 May 1918 the forehead flap had lost its attachment because of infection but
it remained attached to the nose. An operation then was undertaken to correct this by
detaching the pedicle of the forehead flap and turning it into the nasal cavity.

It was noted on 10 June that the wounds had healed and the contour was good. On
2 October 1918 it was noted that George was discharged permanently unfit and it was
not possible to fit an eye into the socket. The suggestion was made that an eye patch
should be worn.

After the War various further operations were performed by Gillies himself to
improve the function and thus his appearance.

George continued to wear a flesh-coloured eye patch for the rest of his life. He also
carried a piece of shrapnel in his buttock. In March 1918 he married a nurse/nursing
assistant/volunteer, Queenie Coleman, who was possibly working at the Royal Herbert
Hospital. His wife was the only person allowed to see George without his eye patch. He
lived in Aberdeen and died in 1964 from a coronorary thrombosis (heart attack) after
years of angina.

George's son, James, emigrated to the USA and was looking for a house. In
conversation with the vendor it turned out that he, the vendor, was a direct descendant
of Harold Gillies. James bought the house and eventually died there. George's wife,
Queenie, also died there when visiting her son in 1986.

In the early days of the Great War, local flaps were the mainstay of reconstruction.
On the whole they were simple enough to be done under local anaesthetic, and this
helped in the management of the sheer numbers of casualties that arrived initially at the
Cambridge Hospital. General anaesthetics at this time were difficult and were largely

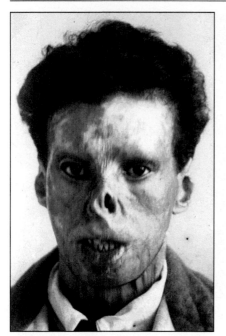

Figure 10.16   A.B. Vicarage
on arrival at Queen's Hospital.
(Courtesy of the Gillies Archives)

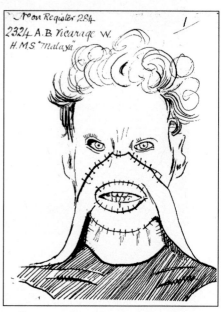

Figure 10.17   Diagram of neck/chest
flap. (Courtesy of the Gillies Archives)

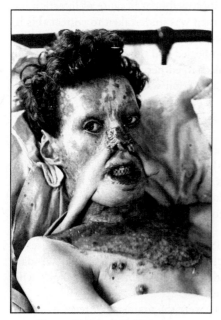

Figure 10.18   A.B. Vicarage –
flaps in position with some loss
around the nose. Note the tubing.
(Courtesy of the Gillies Archives)

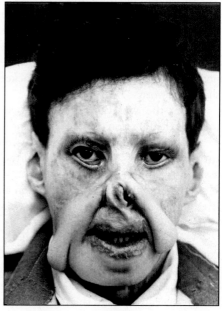

Figure 10.19   A.B. Vicarage – flaps
now swung to reconstruct the nose.
(Courtesy of the Gillies Archives)

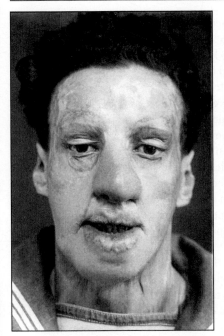

Figure 10.20   A.B. Vicarage after reconstruction. (Courtesy of the Gillies Archives)

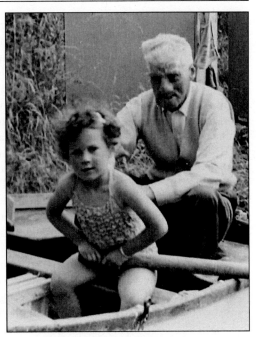

Figure 10.21   A.B. Vicarage many years later. (Private collection)

unsuitable for use in work on large facial wounds. These local flaps, raised and moved in many forms from adjacent areas of the face and neck, were used to fill relatively discreet defects of the face (as above). These could be quite large if there was normal skin nearby that could be utilised. For larger defects or injury affecting more of the face, such as burns, then tissue from outside the area needed to be imported to avoid undue distortion of the local normal tissue. This could be in the form of a skin graft, but the limitations of this have already been mentioned. Other solutions were required.

Tube pedicles

A breakthrough came with the treatment of a seaman, one of 33 wounded, who had received burns to the face and neck whilst serving on HMS *Malaya* at the Battle of Jutland in May 1916. Casualties with burns were at this time initially treated in general hospitals, so it was not until August 1917 that he was admitted to Gillies' unit with extensive scarring to the face, lips, nose and eyelids.

To release the contractures around the lips and chin, a bi-pedicled flap (see figures 10.16 to 10.21) was designed on the anterior neck and shoulders. This was brought up to the lower face and a slit made for the mouth. It was noticed that the skin near the base at both ends of the flap naturally formed itself into tubes. The edges were therefore sutured together to form a sausage-like tube. Some of the flap moved onto the face did not survive but it was noted that the "tubes" remained viable, soft and uninfected. Enough of these flaps survived to be swung up onto the face to resurface the cheeks and nose. Grafts were used to reconstruct the eyelids.

This observation gave rise to the development of the tube pedicle flap. The tubing was thought to stimulate the blood supply to run in a longitudinal direction within the flap. After three or so weeks this was sufficient for one end to be detached and for the whole flap still to be vascularised. One end could be detached and transported elsewhere. From there it picked up a new blood supply which joined on to the already longitudinal vessels within the flap. Again after a few more weeks the remaining original attachment could be lifted and that end moved. Tissue could thus be transported ("waltzed") from remote uninjured areas to fill defects virtually anywhere else.

This concept had in fact already been used in September 1916 in Russia by Vladimir Filatov, an ophthalmic surgeon working in Odessa. The technique, however, was only published in May 1917 in Russian.[33] There has been much argument about the originator of the tube pedicle.[34] Gillies would not have been aware of the Russian account appearing just a few months before he "discovered" it, and it has to be considered that the two invented the concept at much the same time and independently. After all, necessity is the mother of invention.

A previous problem of distant flaps had been the exposed raw under-surface becoming over-granulated and infected. By forming the flap into a tube there was a completely enclosed skin pedicle which healed, so avoiding these complications. Reliability of these flaps therefore improved and they became more dependable. They were then able to be developed and became more refined, and, by the end of the Great War it was said that:

> The wards at Sidcup resembled the jungles of Burma, teeming with dangling pedicles.[35]

Further advancements included raising flaps with attached bone for reconstruction of the mandible. Reconstruction using these techniques took time, and as can be seen from the narrative of George Florence, sometimes several years. The Queen's Hospital was ideal for convalescence between operations. Patients had access to the large grounds of the Frognal Estate and many pursuits were set up to keep them occupied. Other local properties were also used for rehabilitation. In spite of this not all patients felt able to undergo the multiple operations required to complete reconstruction and they were discharged with other means to deal with their facial wounds (such as prosthetic masks).

The importance of lining

The Indian forehead flap much used in the early days of the unit for nasal reconstruction was usually brought down as a skin flap without any inner lining at all. It may have been draped over a bone or cartilage graft for support and was made 30% larger than the defect to allow for subsequent shrinkage. It was noticed that one patient in whom the turbinates (part of the lining of the nose) had been turned upwards for support maintained the reconstruction without this post-operative shrinkage. It was realised that this was because the turbinates had provided a mucosal lining for the nose and prevented its collapse. The understanding of this concept of reconstructing all layers, "cover, support and lining", is a principle underlying the practice of plastic surgery to this day.

After restoring the facial skin in these patients there remained the problem of the defects in the underlying facial skeleton, mandible (lower jaw), maxilla (upper jaw), nose

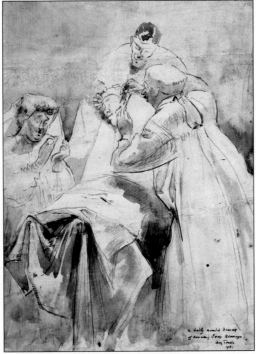

Figure 10.22   A sketch by Tonks of Gillies operating. (Courtesy of
the Hunterian Museum at the Royal College of Surgeons)

and orbits (eye sockets). The unit evolved to treat these injuries as a result of co-operation between dentists (Gillies' initial interest, it must be remembered, had been stimulated by his contact with the dentist Valadier) and, mostly, ENT surgeons. Restoration of facial appearance could only be effective if the reconstructed skin had an intact skeletal framework on which it could sit.

This co-operation was confirmed with the appointment of Captain (later Sir) William Kelsey Fry, a medical officer in the 1st Battalion Royal Welch Fusiliers, to the Cambridge Hospital. He had been wounded twice and awarded the Military Cross, and was on "home service". The suggestion was made by Fry to Gillies that, as a dentist, he would "take the hard bits and that Gillies should take the soft bits". Prosthetic appliances were developed to hold the skeletal structures in place whilst soft tissue was restored over it, and bone grafts were then used to consolidate the facial skeleton. It would appear that bone grafts were also taken from other patients, although little detail is given about the techniques used, how rejection was dealt with and the long-term results.

None of these more complex operations could have been performed without the use of general anaesthetic. At the beginning of the war most anaesthetics used ether or chloroform given through a mask applied to the face. For obvious reasons this was not suitable for the type of surgery being undertaken on these patients, as the mask would have hindered the surgeon in gaining access to the area on which the operation was to take place. Various tube mechanisms were devised to administer the anaesthetic gasses to the patient and indeed these developments went on to form the basis of the endo-tracheal tube used in modern anaesthesia (see Chapter 3).

A consequence of anaesthesia during the Great War was the unpredictability of blood pressure control. The face has a very rich blood supply. With too high a blood pressure, excessive bleeding was a problem for the surgeon. Not only was there excessive blood loss, but also, blood obscured the surgical field, thus making any procedure technically more difficult and therefore prolonged. One solution to this problem was to operate with the patient sitting up, a strain on the backs of all concerned.

The Legacy
There is no doubt that the work performed at the Cambridge Hospital in Aldershot, and later at the Queen's Hospital in Sidcup, and at the other hospitals dealing with wounds of the face produced results of far greater quality than anything that had been achieved before. In spite of the relative paucity of information and guidance available at the time, principles of treatment emerged from the sheer numbers of cases treated The analytical approach to diagnosis, on which sound practical management could be based, permitted techniques to be developed on a firm clinical base, very much to the advantage of those treated and for the future of facial reconstruction. It also allowed for the development of plastic surgery as a separate specialty in the field of medical practice.

This experience also allowed other aspects of care of these injured servicemen to be developed. Patients who had lost limbs were often celebrated as heroes. The injured part could be hidden from sight whether or not a prosthesis (artificial limb) was worn. This was not an option for those who had suffered facial loss and the results of the injury would remain open for all to view. Facial deformity represented a loss of identity and with it a loss of humanity.[36] Patients would regard themselves as being socially unacceptable because of their appearance and many were reluctant to return home to their family and friends because of this. It was also difficult for outsiders to look at them without a sense of shame or even revulsion.[37] In Germany, patients were even treated in institutions for the blind so that no-one would see them. Gillies himself noted that,

… only the blind kept their spirits up through thick and thin.[38]

Psychological disturbance was understandably common and comments in the newspapers at the time reported a high incidence of depression. Of course, not all reconstructive procedures went exactly to plan. It was noticed that if the results were not as good as expected, depression was more likely. On the other hand, if the reconstruction went well, patients tended to recover their pre-injury state more quickly.[39] This was recognised and the Queen's Hospital was designed with rooms for psychotherapy. What form this took is not recorded although it perhaps heralded the first formal co-operation of psychologists and surgeons in treating patients with disfigurement as a result of injury. It also demonstrated that a holistic approach to management was taken in which these casualties of war were treated as individuals rather than clinical cases.

The success of the Queen's Hospital owed much to the presence of practitioners from many different specialties and disciplines, but it was the co-operation between dental surgeons and, initially, ear, nose and throat surgeons that formed the basis of the multi-disciplinary team. Added to this were surgeons from around the world, together with others in supporting roles, radiologists and radiographers, artists, sculptors and technicians. The role of nurses and their helpers in caring for all the needs of the patients, both physical and psychological, was acknowledged and much appreciated.

In 1911, Gillies had married Kathleen Jackson, a nurse who was much involved in the care of the patients. Nursing regimes were strict, with prescribed methods for tasks such as dressing changes.[40] Overall, however, a rather informal style of management was encouraged from all staff, in contrast to the necessarily formal environment in the armed forces. This put patients at ease and helped their recovery. This multidisciplinary approach to the care of complex cases was new at the time and is an excellent illustrative model for how complex cases are managed today.

At the start of the war, there was a considerable amount of literature on procedures that might have been described as "plastic surgery". It was, however, rather disorganised and there were no reports of tried and tested methods on which someone faced with patients who arrived in such numbers could turn for guidance. Indeed much of what had been written by then could be described as science fiction.[41] Thus, much of the "plastic surgery" performed by Gillies and others at the time was by definition, innovative, in that it had not been read about or seen by any of the operators.[42] The experience of treating over 5,000 injured servicemen by the time the War had ended led to an organisation of knowledge in the form of two major textbooks by J.S. Davis in 1919 in America[43], and Gillies in Britain in 1920[44]. Both authors commented on the lack of previous useful literature available to them and other surgeons. Although mostly

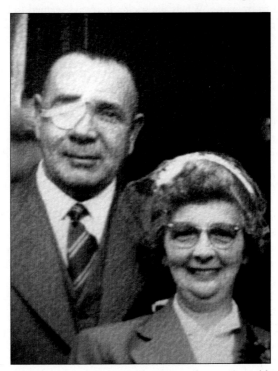

Figure 10.23   George and Queenie Florence at their son's wedding in 1957.
(Courtesy of Diane Florence, the granddaughter of George Florence)

collections of case reports, they were organised and accurate, so forming a base on which future developments could be made.

In one respect, however, with the benefit of hindsight, an opportunity could be said to have been missed. The tube pedicle was a tremendous success in terms of bringing uninjured tissue to restore large facial defects and was a great improvement on other existing reconstructive methods. Much intellectual energy was expended in perfecting the techniques of raising, transferring and dressing this flap and the understanding of its limitations. Davis[45], in his book, included diagrams of Manchot's[46] work describing specific blood vessels supplying the skin but made no mention of it in the text. Gillies described extending the length of a flap taken with the superficial temporal artery in its base for eyebrow reconstruction.[47] This observation was not taken further, and the realisation that all skin was supplied by specific blood vessels and that flaps could be raised on these was not made at the time. Had the connection been made, the tube pedicle would not still have been in use until well after the Second World War.

Perhaps, however the most important legacy was the generation of young wounded servicemen who, as a result of the treatment they received under the care of Harold Gillies and his team, were able to return into society in a manner that would have been impossible before.

Queenie Florence regularly spoke with such pride that George had "been chosen by the King" and for getting such wonderful treatment by Sir Harold Gillies, who was always referred to by name. When she spoke, it always seemed to be on behalf of them both, so one can hopefully assume that George felt the same way.[48]

Notes

1   Tagliacozzi, G., *De curtorum chirurgia per insitionem*. Venice: Gaspar Bindonus, 1597.

2   *The Gentleman's Magazine*, October 1794, p.891.

3   von Graefe, C.F., *Rhinoplastik, oder die Kunst, den Verlust der Nase organisch zu ersetzen*. Berlin: Realschulbuchhandlung, 1818.

4   *Shorter Oxford English Dictionary*. Oxford: Oxford University Press, 1973.

5   Reverdin, J.L., "Greffe épidermique", *Bulletin de la Société de chirurgie de Paris*, Paris, 1869 10: pp.511-515.

6   Klasen, H.J., *History of Free Skin Grafting: Knowledge or Empiricism?* Berlin: Springer Verlag, 1981.

7   Manchot, C., *Die Hautarterien des menschlichen Körpers*. Leipzig Vogel, 1889.

8   Gillies, H.D., *Plastic Surgery of the face based on selected cases of war injuries of the face including burns*. London: Henry Frowde, Oxford University Press, Hodder & Stoughton, 1920.

9   Davis, J.S., *Plastic Surgery – its Principles and Practice*. Philadelphia: P. Blackston's Sons, 1919.

10 McGregor, I.A. & G. Morgan, "Axial and random pattern flaps", *British Journal of Plastic Surgery* 1973; 26: pp.202-213.

11 Taylor, G.I. & P. Townsend, "Composite free flap and tendon transfer: An anatomical study and a clinical technique", *British Journal of Plastic Surgery* 1979; 32: pp.170-183.

12 Taylor, G.I. & J.H. Palmer, "The vascular territories (angiosomes) of the Body: experimental study and clinical applications", *British Journal of Plastic Surgery* 1987; 40: pp.113-141.

13 Valadier, C.A. & H.L. Whale, "A note on oral surgery", *British Medical Journal* 1917; 2: pp.5-6.

14 Colyer, J.F., "A note on the treatment of gunshot injuries of the mandible", *British Medical Journal* 1917; 2: pp.1-3.

15 McAuley, J.E., "Charles Valadier: a forgotten pioneer in the treatment of jaw injuries", *Proceedings of the Royal Society of Medicine* 1974; 8: pp.785-789.

16 Ilizarov, G.A., "The tension-stress effect on the genesis and growth of tissues. Part 1 – The influence of stability of fixation and soft-tissue preservation", *Clinical Orthopaedics* 1989; 238: pp.249-285.

17 Gillies, H.D. & D.R. Millard, *The Principles and Art of Plastic Surgery*. Boston: Little, Brown and Co, 1957.

18 Lalardrie, J.P., "Hippolyte Morestin 1869-1918", *British Journal of Plastic Surgery* 1972; 25: pp.39-41.

19 Martin, N.A., "Sir Alfred Keogh and Sir Harold Gillies: their contribution to reconstructive surgery", *Journal of the Royal Army Medical Corps* 2006; 152: pp.136-138.

20 Brown, R.F., C.W. Chapman & B.C. McDermott, "The continuing story of plastic surgery in Britain's Armed Services", *British Journal of Plastic Surgery* 1989; 42: pp.700-709.

21 Gillies, H.D., *Plastic Surgery of the face based on selected cases of war injuries of the face including burns*. London: Henry Frowde, Oxford University Press, Hodder & Stoughton, 1920.

22 Mitchell, T.J. & G.M. Smith, *History of the Great War based on Official Documents. Medical Services. Casualties and Medical Statistics*. London: HMSO, 1931, pp.40-42.

23 Gillies & Millard, *op.cit.*

24 Pound, R., *Gillies: Surgeon Extraordinary*. London: Michael Joseph, 1964.

25 Gillies, *op.cit.*

26 *Ibid.*

27 Gillies & Millard, *op.cit.*

28 Gillies & Millard, *op.cit.*

29 Morrisey, C., "1st/5th Battalion Gordon Highlanders: A Brief Summary of the Battalion's History 1914–1918", http://gordonhighlanders.carolynmorrisey.com/History.htm accessed 1 April 2011.

30 Falls, C., *The Life of a Regiment: The History of the Gordon Highlanders. Volume 4: 1914-1919*. Aberdeen: The University Press, 1958.

31 Battalion War Diary, 1st/5th Gordon Highlanders, May, 1917.

32 Florence, D., (granddaughter) – personal communication 2011.

33 Filatov, V.P., "Plastic procedure using a round pedicle" [in Russian], *Vestnik Oftalmologii* 1917; 34: p.149. English translation appeared in *Surgical Clinics of North America*, 1959; 39: p.261.

34 Webster, J.P., "The early history of the tubed pedicle flap", *Surgical Clinics of North America*, 1959; 39: pp.261-75.

35 Gillies & Millard, *op.cit.*

36 Gilman, S.L., 1999, cited in S. Biernoff, "The Rhetoric of Disfigurement in First World War Britain", *Social History of Medicine* (in press).

37 Van Bergen, L., *Before my Helpless Sight – Suffering, Dying and Military Medicine on the Western Front 1914-1918*. Aldershot: Ashgate, 2009.

38 Pound, *op.cit.*

39 Gillies & Millard, *op.cit.*

40 Gillies, H.D., "Nursing in plastic surgery and maxillo-facial injuries" in J.M. Mackintosh (ed.), *War-Time Nurse: An Anthology of Ideas about the Care and Nursing of War Casualties*. London: Oliver & Boyd, 1940.

41 Freshwater, M.F., "A critical comparison of Davis' principles of plastic surgery with Gillies' plastic surgery of the face", *Journal of Plastic, Reconstructive and Aesthetic Surgery* 2011; 64: pp.17-26.

42 Obituary, *British Medical Journal* 1960; 2: pp.866-867.

43 Davis, *op.cit.*

44 Gillies, H.D., *Plastic Surgery of the face based on selected cases of war injuries of the face including burns*. London: Henry Frowde, Oxford University Press, Hodder & Stoughton, 1920.

45 Davis, *op.cit.*

46 Manchot, *op.cit.*

47 Gillies, *op.cit.*

48 Florence, D., (granddaughter) – personal communication 2011.

Index

---

1   Numbered casualty stations have been grouped together where this reflects their service activity.

Related titles published by Helion & Company

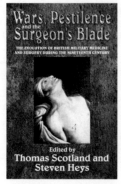

Wars, Pestilence and the Surgeon's Blade. The Evoluton of British Military Medicine and Surgery during the Nineteenth Century
Thomas Scotland & Steven Heys
Hardback
ISBN 978-1-909384-09-5

Praise for the hardback edition of *War Surgery 1914-18*

"… this volume … should be in the hands of all whose concern is with injuries of war and conflict … No reader of this book will fail to realise the impact of the lessons of surgery in the Great War on the progress and advance of the science and art of Surgery itself." *Colonel Michael P M Stewart, CBE, QHS, MBChB (Abdn), FRCS, FRCS Tr & Orth L/RAMC, Honorary Surgeon to H.M.The Queen*

"This is a brilliant book. Considering that the editors and contributors are medical professionals, it reads incredibly well as a history book – much more readable than many a military history text! I recommend it wholeheartedly to any historian of the Great War who wishes to develop a broader understanding of battlefield medicine. It has certainly helped me to broaden mine, and I must confess, I now think that researching casualties of war without looking at surgery in war is simply inadequate. " *James Daly, Daly History Blog*

"… a most interesting book, both from a World War I historical perspective and from the major changes in medicine that are so well outlined."*British Journal of Surgery*

"A most valuabe addition to our knowledge of the war it is also a tribute to the pioneers of many aspects of surgery - the evacuation may now be by helicopter and the modern equivalent of the Casualty Clearing Station full of high-tech equipment, but the basic principles established in the Great War for the treatment of wounds are just as valid today and are still helping to save British soldiers' lives in Afghanistan." *Bulletin of the Military Historical Society*

"The writing is clear, concise, expertly suited to those lacking medical knowledge, yet not passée to the expert. The book's many well-chosen illustrations are greatly aided by printing on high quality coated paper. Although it is far too early to name my Great War book of the year, I have little doubt that *War Surgery 1914-18* will be a major contender. Very highly recommended." *Stand To! Journal of the Western Front Association*

"…an excellent, well presented and well illustrated book, printed on good quality paper... very highly recommended." *Mars & Clio(Newsletter of the British Commission for Military History)*

"…important reading for anyone involved in war and conflict injuries." *Journal of Plastic, Reconstructive & Aesthetic Surgery*

HELION & COMPANY
26 Willow Road, Solihull, West Midlands B91 1UE, England
Telephone 0121 705 3393 | Fax 0121 711 4075
Website: http://www.helion.co.uk
Twitter: @helionbooks | Visit our blog http://blog.helion.co.uk